Case Studies in Family Violence

Case Studies in Family Violence

Edited by
Robert T. Ammerman
Western Pennsylvania School for Blind Children
Pittsburgh, Pennsylvania

and
Michel Hersen
Western Psychiatric Institute and Clinic
University of Pittsburgh School of Medicine
Pittsburgh, Pennsylvania

Plenum Press • New York and London

Library of Congress Cataloging-in-Publication Data

Case studies in family violence / edited by Robert T. Ammerman and
  Michel Hersen.
        p.   cm.
    Includes bibliographical references and index.
    ISBN 0-306-43622-1. -- ISBN 0-306-43649-3 (pbk.)
    1. Family violence--United States--Case studies.   I. Ammerman,
  Robert T.   II. Hersen, Michel.
  HQ809.3.U5C37   1990
  362.82'92--dc20   90-49558
                                                                  CIP

© 1991 Plenum Press, New York
A Division of Plenum Publishing Corporation
233 Spring Street, New York, N.Y. 10013

Printed in the United States of America

From Robert to his father
From Michel to Victoria

Contributors

Robert T. Ammerman, Department of Research and Clinical Psychology, Western Pennsylvania School for Blind Children, Pittsburgh, Pennsylvania 15213

Susan M. Andersen, Department of Psychology, New York University, New York, New York 10003

Teresa Ramirez Boulette, Santa Barbara County Mental Health Care Services, Santa Barbara, California 93110

Marla R. Brassard, Office for the Study of the Psychological Rights of the Child, University of Massachusetts–Amherst, Amherst, Massachusetts 01030

Susan E. Briggs, Harvard Medical School, Massachusetts General Hospital, Boston, Massachusetts 02114

Angela Browne, Department of Psychiatry, University of Massachusetts Medical School, Worcester, Massachusetts 01655

Robert L. Burgess, Department of Human Development and Family Studies, Pennsylvania State University, University Park, Pennsylvania 16802

Naomi R. Cahn, Sex Discrimination Clinic, Georgetown University Law Center, Washington, D.C. 20001

Barbara A. Carson, Department of Criminal Justice and Criminology, Ball State University, Muncie, Indiana 47306

Judith A. Cohen, Department of Psychiatry, Western Psychiatric Institute and Clinic, University of Pittsburgh School of Medicine, Pittsburgh, Pennsylvania 15213

Paul Cohen, Hutchings Psychiatric Center, Syracuse, New York 13210

Karen F. Drudy, John Merck Program, Western Psychiatric Institute and Clinic, University of Pittsburgh School of Medicine, Pittsburgh, Pennsylvania 15213

Ellen R. Fisher, La Casa de las Madres, San Francisco, California 94103

Barbara Forsstrom-Cohen, Syracuse Public Schools, Syracuse, New York 13210

Ronita S. Giberson, Graham B. Dimmick Child Guidance Service, Comprehensive Care Center, Lexington, Kentucky 40507

Edward W. Gondolf, Western Psychiatric Institute and Clinic, University of Pittsburgh School of Medicine, Pittsburgh, Pennsylvania 15213; and Department of Sociology, Indiana University of Pennsylvania, Indiana, Pennsylvania 15705

Arthur H. Green, Department of Psychiatry, Columbia University College of Physicians and Surgeons, Columbia Presbyterian Medical Center, New York, New York 10032

David B. Hardy, Office for the Study of the Psychological Rights of the Child, University of Massachusetts–Amherst, Amherst, Massachusetts 01030

Stuart N. Hart, School of Education, Indiana University–Purdue University at Indianapolis, Indianapolis, Indiana 46202

Michel Hersen, Department of Psychiatry, Western Psychiatric Institute and Clinic, University of Pittsburgh School of Medicine, Pittsburgh, Pennsylvania 15213

Richard L. Judd, Emergency Medical Sciences, Central Connecticut State University, and Allied Medical Staff, New Britain General Hospital, New Britain, Connecticut 06050

Cheryl Carey Kent, Children's Evaluation Center, Los Angeles, California 90020

Dean G. Kilpatrick, Department of Psychiatry and Behavioral Sciences, Crime Victims Research and Treatment Center, Medical University of South Carolina, Charleston, South Carolina 29425

David J. Kolko, Department of Psychiatry, Western Psychiatric Institute and Clinic, University of Pittsburgh School of Medicine, Pittsburgh, Pennsylvania 15213

Lisa G. Lerman, Columbus School of Law, Catholic University of America, Washington, D.C. 20064

Martin J. Lubetsky, John Merck Program, Western Psychiatric Institute and Clinic, University of Pittsburgh School of Medicine, Pittsburgh, Pennsylvania 15213

Bruce K. Mac Murray, Department of Sociology, Social Work, and Criminal Justice, Anderson University, Anderson, Indiana 46012

Anthony P. Mannarino, Department of Psychiatry, Western Psychiatric Institute and Clinic, University of Pittsburgh School of Medicine, Pittsburgh, Pennsylvania 15213

Edward R. McCarthy, Elder Home Care Services of Worcester Area, Worcester, Massachusetts 01603

R. Kim Oates, Department of Pediatrics and Child Health, University of Sydney, and Division of Medicine and Child Protection Unit, The Children's Hospital, Camperdown, Sydney 2050, Australia

Heidi S. Resnick, Department of Psychiatry and Behavioral Sciences, Crime Victims Research and Treatment Center, Medical University of South Carolina, Charleston, South Carolina 29425

Alan Rosenbaum, Department of Psychiatry, University of Massachusetts Medical Center, Worcester, Massachusetts 01655

Mindy S. Rosenberg, Private Practice, 1505 Bridgeway, Suite 123, Sausalito, California 94965

Daniel G. Saunders, Department of Psychiatry, University of Wisconsin–Madison Medical School, and Family Service Program to Prevent Woman Abuse, Madison, Wisconsin 53792

Amy H. Schwartz, Department of Psychology, New York University, New York, New York 10003

Janet Stauffer, Department of Psychiatry, Western Psychiatric Institute and Clinic, University of Pittsburgh School of Medicine, Pittsburgh, Pennsylvania 15213

Lois J. Veronen, Human Development Center, Rock Hill, South Carolina 29730

Catherine Walsh, Private Practice, Mt. Pleasant, South Carolina 29464

Rosalie S. Wolf, Institute on Aging, The Medical Center of Central Massachusetts, Worcester, Massachusetts 01605

Preface

The past 20 years have seen the emergence of family violence as one of the most critical problems facing society. The alarming incidence figures of abuse and neglect directed toward family members justify this attention. For example, over 1 million children are thought to be abused and neglected each year. Similarly, almost 2 million women are victims of wife battering each year. Annual rates of elderly mistreatment are thought to be as high as 32 per 1000 population. Accurate epidemiological data only now are being compiled on more recently recognized forms of mistreatment, such as psychological abuse, ritualistic abuse of children, and child witnessing of adult violence. The pervasiveness of domestic mistreatment makes it a priority for clinicians and researchers alike.

For clinicians, intrafamilial violence represents a formidable challenge with respect to assessment and treatment. The etiology of abuse and neglect is multidetermined. There are numerous pathways in the development of family violence, and these interact and converge in a nonlinear fashion. The consequences of family violence are equally complex and divergent. Victims of mistreatment can display a variety of physical injuries and psychological disturbances. No single psychiatric syndrome or symptom constellation has been consistently implicated in any form of family mistreatment. The perpetrators of family violence are equally heterogeneous in their clinical presentations. Illustrative dysfunctions in perpetrators include skill deficits, substance abuse, mental illness, and impulse-control disorders. The clinician must administer a comprehensive assessment battery, select the level of intervention (i.e., individual, family, or group therapy), and choose the appropriate treatment. This is conducted within the context of the involvement of other professionals and organizations, including medical, legal, and social services. Balancing the clinical needs of the family with the sometimes competing interests of other disciplines requires extensive and polished case-management skills.

The purpose of this book is to elucidate and highlight the complex and multidisciplinary issues that face the clinician working with family violence cases. It is our contention that most clinicians will confront families engaged in domestic violence at some point, and it is imperative that they be prepared for the maze of issues and problems encountered in intervening with both victims and perpetrators. The empirical literature in family violence rarely reveals the underlying complications in intervening with such families. Therefore, we determined that a collection of case examples describing the different forms of family violence and the many problems with which the clinician must contend would fill a significant gap in the field. The heterogeneity of family violence precludes any one case from being fully representative of each form of abuse or neglect. Therefore, each chapter in this book combines an illustrative case with a broader discussion of the issues encountered by clinicians working with families that engage in abuse or neglect.

The book is divided into three parts. Part I includes chapters that address the ecological, legal, and medical issues encountered in family violence involving children and adults. The various forms of violence toward children are detailed in Part II. Several types of maltreatment that have only recently been identified or scrutinized are represented in this section, including abuse and neglect of handicapped children, the child witness of family violence, psychological and emotional abuse, and ritual abuse. Family violence toward adults is discussed in Part III. Wife battering and elder maltreatment are addressed here, in addition to psychological mistreatment of spouses, marital rape, and domestic homicide. In order to elucidate the many issues encountered by clinicians, the chapters in Parts II and III follow identical formats, in that medical issues, legal issues, social and family issues, assessment of psychopathology, and treatment options are reviewed.

We wish to acknowledge the help provided to us by many individuals in bringing this book to fruition. We are especially grateful to the contributors for sharing with us their knowledge and expertise. We also thank our editor, Eliot Werner, for his valuable support and encouragement. Special mention is due to Mary Jo Horgan, whose day-to-day assistance greatly facilitated the publication process. Several of our support staff also provided considerable assistance, including Karen Drudy, Mary Anne Frederick, Cheryl Huttenhower, Jennifer McKelvey, Louise Moore, and Mary Newell. Finally, we extend our gratitude to our wives, Caroline and Victoria, for their continued faith and support in our endeavors.

Robert T. Ammerman
Michel Hersen

Pittsburgh, Pennsylvania

Contents

PART II.   VIOLENCE TOWARD CHILDREN

PART III.   VIOLENCE TOWARD ADULTS

I

General Issues

Family Violence

A CLINICAL OVERVIEW

Robert T. Ammerman and Michel Hersen

Few topics have elicited such public and professional interest in the past two decades as family violence. Although the abuse and neglect of other family members has been with us for centuries, and during that time it has often received tacit societal approval, only recently has the outcry against domestic violence resulted in a significant allocation of resources directed toward intervention and research. The expanded awareness of the extent of maltreatment has also led to a dramatic increase in the reported incidence of abuse and neglect. In turn, the clinical intervention with family violence is no longer a specialty practiced by a few professionals. Rather, family violence is so pervasive that most clinicians will confront it at some point in their careers. Indeed, family violence has been linked with such diverse phenomena as physical trauma, dental injuries, depression, anxiety disorders, conduct problems in children, sexual dysfunctions, and multiple personality disorder (see Ammerman, Cassisi, Hersen, & Van Hasselt, 1986; Ammerman & Hersen, 1990). Moreover, several relatively common conditions are associated with family violence, including substance abuse, poverty, unemployment, and stress (see Burgess & Draper, 1988; Wolfe, 1987). It is evident that every clinician must be familiar with the indicators, etiology, and treatment of intrafamilial abuse and neglect.

The likelihood of having professional contact with victims and/or perpetrators of family violence is great and is underscored by the high incidence of abuse and neglect in the population. For example, in the

Robert T. Ammerman • Department of Research and Clinical Psychology, Western Pennsylvania School for Blind Children, Pittsburgh, Pennsylvania 15213.   **Michel Hersen** • Department of Psychiatry, Western Psychiatric Institute and Clinic, University of Pittsburgh School of Medicine, Pittsburgh, Pennsylvania 15213.

case of child maltreatment, it is estimated that almost 1 million children were abused and neglected in 1982 (American Humane Association, 1984). Wife battering also occurs at alarming rates, with an estimated 2 million women battered each year (Straus, Gelles, & Steinmetz, 1980). Approximately 20% of children are victims of sexual abuse (see Walker, Bonner, & Kaufman, 1988). This, in turn, has focused attention on the large number of adults who were sexually mistreated as children, often by other family members (Lundberg-Love, 1990). More recently, recognized forms of family maltreatment have eluded precise epidemiological description, although data are now emerging about such areas as elder abuse and neglect, psychological mistreatment, and child witnessing of intrafamilial adult violence. In fact, evidence suggests that some nonphysical forms of maltreatment (psychological abuse, witnessing adult violence) may have deleterious consequences similar to physically traumatic mistreatment (see Rosenberg & Rossman, 1990).

In addition to the varied types of family violence facing the clinician, the cases are further compounded by the many etiologic influences operating in maltreatment. It is universally acknowledged that causative factors in abuse and neglect interact with each other and can be manifested via multiple pathways. Etiological models in which societal, cultural, family, individual, and contextual variables are represented as contributing factors have predominated in the field. Also, these factors are often thought to combine in nonlinear ways to bring about maltreatment (Ammerman, 1990). Indeed, the search for risk factors in maltreatment that are both sensitive and specific has yielded few consistent findings. There is no one variable that significantly accounts for the development and maintenance of maltreatment. Because intervention should follow directly from etiology, problems have been encountered in designing clinical treatments that are useful for *all* families involved in each type of maltreatment. Finally, a growing literature attests to the divergent causes of various forms of abuse and neglect. For example, although past experience of maltreatment as a child is implicated in subsequent child abuse (Kaufmann & Zigler, 1987), no such relationship has been found to date for elder abuse and neglect. Likewise, alcohol abuse is strongly associated with wife battering, although its role in other forms of maltreatment is less well understood. A unifying theory tying together the various types of family violence under one conceptual umbrella is unavailable, and it is unlikely that such a model can be constructed given the qualitatively unique developmental and life-span issues associated with violence directed towards children, adults, and the elderly.

Numerous factors mediate the extent, severity, and impact of abuse and neglect. These, in turn, determine the level of intervention required for treatment. For example, in the case of child abuse, the following topographical characteristics of abuse are relevant: age of child, age of first abuse, seriousness of abuse, type and frequency of abuse, and duration of abuse. Number of perpetrators, the addition of psychological abuse, whether or not the child is the sole recipient of mistreatment in families with other children, and the medical status of the child further complicate the clinical picture. Indeed, the differential effects of abuse on child victims as a function of past or current abuse and severity of mistreatment has been demonstrated (see Ammerman et al., 1986). Descriptions of the characteristics of abuse and neglect are only now becoming standard practice in the empirical literature. Incidence of concurrent forms of maltreatment, however, has been documented for some time. Thus, almost half of all child maltreatment cases included both physical abuse and neglect (American Association for Protecting Children, 1985). An analogous elucidation of those factors influencing the extent and severity of mistreatment involving adult victims of family violence is clearly needed.

Cases of family violence are among the most challenging a clinician will ever face. Few conditions elicit such powerful emotional responses from professionals. It is difficult to imagine other clinical presentations that so clearly require multidisciplinary intervention. These families cannot be treated in isolation; to the contrary, the active participation of medical, legal, and social services is an essential (if complicating) feature of family violence. Clinicians, therefore, not only must be careful assessors and effective therapists but also need to balance the always present (and sometimes competing) interests of other professionals. Skills in case management are, therefore, crucial ingredients in interventions with family violence.

The chapters in this volume are divided into five primary sections reflecting those areas that must be addressed in intervening with family violence: medical, legal, family and social issues, assessment of psychopathology, and treatment. These will each be briefly discussed below.

Medical Issues

Physicians, nurses, and emergency medical personnel are the first line in the identification and, in many instances, treatment of family violence. Physical trauma is not a necessary consequence of mistreatment of adults and children, but serious injury often brings the victim to the attention of medical services. For example, up to 25% of abused and neglected children suffered physical injuries (American Humane Association, 1984) as a result of abuse. In the case of wife battering, one study found that 42% of victims in a shelter had sought medical care for injuries sustained secondary to maltreatment (Gondolf & Fisher, 1988).

Emergency intervention is the first task of the medical professional who treats victims of family violence. The possible injuries that are sustained as a result of abuse and neglect are limitless (see Chapters 6 and 7, this volume). In physically abused children these range from bruises and abrasions to broken bones. They also may display severe burns, organ damage, head injuries, internal damages, malnutrition, failure to thrive, and developmental delays. Likewise, battered adults may sustain bruises, dental trauma, broken bones, burns, and severe multisystemic injuries. Neglected elderly persons often exhibit poor nutrition and open sores, and may take inadequate or inappropriate medications. All of these conditions require prompt medical attention and treatment. Nonmedical professionals who work with victims of family violence (e.g., shelter workers, social workers, family counselors) must be familiar with the physical signs and consequences of abuse and neglect so that appropriate referrals can be made.

The second role of medical personnel in family violence is the identification of maltreatment. For many victims, their first contact with health and social services is via private or emergency room physicians and other medial professionals. Indeed, up to 20% of battered wives are seen in emergency rooms at some point for injuries secondary to domestic violence (Stark, Flitcraft, & Frazier, 1979). Similarly, a significant proportion of physically abused children are seen in emergency settings. Less seriously injured children and adults may be seen in outpatient clinics or in the offices of private physicians. In all of these instances, medical professionals must be familiar with the telltale signs of mistreatment. Certain injuries are clearly indicative of abuse (e.g., cigarette burns, welts from an electric cord). Others, however, are more elusive. Signs of abuse and neglect include (1) implausible or inconsistent accounts of how the injury occurred, and (2) a pattern of poorly explained injuries and/or accidents over a period of time.

A medical examination may also be important in the identification of child sexual abuse. Tissue damage and the presence of sexually transmitted diseases are compelling evidence for sexual mistreatment. However, absence of such findings does not preclude occurrence of sexual abuse (see Sgroi, 1982).

Medical personnel must be vigilant for signs of abuse or neglect in patients that are at high risk for maltreatment. These consist of medically fragile or handicapped and multihandicapped populations that sometimes exhibit difficult to manage or "abuse-provoking" behaviors (Ammerman, Van Hasselt, & Hersen, 1988). Individuals who significantly add to family stress (and, therefore, may contribute to the development of abuse in already at-risk families) are children with attention deficit-hyperactivity disorder, and elderly adults with dementia. Because these populations often need to be followed by health care professionals continually, medical personnel are in the best position to recognize early indicators of maltreatment.

Legal Issues

Legal and criminal justice systems are involved with family violence at several levels. Child protective service agencies exist in every state of the United States and in many other countries to investigate allegations of child abuse and neglect. In addition, these organizations typically provide emergency shelter to maltreated children, offer remedial programs for families engaged in abuse and neglect, and arrange for foster placement and adoption. Child protection laws vary considerably between states and countries, but most mandate reporting of suspected incidents of maltreatment by professionals who work with children.

Although child protective service agencies provide nonmedical intervention for maltreated children, several problems plague these systems. In general, they suffer from too few resources, too many cases, and overworked staffs with an inordinately high turnover in personnel. These issues are further compounded in developing countries, in which structured child service organizations may be severely compromised or nonexistent. Child protective services have come under increasing criticism in recent years, although it is widely acknowledged that they face a formidable task with limited resources and support.

In family violence directed toward adults, no analogous agency exists similar to that mandated to protect children (although there are county and state organizations in the United States that serve battered wives and mistreated elders). Rather, interactions between families and members of the legal and criminal justice systems occur through law enforcement responses to domestic violence and criminal prosecution of perpetrators. Thus, the police may be the first involved with wife battering in reaction to incidents of domestic assault. In the past, law enforcement personnel infrequently arrested the batterer and pursued the case only if the wife pressed charges. Now, however, numerous police departments utilize a protective strategy in which arrests are usually made. This, in turn, has led to a dramatic reduction in recidivism rates (Sherman & Berk, 1984). Court injunctions of protection orders have also been used to restrict contact between the perpetrator and the woman. Unfortunately, these are often difficult to enforce and are of questionable efficacy.

An additional legal issue for clinicians seeing families engaged in domestic violence is the duty-to-warn requirement. Specifically, recent court decisions (see Koocher, 1988) have stipulated that clinicians must notify potential victims of harmful threats made by clients. Even when such threats are made in the context of therapy, these regulations limit therapist–client confidentiality in favor of notifying the potential victim. The importance of the duty-to-warn requirement is underscored by the alarming number of fatalities in battered women in which numerous indications of abuse existed prior to their death (Browne, 1987).

Because of its relative newness, formal recommendations for law enforcement responses to elder abuse and neglect have not yet emerged. As with wife battering, arrest of the perpetrator and subsequent prosecution are often carried out. Likewise, protection orders may be utilized by victims or legal guardians of the elderly person. These procedures, however, can be difficult for the elderly victim to initiate because of "loyalty" to the perpetrator, dependence on the perpetrator for care and companionship, or confusion and impaired judgment resulting from disease or medication. Many of those impediments also influence arrest and prosecution in wife battering. In such instances, social services, advocacy, and therapeutic interventions are important in using the legal system to the maximum benefit of victims and their families.

Family and Social Issues

Family violence is best understood within the context in which abuse and neglect take place. Indeed, family violence is a symptom of deeper and more extensive problems in the individual (i.e., perpetrator), family, and society. Thus, ecological models describing multilevel contributions to the development and maintenance of abuse and neglect abound. For example, Belsky (1980) and Garbarino (1977) propose conceptualizations of child abuse and neglect that posit four strata of causative influence; ontogenetic, microsystem, exosystem, and macrosystem. Ontogenetic factors consist of individual personality and behavior characteristics (e.g., low intelligence). Microsystem elements comprise family variables that mediate the probability of maltreatment (e.g., marital discord). Exosystem factors pertain to social influence, including unemployment and social isolation. Finally, at the macrosystem level, cultural factors affect the likelihood of abuse and neglect (e.g., cultural acceptance of corporal punishment). Similar multilevel ecological formulations have been proposed for family violence with adults (see O'Leary, 1988).

Pervasive dysfunction is found in many families plagued with family violence. Coercive family processes, marital distress, and maladaptive parent–child interactions have repeatedly been documented in child abuse and neglect, child sexual abuse, and wife battering (see Burgess & Draper, 1988; Wolfe, 1987). For many authors, family violence is viewed as an expression of more intensive and ingrained family pathology (Brunk, Hengeller, & Whelan, 1987). Interventions, therefore, frequently target deficiencies in the family system rather than abuse or neglect per se.

Social and societal factors also must be considered when working with families engaged in domestic violence. Social isolation or inadequate social supports have been found in perpetrators of child abuse and neglect (see Wolfe, 1985) as well as wife battering. Likewise, economic underprivilege and unemployment also have been linked to family violence.

Assessment of Psychopathology

The prevalence of specific psychiatric disorders is relatively infrequent in perpetrators of family violence and their victims. For example, in child maltreatment, only 10% of abusive parents suffer from a diagnosable mental illness (see Wolfe, 1985). Substance abuse, in particular alcoholism, is often associated with wife battering, although spousal mistreatment in the absence of substance abuse is also common. Similarly, no specific pathological syndrome has been consistently found to result from being the victim of physical abuse, sexual abuse, or neglect (see Ammerman *et al.*, 1986). However, both perpetrators and victims display a variety of symptoms and psychopathologies indicative of maladjustment and disturbance. These may contribute to the etiology or maintenance of maltreatment (e.g., marital conflict), precede family maltreatment (e.g., poor parenting skills), or result from abuse or neglect (e.g., depression).

Because so many aspects of family and individual dysfunction can play a role in family violence, it is necessary to administer a comprehensive assessment battery. The purposes of assessment are twofold: (1) to screen for severe forms of psychopathology that may require separate treatment either preceding or in conjunction with interventions for maltreatment, and (2) to identify targets for treatment. There are three assessment strategies that are typically employed. First, a clinical interview of the perpetrator and the victim is required. Second, individual maladjustment is examined using self-report questionnaires. And third, simulated or naturalistic interactions between family members are observed. Time, resources, and/or other clinical limitations may preclude implementation of all of these assessment approaches.

The objectives of the clinical interview are to determine mental status, diagnose psychiatric disorders, and gather information about maltreatment. Regarding the latter, specific details about the abuse and neglect should be delineated, including frequency, severity, and situational precipitants. Formats of the interview vary widely. For example, an unstructured play session is often most appropriate for a young abused child. For adults, formal structured or semistructured interviews are available. In general, the clinical interview will form the basis of continued assessment and subsequent treatment planning.

Self-report questionnaires in family violence abound. The majority of these instruments are borrowed from other specialties, and they are used to evaluate psychopathology, social network, parenting stress, anger responsivity, and knowledge of child development. Several inventories, however, are designed specifically for families engaged in maltreatment. The benefits of utilizing self-report measures are (a) that they are relatively easy to administer and can be completed in a short amount of time, and (b) that they allow for comparisons between the respondent and the normative sample used to develop the measure. The primary drawback of self-report assessments, on the other hand, is that they are prone to distortion and fabrication, and thus should be interpreted cautiously.

Interactional dysfunction is a universal characteristic of violent families. Indeed, maltreatment is often symptomatic of more pervasive family distress. Observation of family interactions permits identification of maladaptive patterns that may contribute to the occurrence of maltreatment. These are best conducted in the natural environment (i.e., the home). However, this is often impossible, necessitating simulated interactions (i.e., mother and child playing together, husband and wife discussing a problem) in the clinical setting. Of course, the private and socially undesirable nature of maltreatment makes it unlikely that specific abusive acts will be observed by the clinician (indeed, eliciting maltreatment is clearly unethical). Rather, the goal of the observational assessment is to identify styles of interactions that may serve to escalate conflict or promote neglectful behavior.

Treatment Options

Given the nascent stage of empirical research in family violence, it is not surprising that treatment strategies have only recently come under careful scrutiny. Recent developments in this area are promising, however. Advances have been made in designing treatments for perpetrators of child abuse, spouse battering, and victims of child maltreatment (see

Ammerman & Hersen, 1990). No single theoretical approach or intervention has emerged as the treatment of choice in any area of family violence. However, it is evident that interventions targeting multiple areas of change are most efficacious. In addition, at least with child maltreatment, skills-based programs appear to be important components of interventions (Kelly, 1983).

The first decision to be made concerns the level of treatment that should be implemented. Choices include individual treatment, couples therapy, or group therapy. In some cases, combinations of these approaches are required. Little consensus has been reached about the optimal format of treatment. There is some indication, however, that group interventions are especially helpful for wife batterers (Gondolf, 1985) and sexually abused children (Mannarino & Cohen, 1990).

The primary goal of treatment is to stop and prevent further instances of maltreatment. The secondary goal is to remediate individual and family dysfunction. It is imperative that the victim receive individual treatment in conjunction with other interventions. The long-term negative impact of maltreatment on victims is well documented (Browne & Finkelhor, 1986; Wolfe, 1987), and their need for extensive treatment is evident (see Ammerman & Hersen, 1990).

Summary

The wide prevalence of family violence all but ensures that clinicians will be faced with maltreatment directed toward children and/or adults. Few clinical phenomena are as complex as family violence. By necessity, it elicits multidisciplinary involvement and intervention. Effective case management is required to balance the often competing needs of the medical, legal, and social systems working with the family. In addition, familiarity with a variety of assessment strategies and treatment approaches is paramount. Above all, the heterogeneity and complexity of family violence requires creativity, flexibility, and patience. These qualities should be apparent in the case descriptions that follow.

Acknowledgments

Preparation of this chapter was facilitated in part by grant No. G008720109 from the National Institute on Disabilities and Rehabilitation Research and the Vira I. Heinz Endowment. However, the opinions reflected herein do not necessarily reflect the position policy of the U.S. Department of Education or the Vira I. Heinz Endowment, and no official endorsement should be inferred. The authors wish to thank Mary

Anne Frederick and Mary Newell for assistance in preparation of the manuscript.

References

American Association for Protecting Children. (1985). *Highlights of official child neglect and abuse reporting 1983*. Denver: American Humane Association.

American Humane Association. (1984). *Highlights of official child neglect and abuse reporting 1982*. Denver: Author.

Ammerman, R. T. (1990). Etiological models of maltreatment: A behavioral perspective. *Behavior Modification, 14*, 230–254.

Ammerman, R. T., & Hersen, M. (Eds.). (1990). *Treatment of family violence: A sourcebook*. New York: Wiley.

Ammerman, R. T., Cassisi, J. E., Hersen, M., & Van Hasselt, V. B. (1986). Consequences of physical abuse and neglect in children. *Clinical Psychology Review, 6*, 291–310.

Ammerman, R. T., Van Hasselt, V. B., & Hersen, M. (1988). Maltreatment in handicapped children: A critical review. *Journal of Family Violence, 3*, 53–72.

Belsky, J. (1980). Child maltreatment: An ecological integration. *American Psychologist, 35*, 320–335.

Browne, A. (1987). *When battered women kill*. New York: Free Press.

Browne, A., & Finkelhor, D. (1986). Impact of child sexual abuse: A review of the research. *Psychological Bulletin, 99*, 66–77.

Brunk, M., Hengeller, S. W., & Whelan, J. P. (1987). Comparison of multisystemic therapy and parent training in the brief treatment of child abuse and neglect. *Journal of Consulting and Clinical Psychology, 55*, 171–178.

Burgess, R. L., & Draper, P. (1988). A biosocial theory of family violence: The role of natural selection, ecological instability, and coercive interpersonal contingencies. In L. Ohlin & M. H. Tonry (Eds.), *Crime and justice—An annual review of research: Family violence* (pp. 59–116). Chicago: University of Chicago Press.

Garbarino, J. (1977). The human ecology of child maltreatment: A conceptual model for research. *Journal of Marraige and the Family, 39*, 721–735.

Gondolf, E. W. (1985). *Men who batter: An integrated approach to stopping wife abuse*. Holmes Beach, FL: Learning Publication.

Gondolf, E. W., & Fisher, E. R. (1988). *Battered women as survivors: An alternative to treating learned helplessness*. Lexington, MA: Lexington Books.

Kaufman, J., & Zigler, E. (1987). Do abusive children become abusive parents? *American Journal of Orthopsychiatry, 57*, 186–192.

Kelly, J. A. (1983). *Treating child abusive families: Intervention based on skills-training principles*. New York: Plenum Press.

Koocher, G. P. (1988). A thumbnail guide to "duty to warn" cases. *Clinical Psychologist, 41*, 22–25.

Lundberg-Love, P. (1990). Adult survivors of incest. In R. T. Ammerman & M. Hersen (Eds.), *Treatment of family violence: A sourcebook* (pp. 211–240). New York: Wiley.

Mannarino, A., & Cohen, J. (1990). Treating the abused child. In R. T. Ammerman & M. Hersen (Eds.), *Children at risk: An evaluation of factors contributing to child abuse and neglect* (pp. 249–268). New York: Plenum Press.

O'Leary, K. D. (1988). Physical aggression between spouses: A social learning theory perspective. In V. B. Van Hasselt, R. L. Morrison, A. S. Bellack, & M. Hersen (Eds.), *Handbook of family violence* (pp. 31–55). New York: Plenum Press.

Rosenberg, M., & Rossman, B. B. R. (1990). The child witness to marital violence. In R. T. Ammerman & M. Hersen (Eds.), *Treatment of family violence: A sourcebook* (pp. 183–210). New York: Wiley.

Sgroi, S. M. (Ed.). (1982). *Handbook of clinical intervention in child sexual abuse.* Lexington, MA: Lexington Books.

Sherman, L., & Berk, R. (1984). The deterrent effects of arrest for domestic assault. *American Sociological Review, 49,* 261–272.

Stark, E., Flitcraft, A., & Frazier, W. (1979). Medicine and patriarchal violence: The social construction of a private event. *International Journal of Health Services, 9,* 461–493.

Straus, M. A., Gelles, R. J., & Steinmetz, S. K. (1980). *Behind closed doors: Violence in the American family.* Garden City, NY: Anchor Books.

Walker, C. E., Bonner, B. L., & Kaufman, K. L. (1988). *The physically and sexually abused child: Evaluation and treatment.* New York: Pergamon Press.

Wolfe, D. A. (1985). Child abusive parents: An empirical review and analysis. *Psychological Bulletin, 97,* 462–482.

Wolfe, D. A. (1987). *Child abuse: Implications for child development and psychopathology.* Newbury Park, CA: Sage.

2

Social and Ecological Issues in Violence toward Children

Robert L. Burgess

Introduction

The issue of parental violence toward children became part of our general social and scientific consciousness over 25 years ago. In a classic paper by Kempe, Silverman, Steele, Droegemueller, and Silver (1962), a group of physicians coined the term *the battered child syndrome*. This work was a result of awareness by these physicians of evidence of repeated multiple bone fractures that were appearing in the X rays of a substantial number of children. Their chief purpose in writing the article was to alert other physicians to the problem in order to facilitate the detection of abuse. Much of the article, as a result, is devoted to detailed descriptions of the syndrome. For example, physicians were warned to suspect the presence of the syndrome in any child showing outward evidence of neglect, contusions to internal organs, soft-tissue swelling or skin bruising, evidence of past or present bone fracture, or clinical symptoms that appear at odds with the mother's description of the child's injury.

The article also marked the initial use of the *medical model*, which emphasized the *pathology* of abusive parents. While noting that research on the personalities of abusive parents was virtually nonexistent, they nonetheless asserted that such parents were typically immature, sexually promiscuous, drug-addicted, and psychopathic. Following this clinical description of child abuse, there was virtually an explosion of

Robert L. Burgess • Department of Human Development and Family Studies, Pennsylvania State University, University Park, Pennsylvania 16802.

publications that addressed the etiology and sequelae of abuse. Just as the first descriptive work was done by physicians, the causal studies were initially carried out by psychiatrists. This work focused attention primarily on the most extreme cases of battery, in which children were beaten, burned, and tortured by their caretakers, and analyses emphasized the pathology of abusive parents. The early trends in the literature were geared toward establishing a conglomeration of personality traits that could be used reliably to characterize the typical abusive parent (e.g., Fischoff, Whitten, & Pettit, 1971; Merrill, 1962; Steele & Pollock, 1968). Abusive parents were described as being psychopathic and emotionally immature (Kempe *et al.*, 1962); irrational, rigid, and compulsive (Merrill, 1962); emotionally disordered; and subject to unresolved dependency needs (Steele & Pollock, 1968).

The second major step in the history of research on violence toward children occurred when scholars from other disciplines began to work on the problem, in part as a reaction to the defects seen in the first wave of studies. Researchers began to design their studies with better samples and with appropriate control groups. From this work, we learned that most of the earlier psychiatric profiles of abusive parents were inaccurate. Of the many psychiatric traits of parents who abuse children, only parental depression and anxiety were largely sustained by later research (Wolfe, 1984). It is worth noting that these traits are common reactions to chronic or sudden stress, a point to which I shall return later.

The focus on stress was a frequent feature of research by social workers and sociologists, who emphasized such correlates of abuse as poverty and unemployment (e.g., Gelles, 1973; Gil, 1970). The idea was that any of us could abuse our children if we were subjected to the stress associated with job loss, poverty, having too many children too early, or being a single parent. Survey research also indicated that while child abuse was to be found in all social strata, it was more prevalent in blue-collar, less well-educated families. For example, Straus, Gelles, and Steinmetz (1980) reported rates of abuse to be 40% higher in blue-collar than in white-collar families and 62% higher in families earning less than $6000 annually.

As soon as scholars from other disciplines turned to the problem of violence toward children, awareness grew that the correlates of abuse were to be found on levels of analysis quite different from the individual personalities of abusive parents. It was realized, for example, that societal values and norms can contribute to the acceptance and even the condoning of child abuse (Gil, 1970). Within our own society, there does appear to be ample evidence that we readily tolerate violence in certain contexts, perhaps especially in the family (e.g., Geis & Monahan, 1975; Stark & McEvoy, 1970).

At a less macrolevel of analysis, it was reported that parents isolated from social support systems in their neighborhoods and elsewhere were especially likely to be violent toward their children (Garbarino & Crouter, 1978). Other research documented the importance of the social organization of the family itself. For example, families with four or more children were overrepresented in child abuse statistics (Burgess, Anderson, Schellenbach, & Conger, 1981). Similarly, higher than expected rates of abuse were found in single-parent households and in families with steprelations (Burgess et al., 1981; Daly & Wilson, 1980).

Matters became even more complicated when it was found that certain children were especially at risk for being victimized. Children with difficult temperaments (Frodi, 1981; Johnson & Morse, 1968) were found to be at risk for maltreatment. So, too, were children suffering from mental retardation (Sandgrund, Gaines, & Green, 1974), as were others who displayed hyperactive and other difficult-to-handle behaviors (Reid, Patterson, & Loeber, 1982).

Having recognized multiple correlates of abuse that operate on different levels of analysis, investigators began to concern themselves with developing explanatory models that would allow them to organize all of the presumed determinants in conceptually meaningful ways (e.g., Belsky, 1978, 1980; Burgess, 1979; Garbarino, 1977; Parke & Collmer, 1975). Both Garbarino (1977) and Belsky (1978, 1980) drew on Bronfenbrenner's (1977) ecological model of human development. With some differences, these writers conceptualized child maltreatment as being multiply determined by forces at work in the individual, the family (the microsystem), the community (the ecosystem), and the culture (the macrosystem). Moreover, they maintained that these multiple determinants are ecologically nested within one another. Such a perspective is important because it explicitly recognizes that the correlates of violence toward children operate at different levels.

In its current state, however, the ecological model has several weaknesses. First, it has never been clear what it means to say that the various correlates of abuse are "ecologically nested" within each other. Second, and perhaps more important, the model by itself does not specify which factors or levels of analysis are most important causally. Third, as currently employed, the ecological model is simply a descriptive or taxonomic system. It alerts us to important correlates of maltreatment, but it does not include the causal mechanisms responsible for the nesting of the correlates at the various levels.

Social and Ecological Factors: A Biosocial Perspective

In a recent essay, Burgess and Draper (1989) have developed a biosocial perspective for understanding both marital violence and violence toward children. In this chapter, I shall draw upon that model as we consider various social and ecological factors implicated in violence toward children.

The biosocial model developed by Burgess and Draper (1989) begins with certain basic assumptions. The first assumption is that, when examined historically and across cultures, the relations between parents and offspring display a great deal more variability than is apparent to social and behavioral scientists whose fields of analysis are limited to complex, stratified Western societies. When considered from our current moral values, behaviors such as child abuse appear to be profoundly pathological. However, our values are entrenched in a stable, centralized political system and economy that distributes huge surpluses with a surprising degree of equity among individuals who are no longer connected to each other by long-standing ties of shared residence and kinship. Looked at historically, humans have not experienced for long the geographical mobility, affluence, and political stability of our current society. Indeed, the industrial revolution and the biomedical advances that have reduced premature mortality are only recent embellishments on earlier inventions that had even more profound consequences for the human social condition. Because of the rapidity of technological advances and the geometric increase in the world population in the last few hundred years, it is easy to forget that social relationships, including family relationships, were typically structured in significantly different ways from those to which we have become accustomed.

Throughout most of history, the individual's "right" to life and to some measure of satisfaction was a function of being born into an established group based on ties of kinship. This preexisting group provided economic and political security for new members; it was also a buffer against other similarly structured groups that, depending on circumstances, could constitute a serious competitive threat. For our ancestors, families or kindreds were a necessity for survival and reproduction (van den Berghe, 1979). In order to maintain a competitive advantage or to expand against the interests of other groups, families (particularly their senior members) had to be able to allocate resources efficiently among kin and other individuals related by marriage. Families both nurtured members and culled from them. Ample examples come from European traditions in the form of primogeniture, of sending surplus children into monasteries and convents, of "selling" children into indentured servitude, and of apprenticing children for periods of years to nonfamily members (Dickemann, 1979). In other, more final, ways, parents discriminated among children, keeping some and "letting go" of others by recourse to distant wet nurses in the notorious rural baby farms of 17th- and 18th-century Europe (Ariès, 1970; DeMause, 1974; Langer, 1972).

I mention these recent practices (which seem abhorrent by modern standards) because in the following pages I will argue that human family relationships cannot be assumed to be inevitably benign. Competition for access to scarce resources is a fact within as well as between families (Trivers, 1974). It is in this context that the cross-cultural record is most valuable. Good ethnographic descriptions are available of societies ranging from technologically simple hunter-gatherers, through tribal economies based on horticulture and animal husbandry, to peasant intensive-land-use systems. Every one of these human societies provides a normative system within which mating, parenting, and ties of kinship develop. By looking at diverse societies, one can see the interplay involving individual behavior, family goals, environment, and social institutions. There are many advantages to broadening one's understanding of family interaction by looking at different cultural settings. In particular, one can analyze how human universals, such as age, gender, competition/hierarchy, and biological kinship, constitute a core around which human families operate. At the same time, one can determine how extrafamilial and nonbiological factors, such as environment, climate, population density, and the economy, affect the expression of these underlying universals.

A second assumption of the Burgess–Draper biosocial model is that there is the potential for violence in us all. In other words, under certain theoretically specifiable conditions, all parents have the capacity to behave in ways that are seriously harmful to their children. A major task before us, then, is to discover what those conditions are. I hope that the present chapter will take at least a modest step toward identifying those conditions. In any event, the model assumes that abusive behavior is a shared potential rather than an aberration that afflicts only those parents suffering from psychopathology (Bolton, 1983).

The third assumption is that parental behavior can best be understood as one manifestation of reproductive effort. It is recognized in evolutionary ecology that any evolutionarily successful organism must balance its allocation of time, energy, risk, and other resources between growth and maintenance (somatic effort) and mating and parenting (reproductive effort) (Daly & Wilson, 1983; Kurland & Gaulin, 1984; Pianka, 1970). What is especially important to note here is that reproductive effort can be conceptualized as a continuum, with one end of the continuum emphasizing mating effort and the other, parental effort. Mating effort is the expenditure of resources in order to obtain access to a sexual partner, while parental effort represents the expenditure of resources in the production and caring of offspring. It is a common part of the parlance in evolutionary ecology to describe patterns of behavior as "strategies"—for example, reproductive, life-historical, or foraging strategies.

This is a convenient metaphor meant to emphasize the nonrandom and functional aspects of alternative behavioral processes. It is not assumed that the individual displaying such a "strategy" either is conscious of its goals or is cognitively deciding the optimal course of action. Some behavioral strategies, however, may necessitate more cognition than we sometimes assume (e.g., Cheney, Seyfarth, & Smuts, 1986).

A fourth assumption is that the behaviors and traits that optimize mating and parental effort represent different interrelated clusters (Draper & Harpending, 1988; Rowe, in press). For example, a reproductive strategy that emphasizes mating effort rather than parental effort places a higher premium on such behaviors as aggressiveness, impulsiveness, deception, a reluctance to form strong long-term emotional bonds, and precocious and promiscuous sexual activity (Rowe, in press). As I shall try to show later, some of the behaviors associated with high mating effort can contribute to a pattern of child abuse and neglect. Conversely, a parenting strategy would emphasize empathy, strong and durable relationships, cooperativeness, high anger control, and the ability and willingness to delay gratification. Admittedly, most individuals tend to be opportunistic and probably pursue some mixture of these pure strategies, and one's strategic emphasis may vary over the life-span (Draper & Harpending, 1987).

In addition to age, reproductive strategies vary as a function of gender, certain ecological conditions, and one's learning history. We shall examine each of these in turn.

The Role of Gender

It has become increasingly apparent in evolutionary ecology that mating systems are related to species characteristics, habitat, resource distribution, and the ease with which resources can be stored or defended (Kleiman, 1977; Kleiman & Malcolm, 1981; Vehrencamp & Bradbury, 1984; Wittenberger, 1980). The key issue in unraveling the associations among these factors is offspring survival. Under some circumstances, females can rear young without direct provisioning from males; for example, where they can independently harvest resources. Another such circumstance is one in which pressure from predators can be handled by the female alone or by associating with other females in protective herds or burrows. In these situations, males may facilitate offspring survival in an indirect manner, as in the case of territorial defense. This ensures the female and her brood the ability to gather food and to give birth to young without intense competition from conspecifics. Most mammals have mating systems of this type.

In other cases, where the sexes form durable pair bonds, it is commonly thought that the paternal role in protecting offspring evolved because it promoted male fitness. According to current evolutionary thinking, high male parental investment cannot evolve (or be "facultatively" expressed) except where benefits to males outweigh costs in terms of forgone mating opportunities (Zeveloff & Boyce, 1980: reviewed in Kurland & Gaulin, 1984). In mammals, the extreme inequality of reproductive investment by the sexes rewards competitive behavior by males for access to multiple mates; for this reason monogamy is rare in mammals. The (infrequent) occurrence of monogamy among mammals is explained in terms of species morphology, characteristics of young, and the distribution of resources, such that the fitness interests of both the male and the female are best served by combining efforts in the form of establishing an exclusive mating relationship, cooperating in nest building or home-territory defense, and rearing young.

Because of the anatomy and physiology of reproduction in mammals, there are asymmetries between the sexes in the amount of time, energy, and risk devoted to reproduction (Dawkins, 1976; Kurland & Gaulin, 1984; Maynard-Smith, 1974; Trivers, 1972). Mammalian physiology requires at minimum almost no parental investment from males, while females must commit much. This asymmetry of parental investment leads to mammalian sex differences in patterns, or strategies, of reproductive behavior. Unlike the male, whose reproductive success (from the perspective of evolutionary biology) may be furthered by mating with as many females as possible, the female's reproductive success is limited by the time, energy, and risk costs of ovulation, conception, successful parturition, and, in the case of relatively helpless (altricial) young, the constraints of nurturing her offspring until they can survive on their own. Given a lower ceiling on ultimate reproductive potential for females than for males, females of most mammalian species are expected to show greater discrimination regarding mate choice and timing of reproduction than is shown by males, and to show greater commitment to parental effort.

Similarly, the sexes differ in their modes of interacting with the opposite sex. The male, in most species, takes the initiative in sexual contact. An example is the establishing of a base from which to attract females by courtship displays and by discouraging other males. The female approach seems in many species to consist of choice and discrimination, whenever this is possible or useful. Where this choice is impossible or pointless, the female may engage instead in passive but powerful signaling, for example, with the pheromones released during estrus.

Males can vary their commitment of resources between the extremes of maximizing mating with a large number of females, the "cad strategy," and maximizing provision of parental care to their offspring, the "dad strategy" (Draper & Harpending, 1982). Among mammals, the empirical correlates of the cad strategy are male dominance hierarchies, male–male aggression and violence, and high morphological dimorphism between the sexes. This is because, in this situation, the fitness of a male seems to be determined primarily by competition with other males. Well-known examples of species with a cad-mating reproductive strategy are elephant seals (LeBouef, 1974), anubis baboons on the savannah (DeVore, 1963), and most herd ungulates. In contrast, when male parental effort is high, the empirical correlates for numerous species are relatively stable male–female monogamous associations, reduced male–male competition for access to females, and reduced dimorphism (Draper & Harpending, 1982). Familiar examples include gibbons, beavers, mongooses, and wolves in some areas (Kurland & Gaulin, 1984).

In conjunction with the extremes of the male strategies, there is a corresponding strategy spectrum for females. In the face of males who will not provide parental effort, females may maximize reproductive success by minimizing time loss; they reproduce early, with little or no concern for their mate or mates. Hrdy (1981) suggests that, in many social species, selection has favored outright promiscuity in females, thus defusing tendencies in males to harm or kill infants in the future. At any rate, in this situation, with her large reproductive commitment and her limited reproductive potential, female investment in each offspring ought to be great relative to that of the male, and this is in fact what is observed.

By contrast, in populations in which males invest heavily in offspring, females delay sexual bonding and tend to refuse any male except the one who promises to be a reliable partner and provisioner for her and the offspring of the mating. This strategy will favor the ability of females to predict the behavior of males, and it will favor sexual reticence and coyness in females. These abilities allow the female to avoid pregnancy without a stable mate and to assure the mate that he is in fact the father of offspring born (Trivers, 1972). In species where such a cautious reproductive style is practiced, there is considerable courtship prior to mating. The female tests the qualities of the male as a potential mate, and the male assures himself during the same period that the female is not already pregnant by some other male.

The perspective of evolutionary ecology on mating, parenting, species morphology, and habitat characteristics can be usefully applied to social processes in humans. In the case of humans, of course, simple knowledge of habitat characteristics does not produce much predictive power because humans remain morphologically quite generalized and "specialize" behaviorally in a variety of adaptive ways (Washburn, 1978).

For humans, technology is one of the critical variables that must be understood in calculating the relationship between human groups and their local environments.

Nonetheless, the central core of my argument in this section is that gender plays an important role in the selection of a person's reproductive strategy. Owing to differences in the anatomy and physiology of reproduction, there are inescapable asymmetries between human males and females such that females tend to emphasize parental effort rather than mating effort to a greater extent than do males. And, as a consequence of greater caution by females in mate selection, females are, in effect, a scarce resource for males (van den Berghe, 1979). These two conditions—low "obligate" parental investment by males and the fact that females are a scarce resource for males—contribute to the tendency for males to emphasize mating effort to a greater extent than females do.

Other circumstances, such as prevailing ecological conditions and learning histories associated with those conditions, will either accentuate or minimize gender-related differences in human reproductive strategies. For example, the socioeconomic conditions found in tribal hunting and gathering societies in resource-rich environments in the Pacific Rim and Polynesia, in low-intensity gardening societies in much of sub-Sahara Africa, and in the "underclass" of technologically advanced societies are associated with especially low male parental effort and high male competition (Harpending & Draper, 1988). Similarly, women in male competitive societies exhibit a pattern of lowered parental care marked by intense care to infants but early weaning followed by the provision of little or no direct care and the reliance upon parent surrogates, such as older siblings or older relatives (e.g., Gallimore, Boggs, & Jordon, 1974; Hippler, 1974). While this child care arrangement clearly can work, it can also set the stage for behavior that we associate with child abuse as well as neglect. In the next section, we will examine two aspects of human ecology that increase the likelihood of such maltreatment: the nature of the operative social norms and the degree of stability in the family's environment.

The Role of Human Ecology

Cultural Norms and Violence toward Children

When examining cultural norms that influence the amount and kind of parental effort, including the maltreatment of children, we must recognize that customs that seem clearly harmful to children are often benign from the parents' perspectives; they are simply following practices that form a part of the traditional ways in which a child becomes a member of the social group. Cassidy (1980), for example, has used the concept of "benign neglect" to emphasize that many weaning customs of nonindustrialized people potentiate malnutrition. Ethnographic studies indicate that there are many customs that contribute to the malnutrition and associated secondary infections of children. Some parenting customs do this indirectly by permitting or encouraging caretakers and toddlers to engage in interpersonal relationships that exacerbate the psychological stress associated with weaning or directly by permitting or encouraging the imposition of dietary restrictions and food competition between age and sex groups (Cassidy, 1980).

In many societies the child is abruptly weaned from the mother's breast. Events surrounding this change in the mother–child relationship include forcible separation of toddler and mother and punishment for the expression of dependency behaviors. The mother may put bitter substances on her nipples, slap her child, burn its arm with caustic plant juice, and ignore the child's cries (Levine & Levine, 1963). Such customs may exacerbate the psychological stress of weaning, including the promotion of the maternal deprivation syndrome. Symptoms following such deprivation include insomnia, anorexia, weight loss, increased susceptibility to infection, and even death (Bowlby, 1951; Rohner, 1975).

Food competition takes many different forms. In some societies, a newly weaned toddler is expected to compete on an equal basis with older siblings and even adults. In Malaya, for example, parents attribute independence and responsibility to young children and explain their extreme thinness by simply saying that the child "refuses to eat" (Wolff, 1965). Wolff attributes high toddler malnutrition and mortality to these practices. In many societies, it is common for toddlers to receive a disproportionately small share of total family food because the traditional food-flow patterns favor adults, especially economically productive males (e.g., Cuthbertson, 1967). These dietary practices usually assume certain predictable patterns. For example, in most societies, the weaning customs favor males (Cassidy, 1980). It is important to note that the child who is weaned later is less at risk of malnutrition.

Several theoretical approaches have been employed to explain these fairly common practices. It has been suggested, for example, that the experience of malnutrition in early childhood may actually be biologically adaptive because it biases developmental plasticity toward hunger resistance in societies where food is often scarce. It has been found that individuals from societies where malnutrition is common grow more slowly, are shorter, and generally require less food (Newman, 1961). Thus, in this case, long-term advantage may accrue despite the short-term damage of malnutrition. Another explanation of these practices is that toddler malnutrition and associated higher mortality rates function as population control mechanisms because they remove individuals from the population directly by causing their deaths (Scrimshaw, Taylor, & Gordon, 1968). This is perhaps best seen in cases where preferential treatment (better or more nutritious foods and delayed weaning) is given to males. Given the "normally" higher mortality rate of male children, such special favors may serve the function of creating adaptive sex ratios (Fisher, 1958; Trivers, 1985) without implying unlikely group-selection mechanisms (Williams, 1966).

Were we to witness similar behavior in our society, we would probably explain it as being due either to "ignorance" of appropriate childrearing techniques or to an underlying lack of affection. To be sure, prescientific conceptions are often at odds with the recent discoveries of Western scientific medicine. Moreover, there is some evidence that, as parents become more educated, the use of traditional methods declines, as does the frequency of malnutrition (Sanjur, Cranoito, Rosales, & vonVeen, 1970).

With regard to a lack of affection, most of the ethnographic literature reports that parents in nonindustrialized societies are generally nurturant and affectionate toward their children (Cassidy, 1980). Moreover, apparent parental rejection may in some societies be common yet not culturally preferred. For example, given a history of malnourishment for both mother and child, a cycle of unresponsiveness may develop in which mother and child display progressively deteriorating behavior patterns. Children of malnourished mothers are found to be of lower birth weight, to demonstrate lower resistance to infection, and to be less responsive to maternal stimulation. By being less responsive, these children may fail to signal their needs to their mothers (Pollitt, 1973).

In a study of 101 societies reported in the Human Relations Area Files, Rohner (1975) finds that both affection and rejection occur in all societies. He suggests a cultural continuum. At one extreme are societies with child care customs that primarily emphasize affection (e.g., Papago), and at the other are those that emphasize rejection (e.g., Ik). But perhaps most important, Rohner distinguishes rejection that is relatively constant, generalized, and expected to have major maladaptive effects on child development from sporadic, short-term rejection that is associated with specific events of childrearing. This concept is important because it illustrates that neglect can simply be a technique for socialization rather than a global parental attitude and tactic indicating disinterest or hostility toward a child.

One interesting feature of harmful dietary and weaning customs is that they illustrate that cultural practices can interpose time and space between actions that are harmful to a child's welfare and the child's actual death. Because of this, the relation between cause and effect can be circuitous and not apparent. For example, systematically denying children access to protein-rich food may produce subclinical malnutrition that may weaken them so that they fall victim to severe diarrhea. In these cases, gastrointestinal disease and dehydration will be recorded as the cause of death instead of the predisposing malnutrition and food practices that are due to parental neglect. Similarly, severe infections may appear several days after puberty rites that ritually inflict wounds. These infections may result in death, especially when ashes or other substances are rubbed into wounds for desired cosmetic effects (Linton, 1936). In addition, Scrimshaw (1984) notes that seeking psychological distance through temporal and spatial distance occurs even among infanticidal parents who often abandon rather than directly murder their children.

There is a considerable amount of evidence that progenicide—action that selectively reduces the probability of survival of children of all ages (McKee, 1984)—has been widely practiced throughout history in many societies. For example, in much of Western Europe throughout the 15th to the 19th centuries, it was customary to send newborn infants to live with rural wet nurses for 9 months to a year or more. Some of these wet nurses were reported to nurse two or three infants at once (Sussman, 1975). Mortality rates for these infants were appallingly high. In Britain in the 1870s, the overall infant mortality rate was approximately 15%, but the mortality rates of infants living with "baby farmers" reached 90% (Sauer, 1978).

While deliberate progenicide may not be a statistically common event, it has been observed for all the major groups of higher primates, including humans (Daly & Wilson, 1983; Dickemann, 1979; Hrdy, 1979). For humans, especially, it has commonly been associated with control of the sex ratio. Drawing on the concepts and principles of evolutionary biology, Dickemann (1979) describes an abundance of historical data that bear on her argument that male preference and the pattern of hypergamy, where females prefer and tend to mate with males of higher status, are ultimately linked to greater variance in male than in female reproductive success. Using ideas from Trivers and Willard (1973), she argues that skewed sex ratios represent the outcome of reproductive strategies that increase the inclusive fitness of the individual parent. For example, differential investment in a high-quality male gains more grandchildren for a mother whose socioeconomic status is high, because that male will be able to compete successfully with other males for access to females. Conversely, investment in daughters is a useful strategy for lower-socioeconomic-status mothers because, while their sons will not fare as well in competition with other males, their daughters may be attractive to higher-status males. Because sex-differential mortality ensures an excess of females at all social levels, it would be predicted that high-status families would be more likely to commit infanticide toward their daughters and find brides for their sons among lower-status families who will pay a dowry for a daughter's alliance with a high-status male. The data fit this model rather well (e.g., Miller, 1981).

The phenomenon of progenicide makes it clear that actions harmful to children are found throughout the historical and cultural record, that such practices do not necessarily imply individual or cultural pathology, and that these practices can be adaptive from an evolutionary perspective (that is, they may contribute to the parents' inclusive fitness under the ecological conditions in which they find themselves). It should not be assumed, however, that we make conscious calculated assessments of actions that may affect our reproductive success. This is probably seldom, if ever, the case. Instead, a multitude of proximate mechanisms undoubtedly bridge the gap between changing ecological conditions and patterns of childrearing. Social norms, values, and beliefs may well rank among these mechanisms. An example would be cultural norms prescribing that male infants should be breastfed longer than female infants. Beliefs may develop around such rules. For instance, in rural Taiwan, mothers apparently believe that earlier weaning assures their daughters of an earlier menopause and a welcome end to the round of childbearing (Wolf, 1972). In the Ecuadorian highlands, there is a widespread belief that if a girl is nursed past 1 year she will, at sexual maturity, become boy-crazy and rebellious (McKee, 1977).

The role of such cultural norms and beliefs may be most useful in explaining normative child maltreatment. They may be of less importance, however, when looking at harm to children that is culturally proscribed. It is not yet known whether there are significant differences between child maltreatment that is prescribed normatively and that which is proscribed. It may even be that one precludes the other.

Ecological Instability and Violence toward Children

Human groups have historically been exposed to ecological changes that signal improvement or degradation of their life situation. Such signals would include changes in the availability of food resources, changes in climatological conditions, and the differential risks associated with war and peace. Given the length of time and amount of effort required for child care, human parents, especially, should be sensitive to turbulence in their environment. Thus, it can be predicted that transition states marked by instability in the environment in which families live will affect the behavioral systems associated with mating and parental effort.

This argument can be appreciated best by viewing the family as an ecosystem—that is, a group interacting with its habitat (Burgess & Youngblade, 1988). Under optimal conditions, an ecosystem will be in a state of dynamic equilibrium so that there is a fairly equal balance, or even an excess, of resources relative to the problems with which the family must cope. To the extent that the resources a family can marshal decrease or are perceived to decrease in proportion to the problems it must solve, stress will occur and the likelihood of conflict and violence will also increase. Actual or perceived decreases in individual and family resources are often observed during transitional periods marked by rapid social change. During these times, there is typically increased uncertainty and an associated disintegration of normal social control mechanisms (e.g., Erlich, 1966).

The critical role of ecological instability for parenting is seen in studies of nonhuman primates. For example, an increased frequency of infanticide has been associated with factors as diverse as increasing population density, changes in the dominance hierarchy, decreased parental control of vital natural resources, uncertain parenthood, and disturbances of the ecology of primate groups by humans (Hrdy, 1979).

These very general issues are related directly to human parenting. Dickemann (1979), in her analysis of infanticide, has also recognized the importance of drastic changes in the ecology. She has argued that periodic catastrophes and resource scarcities typically raise mortality rates for males because of their increased susceptibility to life-threatening birth defects and infectious diseases, particularly those of the digestive and respiratory tracts (Preston, 1976). Because infant mortality rates of males are especially sensitive to economic conditions, females tend to become the more numerous sex whenever environmental conditions for childrearing are less than optimal (Preston, 1976). Under these conditions, preferential treatment for males arises. Thus, male preference may have been the preferred parental strategy for humans given the general unpredictability of the environment (Dickemann, 1979). As McKee (1984) comments, "It is ironic that female biological strength may be one factor promoting the development of social systems oppressive to women" (p. 95). In any case, conditions of ecological instability may produce a postcatastrophe sex ratio highly favoring males owing to more intense female infanticide. This, in turn, may lead to the subsequent need for males to colonize less populated areas, which, in turn, can lead to ecological instability in the new areas (Bigelow, 1969).

Many of the common macro, social-structural correlates associated with violence toward children can be regarded as markers of ecological instability, in that they represent situations in which the level of stress often exceeds the family's resources. Among examples of such situations are the circumstances surrounding low socioeconomic status, including below-average family income, chronic joblessness, and all the problems these conditions produce—such as suboptimal housing in neighborhoods marked by high crime rates and high migration, less than adequate diets, and frequent disputes with creditors. Similarly, at the community level, parents who do not have ready access to the resources associated with effective support systems are going to find themselves experiencing considerable stress. Certain features of family organization, itself, are associated with chronic or periodic stress, such as large family size, single parenthood, and steprelations in a family (see e.g., Belsky, 1980; Burgess *et al.*, 1981; Garbarino & Crouter, 1978; Straus *et al.*, 1980). All of these factors have been found to be predictive of higher rates of child maltreatment (Burgess, 1979).

These indicators of ecological instability do seem to intensify conflicts of interest within families, yet they do not, of course, inevitably lead to violence. Other factors, at a more microlevel of analysis, allow us to explain individual differences in response to accumulating stress. This brings me to the third set of conditions that were postulated to affect reproductive effort—that is, the individual's learning history.

The Role of Learning

The ecological conditions outlined above have been found to be associated with higher frequencies of aversive exchanges with others, outside as well as inside the family. For example, Wahler and Hahn (1984) have found that abusive parents more often interact with others who are experiencing levels of stress similar to their own than with people who form a warm, supportive network, and who provide assistance, empathy, and problem-solving help. Two somewhat different lessons can be learned from these encounters. The first is that as a result of simply swapping "war stories," the parents may encourage, defend, and otherwise reinforce one another's coercive behavior toward their children. The second is that the parent may find these encounters outside the family so aversive that he or she progressively avoids interacting with other people. In this case, the parent may end up being cut off from potentially helpful support and experience fewer opportunities to acquire more socially acceptable forms of parental behavior. Both of these learning conditions will increase the probability of violence.

Other researchers have concentrated on the nature of the interaction that occurs within abusive families and have compared those interactions with the interaction that takes place within families matched on socioeconomic conditions but with no known history of child maltreatment (e.g., Burgess & Conger, 1978). This research suggests that the family itself can function as an important learning environment wherein family members, in essence, train one another to be increasingly coercive and contentious (Patterson, 1982a). For example, abusive parents have been found to behave in ways that suggest that they are rather poor observers of their children's behavior (Burgess *et al.*, 1981). Such failure to monitor the child's behavior may be due either to a lack of skills (Patterson, 1980, 1985) or to a lack of the resources that facilitate effective parental monitoring (Wolfe, 1984), or both. In each of these cases, poor monitoring often results in parents' responding to their children in ways that are functionally noncontingent (Dumas & Wahler, 1985; Patterson, 1979; Wahler & Dumas, 1986).

Apart from making life unpredictable for children, such uncertainty can have serious consequences for the parent–child relationship. It is commonly believed that if rewards are consistently provided on a noncontingent basis, they may eventually lose their capacity to function as positive reinforcers (Bijou & Baer, 1961). To the extent that this happens, parents will be deprived of a major source of influence over their children (i.e., positive reinforcement) (Burgess & Richardson, 1984). This kind of learning experience may account for the fact that abusive parents exhibit lower frequencies of positive behavior toward their children than do nonabusive parents (Burgess & Conger, 1978). In other words, parental attempts to use positive consequences to control a child's behavior may have diminished owing to a lack of success.

Other factors, however, could also account for the low frequency of positive interchanges between parents and children. For example, certain ecological intensifiers, such as loss of job, low income, marital discord, and separation, and other circumstances that imply resource scarcity, may exacerbate the child's role as a competitor with the parent for access to those resources. To put it another way, ecological instability may lead a parent to emphasize the costs rather than the benefits of parental care (Bolton, 1983).

A third possibility follows from my earlier argument that some of the behavioral traits associated with high mating effort as a reproductive strategy (e.g., impulsiveness and low bonding) may adversely affect the formation of a parent–child relationship based on high parental effort and mutual positive reinforcement. Thus, the low frequencies of positive interaction found in abusive families may be due to the fact that the parent (or the child) has a low capacity to form close bonds with others (Bolton, 1983; Draper & Harpending, 1988; Rowe, in press). Under normal circumstances, parent–child attachment is an important proximate mechanism encouraging parental effort. It may do so by reducing the importance of conscious cost–benefit calculations by the parent or by focusing the parent's attention on the benefits of parenthood

(Bolton, 1983). Patterson (1982b), for example, found a strong association between a mother's labeling of her child as deviant and her rejection of the child. Such rejection, whatever its developmental sequence, makes the child a more likely target for abuse (Burgess, Garbarino, & Gilstrap, 1983).

In addition to the breakdown of positive reinforcement processes, another important characteristic of family interaction within abusive families is an unusually high frequency of punitive behavior (Reid, 1984). This, too, can occur for several different reasons. Such a pattern may be a natural consequence of the low rate of positive reinforcement employed by the parent, coupled with the normal conflicts of interest that characterize family life. This parent may have no other option than to turn to aversive measures to control the child's behavior. Once again, learning contingencies may play an important role. There is evidence, for example, that an abusive parent's use of punishment is often a function of events other than the child's behavior. For instance, Dumas and Wahler (1985) have shown that higher rates of punitive behavior are especially common when the parent has had a "bad day." On those days when an abusive mother has had negative interactions with social agencies, neighbors, her husband, or her boyfriend, and is especially irritable, she is most likely to exhibit high rates of punitive behavior, perhaps even abusive behavior, toward her child, regardless of what the child is doing. Punishment that is provided noncontingently becomes increasingly ineffective, at least at levels acceptable to society (Parke, Deur, & Saivin, 1970). Thus, at those times when the parent is very irritable, matters can quickly get out of hand. This would be particularly likely if the child reciprocated the parent's abusive behavior or if there were a flare-up in fighting among siblings. Both possibilities are more common in abusive families (Burgess & Conger, 1978; Burgess et al., 1981; Reid et al., 1982) and can, thereby, contribute to escalating violence.

This high level of aversive interaction might also be due to the direct effect of perceived resource scarcity and the tendency for the parent to see the child as a competitor for those resources. Alternatively, high punitiveness might simply be one exemplar of the behavioral propensity associated with high mating effort and the antisocial behavior that often accompanies it (e.g., impulsiveness, aggressiveness, low anger control) (Harpending & Draper, 1988; Rowe, in press).

Whichever is the case, certain facts seem clear. *One*, abusive parents exhibit high rates of punitive behavior to their children. Reid (1984) reports, for example, that abusive mothers display approximately twice the rate of punitive behavior as nonabusive parents with child management problems and nearly four times the rate found in nondistressed families. Other investigators have found a similar pattern (e.g., Bousha

& Twentyman, 1984). *Two,* as exchanges within the family become increasingly negative (Vasta, 1982), emotions flare and it becomes more and more difficult to terminate the aversive interchanges. *Three,* abusive mothers are much less successful in their child-management efforts than are nonabusive mothers. In one study, it was reported that non-distressed mothers were successful in 86% of their discipline attempts; nonabusive mothers with child-management problems were successful 76% of the time; abusive mothers were effective in only 46% of their discipline attempts (Reid, Taplin, & Loeber, 1981). These abusive parents were also less likely to use positive acts, such as teasing or humor, and were more likely to use physical coercion in their attempts to discipline.

Over time, then, interactions within the family become less and less positive and more negative. Indeed, there is growing evidence of a significant relation between the frequency of mildly aversive interchanges and the rate of intensely aversive interchanges between parents and children (e.g., Reid, 1984). The more often a parent exhibits mild forms of aversive behavior, the more likely it is that significantly abusive behavior will occur. Consequently, violent attacks may result not only from strong situational or personal stress but also from the outcome of progressively aversive exchanges between a child and a parent who is frequently and easily irritated and who is unskilled at quickly resolving conflicts of interests and discipline confrontations. It is possible, of course, that the probability of an abusive assault is greatest on those days where levels of stress are high and the parent's effectiveness at or interest in child management is especially low.

Moreover, because these exchanges become increasingly unpleasant, the impetus for family interaction may be extinguished, except during those occasions when contact is necessary. The overall effect, then, would be lowered frequencies of family interaction, which is another pattern found in abusive families (Burgess & Conger, 1978).

Summary and Future Directions

This chapter began by my noting that violence toward children has been found to be reliably associated with a variety of correlates operating on very different levels of analysis. To explain these complex findings, a model was presented that entails four chief assumptions. The first assumption is that family relations exhibit considerable variation across time and cultures, with some of these variations lying well outside what we, in our own society, consider normative and proper. Second, the model assumes that all parents are capable of treating their children in ways that are seriously harmful. Third, parental behavior was assumed to represent just one of the two principal components of reproductive effort, the other component consisting of mating behavior. Moreover, it was assumed that mating and parenting represent alternative reproductive strategies. Fourth, the model assumes that the behaviors and traits that optimize mating and parental effort represent different interrelated clusters and that these clusters, in turn, are incompatible with each other and differentially related to the likelihood of violence toward offspring. The chapter, thereafter, consists of an examination of the implications of these assumptions and how gender, human ecology, and certain learning conditions guide the selection of a reproductive strategy.

We have seen that, in general, females tend to emphasize parental effort over mating effort more than do males, but that in circumstances where male–male competition is especially prominent, there is reduced parental effort by females as well. We have seen further that certain cultural norms and values can set the stage for the maltreatment of children, particularly in circumstances marked by the ecological disturbances associated with such events as droughts, famines, rapid social change, and other circumstances indicative of real or perceived resource scarcity. The probability of violence toward offspring increases even further if parents rely heavily upon negative forms of communication within the family. Thus, it is possible to think of the model as having the shape of a pyramid. At the base, we are all capable of violence toward children. Our predictive power increases when we recognize that certain cultural norms and values are associated with higher rates of maltreatment. We can predict the occurrence of abuse even better when the family ecology is disturbed and resource scarcity increases. The precision of our predictions increases further when the family's interaction patterns are coercive in nature. One of the advantages of the model presented is that it attempts to specify the mechanisms by which macroindicators of ecological disturbance can lead to microlevel processes that culminate in violence and other forms of maltreatment. Coercive patterns of family interaction represent the principal causal pathway that links ecological instability to violence within families (Burgess & Draper, 1989).

But this is just a beginning. There are undoubtedly other links between the macro and micro correlates of parental effort. For instance, as discussed in this chapter, we do not yet fully understand the determinants of these communication patterns. Are they a product of a learning history within the family (e.g., Burgess et al., 1981; Patterson, 1982b), of experiences outside the family (e.g., Wahler & Hahn, 1984), or of both (e.g., Burgess & Youngblade, 1988)? Or are they, at least in part, genetically determined (Bolton, 1983; Burgess & Draper, 1989; Draper & Harpending, 1988; Rowe, in press)? If so, how does a person's genetic material interact with the environment to produce a particular behavioral phenotype? This process is not well understood at all. These are only some of the important questions we still need to answer.

References

Ariès, P. (1970). *Centuries of childhood: A social history of family life.* New York: Knopf.

Belsky, J. (1978). Three theoretical models of child abuse: A critical review. *Child Abuse and Neglect, 2,* 37–49.

Belsky, J. (1980). Child maltreatment: An ecological integration. *American Psychologist, 35,* 320–335.

Bigelow, R. (1969). *The dawn warriors: Man's evolution toward peace.* Boston: Little, Brown.

Bijou, S. W., & Baer, D. M. (1961). *Child development, Vol. 1: A systematic and empirical theory.* New York: Appleton-Century-Crofts.

Bolton, F. G., Jr. (1983). *When bonding fails: Clinical assessment of high-risk families.* Beverly Hills, CA: Sage.

Bousha, D. M., & Twentyman, C. T. (1984). Mother-child interactional style in abuse, neglect, and control groups: Naturalistic observations in the home. *Journal of Abnormal Psychology, 93,* 106–114.

Bowlby, J. (1951). Maternal care and mental health. *World Health Organization Bulletin, 3,* 355–534.

Bronfenbrenner, U. (1977). Toward an experimental ecology of human development. *American Psychologist, 32,* 513–531.

Burgess, R. L. (1979). Child abuse: A social interactional analysis. In B. B. Lahey & A. E. Kazdin (Eds.), *Advances in clinical child psychology.* New York: Plenum.

Burgess, R. L., & Conger, R. D. (1978). Family interaction in abusive, neglectful, and normal families. *Child Development, 49,* 1163–1173.

Burgess, R. L., & Draper, P. (1989). The explanation of family violence: The role of biological, behavioral, and cultural selection. In L. Ohlin & M. Tonry (Eds.), *Family violence.* Chicago: University of Chicago Press.

Burgess, R. L., Anderson, E. A., Schellenbach, C. J., & Conger, R. (1981). A social interactional approach to the study of abusive families. In J. P. Vincent (Ed.), *Advances in family intervention, assessment, and theory: An annual compilation of research.* New York: Columbia University Press.

Burgess, R. L., & Richardson, R. A. (1984). Coercive interpersonal contingencies of reinforcement as a determinant of child abuse: Implications for treatment and prevention. In R. F. Dangel & R. A. Polster (Eds.), *Behavioral parent training: Issues in research and practice.* New York: Guilford Press.

Burgess R. L., & Youngblade, L. M. (1988). Social incompetence and the intergenerational transmission of abusive parental practices. In R. Gelles, G. Hotaling, D. Finkelhor, & M. Straus (Eds.), *Family abuse and its consequences: New directions in family violence research.* Beverly Hills, CA: Sage.

Burgess, R. L., Garbarino, J., & Gilstrap, B. (1983). Violence to the family. In E. J. Callahan & K. McCluskey (Eds.), *Life span developmental psychology: Non-normative life events.* New York: Academic Press.

Cassidy, C. M. (1980). *Benign neglect and toddler malnutrition: Social and biological predictors of nutritional status, physical growth, and neurological development.* New York: Academic Press.

Cheney, D., Seyfarth, R., & Smuts, B. (1986). Social relationships and social cognition of nonhuman primates. *Science, 234,* 1361–1366.

Cuthbertson, D. P. (1967). Feeding patterns and nutrient utilization: Chairman's remarks. *Proceedings of the Nutrition Society, 26,* 143–144.

Daly, M., & Wilson, M. I. (1980). Abuse and neglect of children in evolutionary perspective. In R. D. Alexander & D. W. Tinkle (Eds.), *Natural selection and social behavior.* New York: Chiron.

Daly, M., & Wilson, M. I. (1983). *Sex, education, and behavior.* North Scituate, MA: Duxbury.

Dawkins, R. (1976). *The selfish gene.* London: Oxford University Press.

DeMause, L. (1974). The evolution of childhood. In L. DeMause (Ed.), *The history of childhood.* New York: Psychohistory Press.

DeVore, I. (1963). Mother-infant relations in free-ranging baboons. In H. L. Rheingold (Ed.), *Maternal behavior in mammals.* New York: Wiley.

Dickemann, M. (1979). Female infanticide, reproductive strategies, and social stratification: A preliminary model. In N. Chagnon & W. Irons (Eds.), *Evolutionary biology and human social behavior.* North Scituate, MA: Duxbury.

Draper, P., & Harpending, H. (1982). Father absence and reproductive strategy: An evolutionary perspective. *Journal of Anthropological Research, 38,* 255–273.

Draper, P., & Harpending, H. (1987). Parent investment and the child's environment. In J. Lancaster, A. Rossi, J. Altmann, & L. Sherrod (Eds.), *Biological perspectives on human parenting.* New York: Aldine DeGruyzer.

Draper, P., & Harpending, H. (1988). A sociobiological perspective on the development of human reproductive strategies. In K. B. MacDonald (Ed.), *Sociobiological perspectives on human development.* New York: Springer-Verlag.

Dumas, J. E., & Wahler, R. G. (1985). Indiscriminate mothering as a contextual factor in aggressive-oppositional child behavior. *Journal of Abnormal Child Psychology, 13,* 1–17.

Erlich, R. S. (1966). *Family in transition: A study of 300 Yugoslav villages.* Princeton, NJ: Princeton University Press.

Fischoff, T., Whitton, C. F., & Pettit, M. G. (1971). Psychiatric study of mothers of infants with growth failure secondary to maternal deprivation. *Journal of Pediatrics, 79,* 209–215.

Fisher, R. A. (1958). *The genetical theory of natural selection.* New York: Dover.

Frodi, A. M. (1981). Contributions of infant characteristics to child abuse. *American Journal of Mental Deficiency, 85,* 341–349.

Gallimore, R., Boggs, J., & Jordon, C. (1974). *Culture, behavior, and education: A study of Hawaiian-Americans.* Beverly Hills, CA: Sage.

Garbarino, J. (1977). The human ecology of maltreatment: A conceptual model for research. *Journal of Marriage and the Family, 39,* 721–735.

Garbarino, J., & Crouter, A. (1978). Defining the community context of parent-child relations: The correlates of child maltreatment. *Child Development, 49,* 604–616.

Geis, G., & Monahan, J. (1975). The social ecology of violence. In T. Likona (Ed.), *Man and mortality.* New York: Holt, Rinehart & Winston.

Gelles, R. J. (1973). Child abuse as psychopathology: A sociological critique and reformulation. *American Journal of Orthopsychiatry, 43,* 611–621.

Gil, D. G. (1970). *Violence against children: Physical abuse in the United States.* Cambridge, MA: Harvard University Press.

Harpending, H., & Draper, P. (1988). *Antisocial behavior and the other side of cultural evolution.* In T. E. Moffitt & S. A. Mednick (Eds.), *Biological contributions to crime causation.* Dordrecht: Martinus Nijhoff Publishers.

Hippler, A. E. (1974). *Hunter's Point: A black ghetto.* New York: Basic Books.

Hrdy, S. B. (1979). Infanticide among animals: A review, classification, and examinations of the implications for the reproductive strategies of females. *Ethology and Sociobiology, 1,* 13–40.

Hrdy, S. B. (1981). *The woman that never evolved.* Cambridge, MA: Harvard University Press.

Johnson, B., & Morse, H. A. (1968). Injured children and their parents. *Children, 15,* 147–152.

Kempe, C. H., Silverman, F. N., Steele, B. F., Droegemueller, W., & Silver, H. K. (1962). The battered-child syndrome. *Journal of the American Medial Association, 181,* 17–24.

Kleiman, D. G. (1977). Monogamy in mammals. *Quarterly Review of Biology, 52,* 39–69.

Kleiman, D. G., & Malcolm, J. R. (1981). Evolution of male parental investment in mammals. In D. J. Gubernick & P. H. Klopfer (Eds.), *Parental care in mammals.* New York: Plenum.

Kurland, J. A., & Gaulin, S. J. C. (1984). The evolution of male parental investment: Effects of genetic relatedness and feeding ecology on the allocation of reproductive effort. In D. M. Taub (Ed.), *Primate paternalism.* New York: Van Nostrand.

Langer, W. L. (1972). Checks on population growth: 1750–1850. *Scientific American, 226*(2), 92–99.

LeBouef, B. J. (1974). Male–male competition and reproductive success in elephant seals. *American Zoologist, 14,* 163–176.

Levine, R. A., & Levine, B. B. (1963). Nyansongo: A Gusii community in Kenya. In B. B. Whiting (Ed.), *Six cultures, studies of child rearing.* New York: Wiley.

Linton, R. (1936). *The study of man.* New York: Appleton-Century.

Maynard-Smith, S. J. (1974). The theory of games and the evolution of animal conflicts. *Journal of Theoretical Biology, 47,* 209–221.

McKee, L. (1977, April). *Differential weaning and the ideology of gender: Implications for Andean sex ratios.* Paper read at the seventy-sixth annual meeting of the American Psychological Association, Houston, TX.

McKee, L. (1984). Sex differentials in survivorship and the customary treatment of infants and children. *Medical Anthropology, 8*(2), 91–108.

Merrill, E. J. (1962). Physical abuse of children: An agency study. In V. De Francis (Ed.), *Protecting the battered child.* Denver: American Humane Association.

Miller, B. (1981). *The endangered sex: Neglect of female children in rural North India.* Ithaca, NY: Cornell University Press.

Newman, M. T. (1961). Biological adaptation of man to his environment: Heat, cold, altitude, and nutrition. *Annals of the New York Academy of Sciences, 91,* 617–633.

Parke, R. D., & Collmer, C. (1975). Child abuse: An interdisciplinary analysis. In M. Hetherington (Ed.), *Review of child development research* (Vol. 5). Chicago: University of Chicago Press.

Parke, R. D., Deur, J. L., & Saivin, M. (1970). The intermittent punishment effect in humans: Conditioning or adaptation? *Psychonomic Science, 18,* 193–194.

Patterson, G. R. (1979). A performance theory for coercive family interaction. In R. B. Cairns (Ed.), *The analysis of social interactions: Methods, issues, and illustrations.* Hillsdale, NJ: Erlbaum.

Patterson, G. R. (1980). Mothers: The unacknowledged victims. *Monographs of the Society for Research in Child Development, 45*(5, Serial No. 186).

Patterson, G. R. (1982a). *Coercive family process.* Eugene, OR: Castalia.

Patterson, G. R. (1982b). The unattached mother: A process analysis. In W. Hartup & Z. Rubin (Eds.), *Social relationships: Their role in children's development.* Harwichport, MA: Harwichport Conference.

Patterson, G. R. (1985). Beyond technology: The next stage in the development of parent training. In L. Abate (Ed.), *Handbook of family psychology and psychotherapy.* New York: Dow-Jones-Irwin.

Pianka, E. R. (1970). On r- and K-selection. *American Naturalist, 104,* 592–597.

Pollitt, E. (1973). Behavior of infant in causation of nutritional marasmus. *American Journal of Clinical Nutrition, 26,* 264–270.

Preston, S. (1976). *Mortality patterns in national populations with special reference to recorded causes of death.* New York: Academic Press.

Reid, J. B. (1984). Social-interactional patterns of families of abused and nonabused children. In C. Zahn-Waxler, M. Cummings, & M. Rake-Yarrow, (Eds.), *Social and biological origins of altruism and aggression.* Cambridge: Cambridge University Press.

Reid, J. B., Taplin, P. S., & Loeber, R. (1981). A social interactional approach to the treatment of abusive families. In R. Stuart (Ed.), *Violent behavior: Social learning approaches to prediction, management, and treatment.* New York: Brunner/Mazel.

Reid, J. B., Patterson, G. R., & Loeber, R. (1982). The abused child: Victim, instigator, or innocent bystander? In D. J. Bernstein (Ed.), *Response structure and organization.* Lincoln: University of Nebraska Press.

Rohner, R. P. (1975). *They love me, they love me not.* New Haven, CT: Human Relations Area Files Press.

Rowe, D. C. (in press). An adaptive strategy of crime and delinquency. In D. Hawkins, (Ed.), *Theories of crime and delinquency.* Beverly Hills, CA: Sage.

Sandgrund, A. K., Gaines, R., & Green, A. (1974). Child abuse and mental retardation: A problem of cause and effect. *American Journal of Mental Deficiency, 79,* 327–330.

Sanjur, D. M., Cranoito, J., Rosales, L., & vonVeen, A. (1970). Infant feeding and weaning practices in a rural preindustrial setting: A sociocultural approach. *Acta Paediatrica Scandinaviea* (Suppl. 200).

Sauer, R. (1978). Infanticide and abortion in nineteenth century Britain. *Population Studies, 32*(1), 81–93.

Scrimshaw, N. S. (1984). Infanticide in human populations: Societal and individual concerns. In G. Hausfater & S. Hrdy (Eds.), *Infanticide: Comparative and evolutionary perspectives.* New York: Aldine.

Scrimshaw, N. S., Taylor, C. E., & Gordon, J. E. (1968). *Interactions of nutrition and infection.* Geneva: World Health Organization Monograph Series 57.

Stark, R., & McEvoy, J., III. (1970). Middle class violence. *Psychology Today, 4,* 52–65.

Steele, B. F., & Pollock, C. B. (1968). A psychiatric study of parents who abuse infants and small children. In R. E. Helfer & C. H. Kempe (Eds.), *The battered child.* Chicago: University of Chicago Press.

Straus, M. A., Gelles, R. J., & Steinmetz, S. K. (1980). *Behind closed doors: Violence in the American family.* Garden City, NY: Doubleday.

Sussman, G. (1975). The wet-nursing business in nineteenth century France. *French Historical Studies, 9*(2), 304–328.

Trivers, R. L. (1972). Parental investment and sexual selection. In B. Campbell (Ed.), *Sexual selection and the descent of man.* Chicago: Aldine.

Trivers, R. L. (1974). Parent-offspring conflict. *American Zoologist, 14,* 244–264.

Trivers, R. L. (1985). *Social evolution.* Menlo Park, CA: Benjamin/Cummings.

Trivers, R. L., & Willard, D. (1973). Natural selection of parental ability to vary the sex ratio of offspring. *Science, 179,* 90–92.

van den Berghe, P. (1979). *Human family systems: An evolutionary perspective.* New York: Elsevier.

Vasta, R. (1982). Physical child abuse: A dual-component analysis. *Developmental Review, 2,* 125–149.

Vehrencamp, S., & Bradbury, J. W. (1984). Mating systems and ecology. In J. R. Krebs & N. B. Davies (Eds.), *Behavioral ecology: An evolutionary approach* (2nd ed.). Oxford: Blackwell Scientific.

Wahler, R. G., & Dumas, J. E. (1986). Maintenance factors in coercive mother-child interactions: The compliance and predictability hypotheses. *Journal of Applied Behavior Analysis, 19,* 13–22.

Wahler, R. G., & Hahn, D. M. (1984). The communication patterns of troubled mothers: In search of a keystone in the generalization of parenting skills. *Journal of Education and Treatment of Children, 7,* 335–350.

Washburn, S. (1978). Human behavior and the behavior of other animals. *American Psychologist, 33,* 405–418.

Williams, G. C. (1966). Natural selection, the costs of reproduction, and a refinement of Lack's Principle. *American Naturalist, 100,* 687–690.

Wittenberger, J. F. (1980). *Animal social behavior.* Boston: Duxbury.

Wolf, M. (1972). *Women and the family in rural Taiwan.* Stanford, CA: Standord University Press.

Wolfe, D. A. (1984, July). *Behavioral distinctions between abusive and nonabusive parents: A review and critique.* Paper presented at the Second Family Violence Research Conference, University of New Hampshire, Durham.

Wolff, R. J. (1965). Meanings of food. *Tropical and Geographical Medicine, 17,* 45–51.

Zeveloff, S. I., & Boyce, M. S. (1980). Parental investment and mating systems in mammals. *Evolution, 34,* 973–982.

3

The Ecology of Domestic Aggression toward Adult Victims

Alan Rosenbaum, Paul Cohen, and Barbara Forsstrom-Cohen

Introduction

Whether or not human beings are inherently aggressive, as some have asserted (Lorenz, 1966), it appears that we are most likely to behave aggressively in our intimate social relationships. Almost one-fourth of all murders occur between relatives, most often involving spouses killing one another (Straus, 1986). Child abuse, spouse abuse, and elder abuse have each become substantial problems in their own right. Date rape and courtship violence occur with distressing frequency. Violence between homosexual couples also has been documented in the literature. No type of interpersonal relationship seems to be immune. Familiarity may breed contempt, but intimacy apparently begets aggression.

The search for the causes of domestic aggression has focused largely on sociocultural and psychological factors. It has been a short search whose primary strategy has been to identify characteristics of the participants that distinguish them from their nonaggressive counterparts. It has been an atheoretical search in which theory is occasionally invoked, post hoc, to explain one or another research finding. Social learning theory, for example, is used as an explanation for the intergenerational

Alan Rosenbaum • Department of Psychiatry, University of Massachusetts Medical Center, Worcester, Massachusetts 01655. **Paul Cohen** • Hutchings Psychiatric Center, Syracuse, New York 13210. **Barbara Forsstrom-Cohen** • Syracuse Public Schools, Syracuse, New York 13210.

transmission of aggression, and female masochism is sometimes employed to account for the battered woman's reluctance to leave an abusive mate.

Efforts to understand domestic aggression have emphasized four sets of factors: intraindividual (the contributions of the background and personality of the participants), interpersonal (marital and familial dynamics), environmental stressors (financial problems, religious or racial influences), and the cultural context in which aggression occurs (including the legislative, law enforcement, and judicial response, as well as literary and media representations). This chapter will examine the contributions of each of these elements in the development of domestic aggression toward adult victims. The primary focus will be on marital aggression, which has been more thoroughly explored than elder abuse.

Marital aggression is recognized to occur in no less than one in every three marriages, and some estimate it to take place in as many as half (O'Leary, Barling, Arias, Rosenbaum, Malone, & Tyree, 1989; Straus & Gelles, 1986). The best available estimates of the incidence of elder abuse are that approximately 4% of the elderly population in the United States are physically abused, suggesting that it is less common than marital aggression but comparable, in frequency, to child abuse (Pillemer & Wolf, 1986). These figures do not include elder neglect, estimated to be more frequent than elder abuse. Incidence estimates for all forms of domestic aggression are typically qualified by sampling problems and suggestions of underreporting. The cliche "tip of the iceberg" often appears alongside such estimates.

Intraindividual Factors

Much of the research in marital aggression has been guided by the question: How are batterers and their victims different from spouses in nonaggressive relationships? The focus has been on differences in upbringing, family environment, personality (broadly defined), and psychopathology (even more broadly defined). Although the research in this area is often flawed by a host of methodological problems (see Geffner, Rosenbaum, & Hughes, 1988; Hotaling & Sugarman, 1986; Rosenbaum, 1988, for reviews of these issues), and the findings have been both inconsistent and inconclusive, numerous studies have found that abusive males often come from violent homes (Caesar, 1988; Hotaling & Sugarman, 1986; Kalmuss, 1984; Rosenbaum & O'Leary, 1981). Several studies have found abusers to have experienced violence (from caregivers) as children (Kalmuss, 1984; Telch & Lindquist, 1984), but it is generally agreed that witnessing interparental aggression is a more significant background factor for batterers (Caesar, 1988; Hotaling & Sugarman, 1986). There is evidence that this may be an important factor for perpetrators of dating aggression (Bernard & Bernard, 1983) and elder abuse (Gold & Gwyther, 1989; Pierce & Trotta, 1986), as well. It should be noted, however, that many batterers do not come from violent backgrounds (Caesar, 1988) and that many nonbatterers do.

The question of whether the wife/victim also experiences a violent family environment is more controversial. The controversy stems, in part, from dissatisfaction with the concept of victim blaming and also from the inconsistencies in the research literature. There appears to be a fine line between blaming an individual for being victimized and suggesting that certain people might be more vulnerable to being victimized. An individual walking through a poorly lit area at night, for example, may be at increased risk of being victimized. This does not justify the attack, nor should the possibility be ignored that such individuals may have limited choices concerning where they walk owing to social and economic circumstances.

Concerning the research, Hotaling and Sugarman (1986) identify interparental aggression in the wife/victim's family of origin as the only consistent risk marker among female victims of marital aggression. Their conclusion notwithstanding, those studies failing to support this relationship (Rosenbaum & O'Leary, 1981; Telch & Lindquist, 1984) have utilized comparison samples of maritally discordant, nonphysically abused women, suggesting that perhaps it is more a feature of severe marital discord than of marital aggression. Alternatively, background violence experiences seem to be more commonly found in community samples (such as those employed by Straus, Gelles, & Steinmetz, 1980) than in clinic or agency samples (such as those examined by Rosenbaum & O'Leary, 1981; Telch & Lindquist, 1984), suggesting perhaps that women who viewed or experienced violence in their parental homes may be more tolerant of it in their own marital relationships and less likely to seek outside assistance from an agency.

Elder abuse has come into the public spotlight even more recently than the other forms of domestic aggression; consequently, there is relatively less empirical research. The relationship between childhood exposure to violence and subsequent approval of violence as an adult (Owens & Straus, 1975), coupled with evidence supportive of intergenerational transmission models for both child and spouse abuse (Straus *et al.*, 1980), prompted Pillemer (1986) to examine this factor in elder abusers. Using a case-control methodology, his data failed to support a relationship between physical punishment as a child and becoming an elder abuser as an adult. Unfortunately, he did not assess whether the abused elder had abused her/his own parent and whether the identified elder abuser might have been exposed to this as a child (i.e., corresponding to the more robust of the findings among wife abusers—namely, witnessing interparental aggression).

The notion that violent people are suffering from some form of psychopathology persists, despite empirical evidence to the contrary (Monahan, 1981). So, too, in the area of domestic aggression there has been an effort to assess whether perpetrators can be characterized as exhibiting some particular psychopathology or personality disorder. In an early investigation with a small sample ($N = 23$), Faulk (1974) reported psychopathology in 16 (70%) of the batterers, with depression being the most common diagnosis, followed by delusional jealousy, personality disorder, and anxiety. In a recent investigation employing the Millon Clinical Multiaxial Inventory (Millon, 1983), Hamberger and Hastings (1985, 1986) reported psychopathology in all but 15% of their batterers. Although studies of batterers have failed to reveal a consistent pattern of psychopathology, several pathological features commonly emerge from the various investigations. These include borderline symptomatology, passive aggressive tendencies, dependency, and pathological jealousy. Since all of these studies are retrospective and correlational, it is unclear whether they predate (and possibly contribute to the production of) or result from the aggressive dynamics. Most of the evidence supportive of psychopathology among abusers suggests that if there is psychopathology, it is typically an Axis II (DSM-III-R) disorder. The high base rate of Axis II symptomatology warrants caution in concluding that this represents a significant etiological factor. In fact, although Hastings and Hamberger (1988) demonstrated significant differences between abusers and controls using the MCMI, the batterers scores were generally within normal limits.

Similarly, there have been numerous attempts to identify psychological disturbances among abused women. It has been reported that victims of marital aggression show elevated MMPI profiles and suffer from a host of problems, including depression and anxiety (Margolin, Sibner, & Gleberman, 1988). Again, the similarity of the behaviors shown by abused wives to the symptoms of posttraumatic stress disorder (PTSD) suggests that these symptoms are a result, rather than a cause, of the aggression.

Elder abuse presents a somewhat different picture. Wolf, Godkin, and Pillemer (1984) found that 31% of elder abusers had a history of psychiatric illness. Pillemer (1986) reported that 79% of the elder victims reported mental or emotional problems on the part of the abuser (compared with 24% of the controls) and further that 36% had been psychiatrically hospitalized (compared with only 7% of controls). Since people are rarely hospitalized for the treatment of personality disorders, the high percentage of elder abusers receiving inpatient psychiatric treatment suggests that Axis I diagnoses are probably more common among elder abusers than they are in groups of either spouse or child abusers. Pillemer (1986) suggests that elder abuse is a more deviant behavior than either child abuse (which is often an exaggeration of legitimate physical punishment) or spouse abuse, and thus we might expect perpetrators to be more deviant.

Alcoholism is one form of pathology that consistently emerges in domestic violence research. Although the operative mechanism is uncertain, a large body of research evidence supports the conclusion that alcohol is a "potent causal antecedent of aggressive behavior" in general (Taylor & Leonard, 1983). Wife abusers are frequently alcoholic, and heavy drinkers are two to three times more likely than moderate drinkers to abuse their wives, yet the majority of alcoholics are not wife abusers, and, even among batterers, the majority of abuse incidents are not alcohol-related (Kantor & Straus, 1986). According to Pillemer (1986), elder abusers were significantly more likely to be identified as alcoholics (45% of abusers compared with 7% of controls), yet more than half of elder abusers were not identified as alcoholic.

A number of studies have demonstrated that wife-abusive males often have defective self-concepts (Goldstein & Rosenbaum, 1985; Neidig, Friedman, & Collins, 1986), undifferentiated sex-role identities (LaViolette, Barnett, & Miller, 1984; Rosenbaum, 1986), spouse-specific assertion deficits (Dutton & Strachen, 1987; Maiuro, Cahn, & Vitaliano, 1986; Rosenbaum & O'Leary, 1981), and high power needs (Dutton & Strachen, 1987). As Hotaling and Sugarman (1986) demonstrate, however, for each of these (and other) factors, there are studies that fail to support the relationship with marital aggression, suggesting that the phenomenon is multidetermined and, thus, stimulating research aimed at identifying subtypes of batterers.

Subtyping strategies typically have focused on either perpetrator behavior or personality. Shields and Hanneke (1983) provide an example of the former, dividing violent men into three categories: those whose violence is restricted to the family, those whose violence is exclusively nonfamily, and generally violent men. Hamberger and Hastings (1986) exemplify a personality-based strategy. They employed the MCMI to classify batterers and identified three personality factors: narcissistic/antisocial, schizoidal/borderline, and passive-dependent/ compulsive. Gondolf (1988) advocates use of a behavior-based typology, suggesting that what batterers "do" is more relevant to the prediction and treatment of marital aggression. It also is less complex and easier to measure. He utilized a cluster analysis to generate three subgroups: the sociopathic batterer, the antisocial batterer, and the typical batterer (this is a behavior-based typology, the names of groups 1 and 2 notwithstanding). The "sociopathic" batterer is extremely abusive of all family members, is likely to have been sexually abusive, is the most likely to have been arrested, and is the most substance-abusive. The "typical" batterer is the largest of the three groups, comprising 51% of the sample and representing the type of batterer most likely to be seen in treatment programs (other than court-mandated programs, which would probably see more "antisocial" and "sociopathic" batterers). Verbal and physical abuse is less severe. Sexual abuse and child abuse is less extensive. He is most likely to be apologetic following abusive incidents and more likely to continue in the relationship with his partner.

There have been relatively few attempts to develop typologies that integrate personality and behavioral factors, and even fewer that examine the pairings between subgroups of husbands and wives. Snyder and Fruchtman (1981) utilized a clustering process to classify abused women into subcategories. Although intended as a typology of abuse victims, they included perpetrator behavior resulting in a typology of couples consisting of five subtypes. Among the factors included in the clustering were the severity and frequency of the abuse, whether there was sexual abuse by the husband, whether the husband had also abused the children, whether there had been aggression by the wife toward the husband, alcohol use by the husband, and whether the couple was cohabitating. Including both husband and wife characteristics (demographic, personality, and behavioral) would appear to merit further consideration by typologists. We are not aware of any attempts to develop typologies of either perpetrators or victims (or the combination) in the elder abuse area.

Biological factors in adult domestic aggression have been virtually ignored. A number of recent investigations (Lewis, Pincus, Feldman, Jackson, & Bard, 1986; Lewis, Pincus, Bard, Richardson, Prichep, Feldman, & Yeager, 1988) have indicated a relationship between head injury and generalized aggressive behavior, in both juveniles and adults. Rosenbaum and Hoge (1989) reported a history of severe head injury in 61% of the male spouse abusers in their sample, suggesting a potential psychophysiological component. Elliott (1977) proposed that episodic dyscontrol syndrome, characterized by explosive rage triggered by minimal provocation, was an important cause of wife and child battery. Interestingly, episodic dyscontrol syndrome often appears as a sequela to head injury, features alcohol intolerance, results in pathological intoxication, and, like spouse abuse, may run in families.

Similarly provocative is the research indicating a relationship between aggression and neurotransmitters. There is evidence, primarily derived from animal analogue studies, linking both predatory and affective aggression with increased levels of acetylcholine and dopamine, and with reduced levels of GABA and serotonin (Eichelman, 1987). Although direct assessment of brain serotonin levels in humans is difficult, a number of studies have found a connection between aggressive and impulsive behavior in humans and reduced levels of serotonin metabolites in the cerebrospinal fluid (Brown et al., 1979). We are not aware of any investigations linking domestic aggression and neurotransmitter dysfunction. However, a variety of neurotransmitters have been implicated in either increasing or decreasing the frequency and intensity of aggressive responses in both humans and animals. Furthermore, the relationship between lowered neurotransmitter levels and depression has been established, and there is some indication that depression is common among abusers (Faulk, 1974), suggesting the value of further research in this area.

The question of whether there are intraindividual demographic factors, such as age, race, and religion, associated with wife battering is difficult to answer because of sampling problems. There is general agreement that wife battering cuts across all races, religions, and social classes. However, there also is evidence that age may be an important factor. Straus and Gelles (1986), reporting on the 1985 resurvey of a nationally representative sample, found that wife batterers were significantly younger than nonbatterers. Controlling for age, Gelles (1988) demonstrated that the association of pregnancy and the onset of spousal aggression, which had previously been reported by a number of investigators (Eisenberg & Micklow, 1977; Gelles, 1974; Helton, 1986; Stacy & Shupe, 1983), was artifactual. These recent findings emphasize the importance of age as a factor in the etiology of spousal aggression.

Attributing behavior, normal and otherwise, to cognitions, rational and irrational, has become so popular that it is not surprising that cognitive mechanisms have been suggested for marital aggression. There are, however, few direct empirical tests of this model (O'Leary, 1988). A recent study by Lohr, Hamberger, and Bonge (1988) demonstrated that certain subgroups of batterers (specifically those with personality disorders) may be characterized as having more irrational beliefs than other subgroups of batterers, although the absence of any nonbattering comparison groups in this study complicates interpretation of the role of cognitions in battering per se. The role of cognitions in battering awaits further explication.

Interpersonal Dynamics

Unlike many other forms of aggression, domestic violence, by definition, assumes a relationship between perpetrator and victim. This has several implications, including differential treatment by law enforcers, the legal system, the helping professions, the media, and the public; increased difficulty of avoiding revictimization for the victim; and a justification for examining victim contribution to the aggressive interaction. It also suggests that we examine the nature of the marital relationship. To begin with, it seems intuitively obvious that abusive couples would report lower levels of marital satisfaction, and there is empirical evidence that this is the case. Research has shown that there is more marital discord, less marital satisfaction, and a less supportive family climate in homes where marital violence has occurred (Resick & Reese, 1986; Rosenbaum & O'Leary, 1981). It also is true, however, that aggression can occur even between relatively satisfied partners. Reporting on a large sample of engaged couples, assessed in the month prior to marriage, O'Leary *et al.* (1989) found 44% of the women and 31% of the men to be physically aggressive with their partners. Although consistently aggressive couples were less maritally satisfied than consistently nonaggressive couples, two-thirds of the men and three quarters of the women in the stably aggressive group scored in the satisfactory range on a standardized measure of marital satisfaction.

Almost every study that has examined the rates of aggressive behavior of both partners has reported higher levels of aggression by women toward their partners (O'Leary *et al.*, 1989; Straus & Gelles, 1986; Straus *et al.*, 1980). This is true of dating couples (Elliott, Huizinga & Morse, 1986; O'Leary *et al.*, 1989), and even among the Quakers (Brutz & Allen, 1986). This is consistent with the reports of abusive husbands in treatment who frequently offer the excuse "she hit me first" (Rosenbaum & Maiuro, in press). Researchers reporting such statistics are quick to point out that the aggression of women toward men is different and less physically and emotionally damaging. While this is no doubt true, it may also be true that aggression by the women is relevant to the development of the aggressive dynamics of the relationship that eventuate in violence by her partner. This is not intended to excuse his aggression, but only to suggest that we not ignore the potential importance of this factor because of fear that it will deflect responsibility away from the abuser.

There is some evidence that ideological and racial differences may be associated with marital aggression. Hotaling and Sugarman (1986) report that religious incompatibility is a consistent risk marker of husband-to-wife aggression. In their study of Quaker families, Brutz and Allen (1986) concluded that religious commitment was a better indicator of the influence of religion on couple aggression. Interestingly, they reported that religious commitment was associated with low levels of marital aggression for wives but with high levels for husbands. There is also some evidence that abusive couples are more likely to be interracial (Wasileski, Callaghan-Chaffee, & Chaffee, 1982).

Hornung, McCullough, and Sugimoto (1981) offer status inconsistency and status incompatibility as couple factors predictive of aggression. They suggest that wife abuse is more probable when the wife is better educated, or employed in a higher status occupation, than her husband. Whereas the ideological and racial differences might operate through increased stress and by contributing more serious (and intense) arguments with a higher probability of provoking an aggressive response, status incompatibility and inconsistency would appear to potentiate the perpetrator's defective sense of self-esteem, perhaps contributing to a shame-induced rage.

A number of investigators have examined components of the marital interaction itself. Margolin, John, and Gleberman (1988) analyzed taped interactions between physically aggressive couples as well as couples in three comparison groups, and reported that husbands in the aggressive group exhibited more overtly negative behaviors, more negative affect, and higher levels of physiological arousal. It has been suggested that couples characterized by physical aggression exhibit marked communications deficits (Neidig & Friedman, 1984). Rosenbaum and Golash (n.d.) examined the communication styles of married couples across the first 18 months of marriage and reported that negative communication styles were characteristic of couples who had experienced aggression. However, when the data were examined longitudinally, the only couple communication factor predictive of aggression was the seriousness of the discussion topic selected. This is congruent with the suggestion that ideological, religious, and racial incompatibilities promote aggression by contributing more serious topics for argumentation—topics that may involve deeply held beliefs and cultural traditions.

There is some evidence that communication deficits may play a role in elder abuse, as well. Hirst and Miller (1986) offer a profile of the individual at high risk to be an elder abuser. According to this profile, the person at high risk is a daughter, experiences marital conflict, and has a lack of communication skills.

Marital dependency has been implicated in the development and maintenance of relationship aggression. Kalmuss and Straus (1982) report that a wife's dependency on her husband is positively related to the extent to which she has experienced violence. They define dependency both objectively (financial and the presence of young children) and subjectively (whether she perceives that things would deteriorate if the marriage broke up). According to Margolin, Sibner, and Gleberman (1988), batterers have also been characterized as dependent upon their wives. Dependency among abusers is less likely to be financial but rather may derive from the sense that his wife and family are "all he has."

Dependency is also recognized to be an important factor in elder abuse, although the directionality of the dependency is unclear. The notion of generational inversion, wherein the parent–child roles are reversed and elderly parents become dependent on their children, has been advocated by some (Steinmetz, 1983). According to this model, aggression erupts when the caretaker cannot cope with the stress of providing care to the elderly parent. This may interact with the guilt evoked by the perceived obligation coupled with the financial strain of providing adequate care. The family disruption engendered by the intrusion of an elderly parent into the home, and the diversion of temporal and emotional resources from the children of the caretaker to the parent of the caretaker, can be a further source of stress, guilt, and, consequently, anger.

Although the generational inversion model is intuitively sensible, there is evidence that it is the dependency of the abuser on the abused that is more relevant to the production of aggression. According to Wolf, Strugnell, and Godkin (1982), the abuser was financially dependent upon the abused elder in two-thirds of their sample, a finding supported by Hwalek, Sengstock, and Lawrence (1984). Pillemer (1986) reported that elder abusers were significantly more dependent on the elder in the areas of housing, household repair, finances, and transportation than were the nonabusive controls. He found fewer than 36% of elder abusers to be financially independent of their elderly victims, and concluded that financial dependence of an adult child on an elderly parent "may be an important predictor of violence" (p. 254).

It has been suggested that powerlessness or perceived powerlessness may be a causal factor common to all forms of family violence (Finkelhor, 1983). According to Pillemer (1986), "it may be that the feeling of powerlessness experienced by an adult child who is still dependent on an elderly parent is especially acute, because it goes so strongly against society's expectations for normal adult behavior" (p. 244).

Environmental Stressors

If financial dependence of abuser on victim is an important cause of elder abuse, it suggests that factors that produce economic stress would promote elder mistreatment. Since it has been established that both child abuse and spouse abuse are associated with unemployment and economic stress (Straus & Gelles, 1986), the addition of elder abuse means that this factor is common to all forms of domestic aggression. Despite the earlier statement that marital aggression cuts across all socioeconomic strata, every study that has shown a relationship between social class and aggression has shown it to be a negative one. Even taking sampling problems into account, it seems clear that there is more marital aggression among the poorer socioeconomic groups.

Job dissatisfaction and work stress have also been associated with marital violence. Barling and Rosenbaum (1986) examined work involvements, organizational commitment, job satisfaction, and work stress in three groups of men: wife abusers, nonabusive maritally dissatisfied, and satisfactorily married. The results indicated that the occurrence of stressful work events and their negative impact were related to wife abuse. This is consistent with studies indicating a relationship between parental work stress and child abuse (Agathanos & Stathakopolou, 1983). In addition to work stress, it has been reported that life stress, in general, is strongly related to marital aggression. Straus *et al.* (1980) counted the number of life (including work) stressors experienced by their subjects and reported that as the number of stressors increased, so did the probability of marital abuse. Women reporting the occurrence of 10 or more life stressors were husband-abusive more than 50% of the time. Husbands reporting 10 or more life stressors were wife-abusive about 25% of the time.

Many of the stressors experienced by couples and families may be moderated by social support networks. The stress of multiple children, for example, can be reduced by the availability of extended family caretakers. Sending the kids to Grandma's house for the weekend may provide a needed respite for overextended parents. Similarly, close relatives can often be counted on for financial support (sometimes in the form of a free meal or the "goody-bag" of groceries), for a place to stay (if the wife has to leave), for moral support, and even as an insurance policy against aggression (negative consequences threatened if you "touch my sister/daughter again"). It is not surprising that domestic aggression is often characterized by social isolation. There is research supporting the relationship between social isolation and both marital aggression (Stark, Flitcraft, Zuckerman, Gray, Robinson, & Frazier, 1981) and elder abuse (Pillemer, 1986). In the case of wife abuse, social isolation may be both a cause and an effect of aggression. Abused wives often withdraw from social interaction because of the stigma attached to being victimized, the embarrassment of visible injuries, and/or constant scrutiny by the husband regarding how they spend their time. It has been suggested that the husband may inflict visible injuries in order to isolate his wife from others, especially other men, who he fears may be more desirable mates than he.

Cultural Context

Several years ago, a superior court judge in Massachusetts heard a case involving a battered woman who was seeking protection from a severely abusive husband. The judge rebuked the woman, in the presence of the husband, for wasting the court's time. A short time later the woman was murdered by her husband. The judge was blamed, by feminist groups, for the woman's death and was criticized by the media. The chief justice promised an inquiry and, under intense pressure, initiated a program of educating the Massachusetts judiciary with regard to domestic violence. The judge was not removed from the bench, although he was, at least temporarily, prevented from hearing marital aggression cases. This is but one example of the way society legitimizes and thereby perpetuates domestic aggression.

Numerous writers have chronicled the historical legitimization of domestic aggression (see, for example, Pleck, 1987). Only recently has society proscribed the use of aggression between family members, yet even today, family violence is treated differently from assault and battery between unrelated parties. As an example, many states currently recognize a marital rape exemption that prohibits the prosecution of a husband for raping his wife.

Despite recent attempts to "enlighten" police officers, the police response is often inadequate. Police officers, like the military, are well represented among the population of abusers and are often more sympathetic to the batterer than to his victim. This, coupled with the dangerousness of intervention in family disputes, contributes to the reluctance of police to intervene in domestic violence situations. It is important to point out that there is research showing that arresting the abuser for his first offense effectively reduces the reoccurrence of battering (Sherman & Berk, 1984).

Sociocultural factors contribute in other ways, as well. Pornography sexualizes aggression toward women and may promote their victimization, by strangers and within the family. Sommers and Check (1987) found that abusive husbands read more pornography than nonabusive husbands (according to wife report). Abused wives also reported that their husbands were more likely to ask them to perform sexual acts depicted in the pornography. Sexual aggression is characteristic of the more severe cases of marital aggression and has been identified as a risk marker for interspousal homicide (Browne, 1987).

There has been a very gradual change in the marital norm from a traditional male-dominated structure to a more equalitarian one (Thornton, Alwin, & Camburn, 1983). This change is also evident in the television and cinematic representations of the typical American family as dramatized by the differences between the family structure depicted in "Father Knows Best" and that portrayed in "The Cosby Show." According to Straus and Gelles (1986), male-dominant marriages are the most violent and equalitarian marriages the least violent. They attribute the observed decreases in rates of marital aggression from 1975 to 1985 in part to this social change.

Another important social change concerns the number of women employed outside the home. Although far from equal to men in terms of salary, women are far more likely to be employed outside the home than they were even as recently as 10 years ago. Since full-time housewives are more likely to be abused (Straus *et al.*, 1980), and more likely to remain in an abusive relationship (Gelles, 1976), changes in cultural norms that encourage women to pursue careers and paid employment should have a favorable impact on rates of marital aggression.

Elder abuse similarly flourishes in a sociocultural environment that glorifies youth and treats aging as a disease. Studies have shown that young people have generally negative views of the elderly. Children tend to describe older people as tired, ill, and ugly (Seefeldt, 1984). In today's mobile society, children are often cut off from contact with aging grandparents and are unable to develop positive relationships with the elderly, thus reducing the likelihood of children learning to care for, care about, or learn from the older generation. Agism, the age equivalent of racism, is a serious problem and one that may contribute to elder abuse (Galbraith, 1986). According to a 1975 Harris Poll, the public image of the elderly is negative and possibly damaging: "The media, with coverage of the elderly poor, the elderly sick, the elderly institutionalized and the elderly unemployed or retired, may be protecting and reinforcing the distorted stereotypes of the elderly. . ." (p. 193). The significance of this negative image for elder abuse can be better appreciated if we consider de Beauvoir's (1973) historical, cross-cultural observation that nations and cultures that perceive the elderly negatively tend to treat them accordingly. According to Viano (1983), "There is no doubt that in American society becoming old means becoming less of something on the way to losing everything. If, in the eyes of many, becoming old means becoming less human, it is easy to see how a wide spectrum of victimization of the elderly can take place and be justified" (p. 13).

One reason for the sudden emergence of elder abuse as a significant problem concerns a phenomenon known as the "graying of America" (Quinn & Tomita, 1986). This refers to the fact that as the life expectancy of Americans increases, the elderly constitute an increasing proportion of the population. This strains a host of social institutions and has a dramatic economic impact on the nation. In recent years this has been seen most clearly in the form of threats to the economic stability of the social security system, a shortage of nursing-home beds, dramatic increases in health insurance costs, and the portion of the economy devoted to health care, Medicare, and other services to the elderly. Burdened with a national deficit that threatens the fiscal foundations of the country, the federal government has been cutting the funds and services provided to the elderly. In 1985 the House Select Committee on Aging, prepared a report entitled "Elder Abuse: A National Disgrace" (*Elder Abuse*, 1985). In that report they noted that while 40% of reported abuse cases involve adults and elderly adults, only 4.7% of state budgets for protective services are devoted to elderly protective services. Since 1981 the primary source of federal funding for protective services has been cut by nearly one-fifth. Three-quarters of the states reported that elder abuse is increasing, yet in the face of a clear need to increase services, the federal government is instead decreasing them.

With the federal and state governments doing less, the burden of caring for the elderly falls to their families. This not only increases stress on the family system, which, as we have discussed, is a major contributor to all forms of domestic violence; it also represents a societal devaluation of the elderly. It would be unfair to close this section without mentioning that governmental support for shelters and other programs for battered woman, batterers' treatment programs, and services to families afflicted by violence is also inadequate. Shelters, in particular, are more and more often forced to appeal to the private sector for needed operating funds or to compete for an ever-shrinking pool of resources. Lack of services for abuse victims and their children forces many victims to remain in abusive situations and perpetuates the aggression.

Summary

Surely it is clear by now that domestic aggression is complex and multidetermined. In trying to understand it we must consider the individuals involved, their histories, and their psychological makeup. We must consider the nature of the relationship between abuser and victim, as well as the family environment. Financial, work, and other life stressors must be taken into account. Finally, we must consider the sociocultural milieu that either tolerates and legitimizes aggression or prohibits and punishes it, that either devalues segments of the population (women and the elderly, for example) or preaches and practices respect and equality for all segments of the population.

References

Agathanos, H., & Stathakopolou, N. (1983). Life events and child abuse: A controlled study. In J. Leavitt (Ed.), *Child abuse and neglect: Research and innovations in NATO countries* (pp. 83–91). Netherlands: Kluver.

Barling, J., & Rosenbaum, A. (1986). Work stressors and wife abuse. *Journal of Applied Psychology, 71*, 346–348.

Bernard, M. L., & Bernard, J. L. (1983). Violent intimacy: The family as a model for love relationships. *Family Relations, 32,* 283–286.

Brown, G. L., Ballenger, J. C., Minichiello, M. D., & Goodwin, F. K. (1979). Human aggression and its relation to cerebrospinal fluid, 5-hydroxyindole acetic acid, 3-methoxy-4-hydroxyphenylglycol and homovanillic acid. In M. Sandler (Ed.), *Psychopharmacology of Aggression.* New York: Raven Press.

Browne, A. (1987). *When battered women kill.* New York: Free Press.

Brutz, J. L., & Allen, C. M. (1986). Religious commitment, peace activism, and marital violence in Quaker families. *Journal of Marriage and the Family, 48,* 491–502.

Caesar, P. L. (1988). Exposure to violence in the families-of-origin among wife abusers and maritally non-violent men. *Violence and Victims, 3,* 49–63.

de Beauvoir, S. (1973). *The coming of age.* New York: Warner.

Dutton, D. G., & Strachen, C. E. (1987). Motivational needs for power and spouse-specific assertiveness in assaultive and non-assaultive men. *Violence and Victims, 2,* 145–156.

Eichelman, B. (1987). Neurochemical bases of aggressive behavior. *Psychiatric Annals, 17,* 371–374.

Eisenberg, S., & Micklow, P. (1977). The assaulted wife: "Catch-22" revisited. *Women's Rights Law Reporter, 3,* 138–161.

Elder abuse: A national disgrace. (1985, May 10). Submitted by the House Select Committee on Aging, Claude Pepper, chair. (Summary published in *Caring,* January 1986)

Elliott, D. S., Huizinga, D., & Morse, B. J. (1986). Self-reported violent offending: A descriptive analysis of juvenile violent offenders and their offending careers. *Journal of Interpersonal Violence, 4,* 472–514.

Elliott, F. A. (1977). The neurology of explosive rage: The dyscontrol syndrome. In M. Roy (Ed.), *Battered women.* New York: Van Nostrand Reinhold.

Faulk, M. (1974). Men who assault their wives. *Medicine, Science and the Law, 14,* 180–183.

Finkelhor, D. (1983). Common features of family abuse. In D. Finkelhor, R. J. Gelles, G. Hotaling, & M. A. Straus (Eds.), *The dark side of families: Current family violence research.* Beverly Hills, CA: Sage.

Galbraith, M. W. (1986). Elder abuse: An overview. In M. W. Galbraith (Ed.), *Elder abuse: Perspectives on an emerging crisis.* Kansas City: Mid-America Conference on Aging.

Geffner, R., Rosenbaum, A., & Hughes, H. (1988). Research issues concerning family violence. In V. B. Van Hasselt, R. L. Morrison, A. S. Bellack, & M. Hersen (Eds.), *Handbook of family violence.* New York: Plenum.

Gelles, R. J. (1974). *The violent home: A study of physical aggression between husbands and wives.* Beverly Hills, CA: Sage.

Gelles, R. J. (1976). Abused wives: Why do they stay? *Journal of Marriage and the Family, 38,* 659–668.

Gelles, R. J. (1988). Violence and pregnancy: Are pregnant women at greater risk of abuse? *Journal of Marriage and the Family, 50,* 841–847.

Gold, D. T., & Gwyther, L. P. (1989). The prevention of elder abuse: An educational model. *Family Relations, 38,* 8–14.

Goldstein, D., & Rosenbaum, A. (1985). An evaluation of the self-esteem of maritally violent men. *Family Relations, 34,* 425–428.

Gondolf, E. W. (1988). Who are those guys? Toward a behavioral typology of batterers. *Violence and Victims, 3,* 187–203.

Hamberger, L. K., & Hastings, J. E. (1985, March). *Personality correlates of men who abuse their partners: Some preliminary data.* Paper presented at the meeting of the Society of Personality Assessment, Berkeley, CA.

Hamberger, L. K., & Hastings, J. E. (1986). Personality correlates of men who abuse their partners: A cross-validation study. *Journal of Family Violence, 1,* 323–341.

Hastings, J. E., & Hamberger, L. K. (1988). Personality characteristics of spouse abusers: A controlled comparison. *Violence and Victims, 3,* 31–48.

Helton, A. (1986). Battering during pregnancy. *American Journal of Nursing, 86,* 910–913.

Hirst, S. P., & Miller, J. (1986). The abused elderly. *Journal of Psychosocial Nursing and Mental Health Services, 24,* 28–34.

Hornung, C. A., McCullough, B. C., & Sugimoto, T. (1981). Status relationships in marriage: Risk factors in spouse abuse. *Journal of Marriage and the Family, 43,* 675–692.

Hotaling, G. T., & Sugarman, D. B. (1986). An analysis of risk markers in husband to wife violence: The current state of knowledge. *Violence and Victims, 2,* 101–124.

Hwalek, M. A., Sengstock, M. C., & Lawrence, R. (1984, November). *Assessing the probability of abuse of the elderly.* Paper presented at the annual meeting of the Gerontological Society of America.

Kalmuss, D. (1984). The intergenerational transmission of marital aggression. *Journal of Marriage and the Family, 46,* 11–19.

Kalmuss, D., & Straus, M. A. (1982). Wife's marital dependency and wife abuse. *Journal of Marriage and the Family, 44,* 277–286.

Kantor, G. K., & Straus, M. A. (1986, April). *The drunken bum theory of wife beating.* Paper presented at the National Alcoholism Forum Conference on Alcohol and the Family, San Francisco.

LaViolette, A. D., Barnett, O. W., & Miller, C. L. (1984, July). *A classification of wife abusers on the BEM Sex-Role Inventory.* Paper presented at the Second National Conference of Research on Domestic Violence, Durham, NH.

Lewis, D. O., Pincus, J. H., Feldman, M., Jackson, L., & Bard, B. (1986). Psychiatric, neurological, and psychoeducational characteristics of 15 death row inmates in the United States. *American Journal of Psychiatry, 143,* 838–845.

Lewis, D. O., Pincus, J. H., Bard, B., Richardson, E., Prichep, L. S., Feldman, M., & Yeager, C. (1988). Neuropsychiatric, psychoeducational, and family characteristics of 14 juveniles condemned to death in the United States. *American Journal of Psychiatry, 145,* 584–589.

Lohr, J. M., Hamberger, L. K., & Bonge, D. (1988). The nature of irrational beliefs in different personality clusters of spouse abusers. *Journal of Rational-Emotive and Cognitive-Behavior Therapy, 6,* 273–285.

Lorenz, K. (1966). *On aggression.* New York: Harcourt, Brace & World.

Maiuro, R. D., Cahn, T. S., & Vitaliano, P. P. (1986). Assertiveness deficits and hostility in domestically violent men. *Violence and Victims, 1,* 279–289.

Margolin, G., John, R. S., & Gleberman, L. (1988). Affective responses to conflictual discussions in violent and non-violent couples. *Journal of Consulting and Clinical Psychology, 56,* 24–33.

Margolin, G., Sibner, L. G., & Gleberman, L. (1988). Wife battering. In V. B. Van Hasselt, R. L. Morrison, A. S. Bellack, & M. Hersen (Eds.), *Handbook of family violence.* New York: Plenum.

Millon, T. (1983). *Millon Clinical Multiaxial Inventory Manual.* Minneapolis: Interpretive Scoring Systems.

Monahan, J. (1981). *The clinical prediction of violent behavior.* Rockville, MD: NIMH.

Neidig, P. H., & Friedman, D. H. (1984). *Spouse abuse: A treatment program for couples.* Champaign, IL: Research Press.

Neidig, P. N., Friedman, D. H., & Collins, B. S. (1986). Attitudinal characteristics of males who have engaged in spouse abuse. *Journal of Family Violence, 1,* 223–234.

O'Leary, K. D. (1988). Physical aggression between spouses: A social learning theory perspective. In V. B. Van Hasselt, R. L. Morrison, A. S. Bellack, & M. Hersen (Eds.), *Handbook of family violence.* New York: Plenum.

O'Leary, K. D., Barling, J., Arias, I., Rosenbaum, A., Malone, J., & Tyree, A. (1989). Prevalence and stability of physical aggression between spouses: A longitudinal analysis. *Journal of Consulting and Clinical Psychology, 57,* 263–268.

Owens, D. S., & Straus, M. A. (1975). The social structure of violence and approval of violence as an adult. *Aggressive Behavior, 1*, 193–211.

Pierce, R. L., & Trotta, R. (1986). Abused parents: A hidden family problem. *Journal of Family Violence, 1*, 99–110.

Pillemer, K. A. (1986). Risk factors in elder abuse: Results from a case-control study. In K. A. Pillemer & R. S. Wolf (Eds.), *Elder abuse: Conflict in the family*. Dover, MA: Auburn House.

Pillemer, K. A., & Wolf R. S. (1986). *Elder abuse: Conflict in the family*. Dover, MA: Auburn House.

Pleck, E. (1987). *Domestic tyranny*. New York: Oxford University Press.

Quinn, M. J., & Tomita, S. K. (1986). *Elder abuse and neglect: Causes, diagnosis, and treatment strategies*. New York: Springer.

Resick, P. A., & Reese, D. (1986). Perception of family social climate and physical aggression in the home. *Journal of Family Violence, 1*, 71–83.

Rosenbaum, A. (1986). Of men, macho, and marital violence. *Journal of Family Violence, 1*(2), 121–129.

Rosenbaum, A. (1988). Methodological issues in marital violence research. *Journal of Family Violence, 3*, 91–104.

Rosenbaum, A., & Golash, L. R. (n.d.) *Communication and aggression in beginning marriages*. Unpublished manuscript, University of Massachusetts Medical School.

Rosenbaum, A., & Hoge, S. K. (1989). Head injury and marital aggression. *American Journal of Psychiatry, 146*(8), 1048–1051.

Rosenbaum, A., & Maiuro, R. D. (in press). Treatment of spouse abusers. In R. T. Ammerman & M. Hersen (Eds.), *Treatment of family violence: A sourcebook*. New York: Wiley.

Rosenbaum, A., & O'Leary, K. D. (1981). Marital violence: Characteristics of abusive couples. *Journal of Consulting and Clinical Psychology, 49*, 63–71.

Seefeldt, C. (1984). Children's attitudes toward the elderly: A cross-cultural comparison. *International Journal of Aging and Human Development, 19*, 319–328.

Sherman, L. W., & Berk, R. A. (1984). The specific deterrent effects of arrest for domestic assault. *American Sociological Review, 49*, 261–271.

Shields, N. M., & Hanneke, C. R. (1983). *Violent husbands: Patterns of individual violence*. Unpublished manuscript submitted to NIMH.

Snyder, D. K., & Fruchtman, L. A. (1981). Differential patterns of wife abuse: A data-based typology. *Journal of Consulting and Clinical Psychology, 49*, 878–885.

Sommers, E. K., & Check, J. V. P. (1987). An empirical investigation of the role of pornography in the verbal and physical abuse of women. *Violence and Victims, 2*, 189–209.

Stacy, W. A., & Shupe, A. (1983). *The family secret: Domestic violence in America*. Boston: Beacon Press.

Stark, E., Flitcraft, A., Zuckerman, D., Gray, A., Robinson, J., & Frazier, W. (1981). *Wife abuse in the medical setting: An introduction to health personnel*. Washington, DC: National Clearinghouse on Domestic Violence. (Monograph series #7)

Steinmetz, S. (1983). Dependency, stress and violence between middle-aged caregivers and their elderly parents. In J. I. Kosberg (Ed.), *Abuse and maltreatment of the elderly*. Littleton, MA: Wright.

Straus, M. A. (1986). Medical care costs of intrafamily assault and homicide. *Bulletin of the New York Academy of Medicine, 62*, 556–561.

Straus, M. A., & Gelles, R. J. (1986). Societal change and change in family violence from 1975 to 1985 as revealed by two national surveys. *Journal of Marriage and the Family, 48*, 465–479.

Straus, M. A., Gelles, R. J., & Steinmetz, S. K. (1980). *Behind closed doors: Violence in the American family*. New York: Anchor/Doubleday.

Taylor, S. P., & Leonard, K. E. (1983). Alcohol and human physical aggression. In R. G.

Green & E. I. Donnerstein (Eds.), *Aggression: Theoretical and empirical reviews.* New York: Academic Press.

Telch, C. F., & Lindquist, C. U. (1984). Violent vs. non-violent couples: A comparison of patterns. *Psychotherapy, 21,* 242–248.

Thornton, A., Alwin, D. F., & Camburn, D. (1983). Causes and consequences of sex-role attitudes and attitude change. *American Sociology Review, 48,* 211–227.

Viano, E. (1983). Victimology: An overview. In J. I. Kosberg (Ed.), *Abuse and maltreatment of the elderly.* Littleton, MA: Wright.

Wasileski, M., Callaghan-Chaffee, M. E., & Chaffee, R. B. (1982). Spousal violence in military homes: An initial study. *Military Medicine, 147,* 761–765.

Wolf, R. S., Strugnell, C., & Godkin, M. (1982). *Preliminary findings from three model projects on elderly abuse.* Worcester, MA: University of Massachusetts, University Center on Aging.

Wolf, R. S., Godkin, M., & Pillemer, K. A. (1984). *Elder abuse and neglect: Report from three model projects.* Worcester, MA: University of Massachusetts, University Center on Aging.

4

Legal Issues in Violence toward Children

Bruce K. Mac Murray and Barbara A. Carson

Introduction

Contemporary work examining legal issues of violence toward children tends to focus on two basic questions. First, when is it appropriate for the state to intervene in situations of child maltreatment? And second, when the state does intervene, how should it respond to these cases? This chapter will review these two questions, presenting a variety of viewpoints, and, when possible, discussing empirical findings regarding the role of the legal system in cases of child physical abuse, neglect, and sexual abuse.

In the 1970s considerable effort was put into legal reform focusing upon the creation of laws making child maltreatment illegal and mandating the reporting of suspected cases. During the debates to create these early laws, concern was expressed about the relationship of the rights of parents, the rights of children, and the role of the state. Beginning with common law and according to legal precedence, parents have the freedom of choice in the guidance and direction of their family (Duncan, 1973). The U.S. Supreme Court has determined that the right to bring up children is one aspect of liberty as stated in the Fourteenth Amendment (*Cleveland Board of Education v. Lafleur*, 1974; *Meyer v. Nebraska*, 1923). Today, however, children have some rights as well. All 50

Bruce K. Mac Murray • Department of Sociology, Social Work, and Criminal Justice, Anderson University, Anderson, Indiana 46012.   **Barbara A. Carson** • Department of Criminal Justice and Criminology, Ball State University, Muncie, Indiana 47306.

states now have laws prohibiting child maltreatment. If parents abuse or neglect their children, or if they provide a life-style that is inappropriate for the upbringing of their children, the state, under *parents patriae*, has the right to intervene and protect the children.

With the accumulation of knowledge regarding what happens to abusive families when their maltreatment is made public, and additional information about how the criminal justice system responds to these cases, there is renewed debate regarding the appropriate role of the state and the determination of precisely at what point the criminal justice system should intervene. Besharov (1986) claims that during the last 20 years there has been a steady decriminalization of physical abuse cases, meaning that more and more cases are being responded to by social service agencies rather than the criminal justice system. Nationwide, less than 5% of all substantiated cases of child maltreatment result in criminal prosecution (American Humane Association, 1986). Undoubtedly, part of the reason for the low prosecution rates for child maltreatment revolves around the difficulties in processing these cases. Nevertheless, Besharov (1986) believes that there should be more involvement by the criminal justice system, primarily because of the basic ineffectiveness of treatment programs for stopping repeated offenses, and the harms associated with foster care or other out-of-home placements.

Other scholars argue that the real problem is that there is *too much* involvement by the legal system in the management of cases involving violence toward children. The primary complaint made by these critics is that children and families are revictimized by the criminal justice system in the investigation of legal processing of these cases. They state that a variety of negative consequences are associated with legal system involvement, including repeated telling of the story and court testimony causing extreme trauma for the victimized child witness (Wolfe, Las, & Wilson, 1987), family relations becoming strained after the official investigation and criminal proceedings get under way (Tyler & Brassard, 1984), and some mandated treatment programs possibly causing further harm to the involved family members (Kent, 1976). In addition, it is argued that child maltreatment cases have become so tied to the legal system that frequently the only way for families to receive services is to have an official report made against them (Newburger, 1985). Generally, there is agreement that some cases need to be referred to the criminal justice system, particularly situations involving serious harm, rape, pornography, forced prostitution, or severe reinjury (Bourne, 1985). However, there is little consensus regarding the appropriate response called for with other types of maltreatment.

Complaints against the legal system are further fueled by its difficulty in responding to child maltreatment cases. These cases are different from most handled by the criminal justice system in two important ways. First, the victims are children who frequently are the only witnesses to the abuse. Prior research suggests that prosecutors are reluctant to use victims as witnesses in general (Littrell, 1979), but this reaction is even more intensified when the only witness is a victimized young child. The second distinction is that these acts are familial in nature. Crimes within the family are traditionally responded to differently than stranger crimes by the legal system. However, in cases of child abuse or neglect, the state must not only attempt to mediate between the rights of parents and the rights of children but must also maintain a commitment, where possible, to do no further harm to the family unit (Duncan, 1973).

As this chapter will document, many new innovations are currently being explored and tried by the legal system. Yet it is unclear whether or not these innovations will necessarily reduce the complaints leveled against the criminal justice system in terms of the harm it creates for children and for families. In addition, other concerns suggest that while attempting to provide a benevolent yet protective approach to maltreatment cases, the state may actually be restricting children's access to justice by not letting them testify in court (Melton, 1980).

The remaining sections will trace the processing of child abuse and neglect cases through the criminal justice system from the beginning stage of reporting to final disposition. Points at which the legal system has difficulty in processing child maltreatment cases will be reviewed, as will some of the innovative procedures now being implemented in an attempt to improve the process.

Reporting Laws and Procedures

Since 1964, all U.S. states have enacted laws requiring reports to be made for incidents of suspected child abuse (both physical and sexual) and neglect. All states mandate physicians, teachers, and social workers to report suspected cases of maltreatment. Some states require additional groups to report, and some (e.g., New Hampshire) have gone so far as to require all adults, be they lawyers, therapists, priests, rabbis, ministers, or others, to report. The majority of states provide specific criminal penalities for the failure to report, with the remaining states specifying general statutory provisions that can establish criminal liability with a fine of from $100 to $1000 and/or imprisonment. A few states have even specified statutory provisions establishing civil liability for failure to report maltreatment cases, resulting in several successful lawsuits against hospitals, police departments, and residential homes.

The justification for mandatory reporting is based upon the view that children, either because of their physical immaturity or because of powerlessness, are unable to make reports for themselves. As such, the burden is placed upon other members of society to notify authorities of improper treatment. According to Besharov (1977), the intent of mandatory reporting is to provide protection to the child, not to punish the offender.

Despite the passage of mandatory reporting laws, there are still problems in the reporting process. Some involve procedural issues. For example, Saltzman (1986) discusses how social workers who work with alcohol or drug users are prohibited by federal law from disclosing the identity of their clients under penalty of criminal liability, and yet every U.S. state specifically requires social workers to report suspected cases of child abuse. It is possible that the substance-abusing client may also be a suspected abuser of children, but there is no clear-cut legal procedure for how social workers should respond to this legal dilemma. Similarly, a recent survey of therapists found that many believe they should not always be required to report suspected cases of child abuse (Miller & Weinstock, 1985), arguing that when the offender is undergoing treatment and the abuse has stopped, there is no need to violate confidentiality between a therapist and a client by filing a report of abuse.

Other procedural issues revolve around deciding the most appropriate agencies to receive reports of suspected cases. In some jurisdictions reports are made to police, while in others they are submitted to social or child protective service agencies, and in still others they are made to both. In some states, serious cases (e.g., sexual assault, deaths, and serious physical injuries) must be reported to the prosecutor's office (Mac Murray, 1988) or to medical examiners. As yet, there has been little systematic evaluation of what is the most effective agency to receive mandatory maltreatment reports and referrals.

Besides procedural concerns, other analysts are critical of the mandatory reporting laws because of the extreme involvement of the legal system and the lack of intervention by helping services. The major concern here is that the legal system has taken over society's primary reaction to violence toward children and that this is not necessarily an appropriate response (Newburger, 1985; Valentine, Stewart-Acuff, Freeman, & Andreas, 1984). The legal response to child maltreatment has the potential to create severe harm to family units once a case of abuse or neglect is reported. For example, Tyler and Brassard (1984) found that many families, including noninvolved family members, suffer from intense public stigma once a report of maltreatment is made, and that internal family relations are also severely strained. Although these families are already suffering major problems related to the abuse and other forms of maladjustment, professionals also are concerned that the involvement of the criminal justice system may actually worsen the home situation.

Another important issue relates to the preeminence of the legal system in processing maltreatment cases. All states have laws stating that emotional or psychological abuse is illegal, but few states have precise definitions as to what this means. As such, it is difficult for the criminal justice system to pursue legal charges in these cases. Thus, even though instances of psychological abuse get reported, few are responded to by the criminal justice system (Melton & Corson, 1987; Melton & Davidson, 1987). This means that when a case is reported but there are difficulties in demonstrating that it meets the legal definition, it often is dropped by the criminal justice system. The implications of this process become even more profound when it is realized that frequently services to abusive families are available only to those families where a formal complaint has been reported (Newburger, 1985). As a consequence, unless there is sufficient evidence to prosecute the offender, a case frequently will receive no further intervention from the legal system or from any other public service agency. This has led one expert in the field (Newburger, 1985) to conclude that, contrary to Besharov's (1977) idea that mandatory reporting is designed to protect the child, the effect of such reporting is rather to control the offender. As a result, often little is said or done about trying to provide a solution to the involved family's problems.

Investigation

The investigation of child maltreatment plays a key role in how the case will proceed through the criminal justice system. At the same time, such investigations also pose the risk of increasing the trauma experienced by children, depending upon how the inquiry is handled (Whitcomb, Shapiro, & Shellwagen, 1985). As in reporting procedures, states vary in who conducts investigations of violence against children. In many states the investigation is carried out by child protective service agencies, in some states it is conducted by the police, and in others by both. In many jurisdictions, multidisciplinary teams comprising social service, legal, and/or clinical professionals have been created to help reduce the trauma experienced by children and families. These teams often coordinate investigative efforts and hold regular meetings to confer on cases and recommend courses of action related to the provision of services, prosecution, custody, and treatment. However, there also is concern about joint endeavors in that police officers, lawyers, and social workers often differentially approach the problem of maltreatment and have their own preferred courses of action (Craft & Clarkson, 1985; Whitcomb et al., 1985). At the present time, there is little empirical research on which approach is most appropriate.

Furthermore, there is variation between states as to whether child maltreatment cases are processed in criminal court, where the highest standard of proof is needed to substantiate a case, or if these cases proceed through civil court, where only a preponderance of evidence is needed (Duncan, 1973). Obviously, it is easier to substantiate cases if they are processed by civil proceedings, but there is as yet no systematic comparison as to which may be the more appropriate process for legal proceedings.

In a number of jurisdictions, innovations involving special facilities and equipment (e.g., special playrooms, anatomically complete or correct dolls, and art materials) have been utilized to facilitate investigations (see Cramer, 1986; Wolfe et al., 1987). Another important effort involves the creation of child/victim/witness advocate or assistant positions (Libai, 1969) filled by personnel specially trained to conduct interviews and work with children and families throughout a case's criminal justice history. Although these efforts appear to be effective, little has been directed toward empirical evaluation of such approaches.

During the investigation of serious cases of child maltreatment, it is possible to temporarily remove the child from the home on an emergency basis. All states have policies authorizing the police to take this action without court order, and approximately 25 states allow child protective service workers to do so as well. This action may be essential to ensure the protection of the child, but it also is a drastic move for several reasons. First, cases of abuse do take place within foster or group homes as well as in natural family settings. Second, a more frequent concern involves the mismanagement of cases. The primary issue here is that sometimes children appear to be forgotten by protective agencies and are left in foster care for too long a time. At the other extreme, some children in foster care are frequently moved, resulting in the related fear that such constant disruption in living arrangements is harmful to the child, especially one who is already coping with being a victim of parental maltreatment (Besharov, 1977; Kent, 1976). The ultimate concern in this regard, of course, is that out-of-home placement may actually cause more harm to the child than the original abuse that instigated official involvement and intervention. Newburger (1985) expresses additional concern that out-of-home placement is too often seen as a first reaction by authorities rather than as an alternative of last resort. Others express concern that decisions to withdraw custody may be made for unwar-

ranted reasons, such as diversity of life-style (Valentine *et al.*, 1984) or because of poverty (Bourne, 1985).

Prosecution Decisions

Implicit within the discussion of criminal proceedings is the question of prosecutorial decision making. Although issues of prosecutorial discretion, plea bargaining, and diversion have been sources of considerable attention in discussions of the criminal justice system in general, relatively little work has been specifically directed to the application of these issues to cases involving violence against children.

One aspect of the criminal justice system's handling of maltreatment that has received substantial empirical evaluation is that concerning prosecutors' decisions about whether or not to press charges in child sexual abuse cases. Finkelhor (1983) found in a national study that criminal action occurred in only 24% of the reported cases, with considerable variability between jurisdictions. Similarly, Rogers (1982) reports that in Washington, D.C., only 38% of those cases referred for prosecution eventually ended up in court. Finally, Mac Murray (1988) reveals that, in two metropolitan Boston counties, almost half of those cases referred under a mandatory prosecutor reporting law were dropped at the point of case screening.

Research on sexual abuse further suggests that a decision to prosecute is less likely in cases (a) with younger victims, (b) where the nature of the relationship between the prepetrator and victim is intra- rather than extrafamilial, (c) where the length of the abuse is quite short, (d) where the case is first reported to the police rather than some other agency, and (e) where the offender has a prior history of drug, alcohol, or spouse abuse (Finkelhor, 1983; Mac Murray, 1989; Rogers, 1982). In short, this empirical work indicates that many cases referred to prosecutors and the criminal justice system "fall between the cracks" and fail to receive any formal action owing to evidentiary and related problems. However, the study by Mac Murray (1988) also found that the vast majority of those cases dropped by prosecutors were ultimately disposed by means of noncriminal judgments designed to reduce the at-risk situation for the child victim. Such actions included the perpetrator's leaving the home or being formally processed on other charges, a restraining or no visitation order against the offender, foster home placement for the victim and other children, or the voluntary participation of the victim and/or the alleged perpetrator in counseling or treatment programs.

Court Testimony

As a result of investigations and prosecutorial screenings, few cases of violence toward children make it to criminal court proceedings. However, for those that do, there are high stakes in case outcomes resting upon court testimony. As such, considerable attention has focused upon issues of children's competency to qualify as witnesses and related concerns about the credibility of their testimony. Current thought regarding the competency issue begins with a recognition that there are different standards of competency (see Davidson & Bulkley, 1982; Melton, Bulkley, & Walkan, 1981; Quinn, 1986). For some states, specific minimum age requirements are delineated, while in a number of other states, the determination of competence is left up to the presiding judge in the case. The primary standard for a judge's determination of competency is based upon the Supreme Court ruling in the murder case of *Wheeler v. United States* (1895). This standard is typically implemented through a *voir dire* questioning dealing with the child witness's capacity and intelligence, his/her appreciation of the difference between truth and falsehood, and the child's duty to tell the truth.

Recent work within developmental psychology, however, has suggested that the testimony of very young children (as young as 4 years of age, according to Melton, 1985) can be as reliable and valid as that of adults. In general, research on memory, suggestability, and cognitive abilities as they relate to legal testimony suggests far greater similarity than important differences between children and adults (see Goodman, 1984; Melton, 1985; Nurcombe, 1986). In reviewing these research findings, Melton (1985; in agreement with Wigmore, 1940, four decades earlier) contends that there may be reason to simply admit the testimony of children without establishing or questioning their competency. Afterwards, through the trial process, an evaluation of the child's credibility by the trier of fact can be made, as it is with any witness's testimony. This standard is basically the same as that adopted by Federal Rule of Evidence 601, which presumes that all witnesses are competent to testify and focuses questions upon credibility assessment (Quinn, 1986).

At the same time, the clinical literature also raises questions regarding retardation, developmental immaturity, language and learning disabilities, fabrication, parental indoctrination, and posttraumatic stress disorder symptoms for child witnesses, particularly in cases involving disputes (e.g., concerning divorce, custody, or visitation issues) between parents or guardians (see Nurcombe, 1986; Quinn, 1986; Terr, 1986; Yates, 1987). One possible remedy to this problem is the involvement of the psychiatrist, therapist, or other qualified professional in the criminal court process as an expert witness on questions related to child

abuse (especially sexual abuse) and the competency and/or credibility of victim witnesses (Gothard, 1987). Indeed, as Terr (1986) points out, in some cases the therapist may have to serve as the child's witness, in effect, on the basis of clinical observations (including hearsay statements) and a professional evaluation of the child.

While much concern has dealt with questions of credibility and competency for child witnesses, even greater attention has been devoted to the potential trauma for child victims related to the criminal court process. This concern with so-called secondary victimization or system-induced trauma (Wolfe et al., 1987) has resulted in a number of proposed and/or implemented innovations to the criminal justice process (Berliner & Barbieri, 1984; Bernstein & Claman, 1986; Colby & Colby, 1987). The stages in the processing of a case that have received the greatest attention in this area are (1) the actual testimony of the child in court, and (2) the delays and generally slow speed by which cases are typically handled in the criminal court.

For the testimony of a child witness in court, the primary concern with trauma centers upon the accused's constitutional right, based upon the Sixth and Fourteenth Amendments, to face and confront all witnesses, related cross-examination by the defense counsel, and the general foreignness of the court setting. A major issue in this latter vein is the unfamiliarity of the child with the criminal courtroom and its procedures. To help remedy this circumstance, a number of publications have been created, often in the form of story or comic books, to explain to children the criminal court's operation and function. In addition, a number of suggestions appear in the professional literature regarding other ways of helping to prepare children for court testimony (Bernstein, Claman, Harris, & Samson, 1982; Claman, Harris, Bernstein, & Lovitt, 1986). Included among these various techniques are courtroom tours and visits (Pynoos & Eth, 1984), efforts to "demystify" the court and its procedures (Whitcomb et al., 1985), the use of role-playing or mock trial simulations (Bauer, 1983), the preparation of children for court testimony via therapeutic evaluation and debriefing (Terr, 1986), and the use of "vertical case management" where the child works with the same professional from the time the case first enters the criminal court through to final disposition and meetings between the prosecutor and witness in preparation for the child's testimony in court (Davidson & Bulkley, 1982; Wolfe et al., 1987).

Similar concerns relate to the issue of preparing the child for facing the accused perpetrator in open court and cross-examination by the defense. The major reforms that have been suggested in this area consist of the use of audio or video closed-circuit depositions or tape testimony, and use of closed courtroom trials or special closed session where children testify (Colby & Colby, 1987; Melton, 1985; Wolfe *et al.*, 1987; Yates, 1987). However, many of these innovations are controversial and have not been fully tested by the courts as they relate to constitutional questions regarding the defendant's trial rights (see *Globe v. Supreme Court*, 1982; Melton, 1985).

A final issue with the criminal court process concerns the considerable time involved in the formal handling of a criminal case through disposition at trial. The problem of delay, based upon postponements, continuances, and the often plodding and methodical way in which the criminal court operates, creates an experience that one group describes as being similar to "an emotional 'roller coaster,' with periods of heightened anxiety before the court date followed by a conflicting disappointment of not testifying and the relief of postponing a stressful encounter" (Wolfe *et al.*, 1987, p. 110). Remedies to this situation have been established in some jurisdictions via policies restricting continuances and other unnecessary court delays, or by witness assistants providing early notification of such events to child witnesses.

Finally, several observers (Pyroos & Eth, 1984; Terr, 1986) point out that while there are clearly threats to the emotional health of child victims resulting from criminal court actions, there also is considerable potential for healing and rehabilitative effects from such involvement. Thus, Terr (1986) states that "fully participating in the courtroom process may help some previously overwhelmed children to feel more potent" (p. 469). Such court involvement may also highlight for the children that justice can be done when they are victims, and that their truthful testimony can be as important and consequential as that of adults.

Final Disposition and Case Outcomes

Formal court dispositions can range along a continuum from punishment to treatment, and may even involve no action at all. Formal punishment for serious offenses involving violence against children in some states can include a fine, incarceration, and/or termination of child custody. Yet the criminal justice system does not limit itself to punitive actions.

As Gelles and Straus (1988) have pointed out, the criminal justice system fluctuates between control and compassion concerns that lead to a focus on treatment in the processing of domestic violence cases. Mandated treatment programs can result either from an informal disposition (e.g., resulting from plea bargaining or pretrial diversion) or as part of a formal criminal sentence handed down at trial. One problem in this regard is that there is the expectation that treatment will be effective, without supporting evaluations that this is in fact the case. Similarly, without careful monitoring, offenders may not follow through on such assigned treatment programs to completion. Furthermore, while there may appear to be a wealth of diverse resources in treatment programs available in a community, practical problems of long waiting lists or strict financial conditions may constrain the full and regular participation by some offenders. As such, this situation may create some liability on the part of the criminal justice system in terms of recidivism and the risk of repeated maltreatment later on.

Weiner (1985) further elaborates on the implications of mandating treatment as an official decree of the criminal justice system. She argues that, in general, competent individuals have the right to refuse treatment, even if these individuals are prisoners. Yet the criminal justice system frequently mandates consent and involvement in treatment as a condition of avoiding criminal prosecution or as a condition for being granted probation or parole. Weiner points out problems in the processing of child maltreatment offenders given the ethical requirement of informed consent for treatment procedures. As yet, there appears to be little concern about the right of convicted perpetrators to refuse treatment or even to demand treatment, although this may become a more significant issue in the future.

It is difficult to determine how many convicted abusers are fined, sent to prison, or receive some other form of punishment. Probably the most frequent punitive measure is the permanent removal of the child's custody from the parents. Previously discussed problems associated with temporary out-of-home placements are even more intensified when permanent termination of parental rights is considered. In custody proceedings, the judge or jury may make a rebuttable presumption that if a child is in the custody of an adult and a nonaccidental injury occurs, it can be assumed that the adult is responsible, even if no direct evidence is presented (Duncan, 1973). While this procedure helps ensure the rights of nonverbal, immature children, several analysts have suggestd that a child should also have access to an adult advocate or even legal counsel (Duncan, 1973; Duquette & Ramsey, 1986; Whitcomb, 1988). There is precedent for this in other legal procedings such as juvenile court, and the argument is basically the same in custody proceedings. The child needs an advocate to consider future protection as well as the child's right to stay in the home. In fact, this proposal for advocacy has been expanded to suggest that children should have an appointed advocate at the commencement of investigations of maltreatment cases (Whitcomb, 1988).

Summary and Future Directions

This review of the literature points out that the legal system is still trying to determine the most effective and least harmful way of processing cases involving the maltreatment of children. It also outlines concerns that professionals have about how beneficial and effective the involvement of the legal and criminal justice system has been in these cases. In light of knowledge of current procedures and the limited research available on this topic, the following suggestions are offered for what the role of the state should be in regard to cases of violence against children.

When the State Should Intervene in Cases of Child Maltreatment

When cases of child maltreatment are discovered, all efforts should be made to work with families to stop the violence. By definition, the family is an institution that exists throughout a person's lifetime, so the optimal solution to child abuse would be to help the family become a better-functioning unit. If it is agreed that this is the primary goal for responding to abusive families, then it is clear that skilled social welfare officials are beset suited to the task of helping families. As such, we suggest that mandatory reports of child abuse be made to child protective agencies rather than to the criminal justice system.

Criminal proceedings should be reserved for only the most serious cases—namely, those in which there is the potential for permanent harm or injury to the child or repeated incidents of serious violence (see Bourne, 1985). In a related sense, the criminal justice system should be involved in all cases where the temporary or permanent termination of parental rights is being considered. In those cases referred to criminal justice agents, such contact should be swift and consistent, both to protect the interests of the child and in order to provide appropriate legal action against accused offenders.

We further suggest that the state should require that all nonserious cases of child maltreatment be handled by social service agencies. Nonserious cases must not be allowed to disappear and be ignored by society simply because they do not meet the legal criteria for criminal processing. As was mentioned earlier as an example, the lack of quality legal evidence in a particular case should not determine whether or not a family receives help and needed services. In addition, social services should be authorized and funded to provide services to families or to individual children who ask for help regardless of whether or not incidents of child maltreatment have been reported to official agencies (Myers, 1985; Newburger, 1985).

The Role of the State When It Does Intervene
in Cases of Violence toward Children

In light of this review of the literature, it is evident that many of the concerns about the legal system's involvement in cases of child maltreatment center around the rights of children and the rights of families. In addition, there are concerns about preventing the criminal justice system from creating further harm while pursuing the state's interests in justice.

It is clear that the continued use of experimentation with creative and innovative options for legal processing and sentencing in child maltreatment cases must be encouraged. Efforts are needed to reduce the trauma experienced by children and, if possible, to help families resolve their conflicts. In addition, there need to be systematic evaluations of these programs to determine their usefulness in reducing revictimization, as well as in ensuring that they are not overstepping the constitutional protections provided to accused defendants.

To help prevent further harm to children, as well as to help protect their legal rights, the use (or expanded use) of child advocates or guardians ad litem appears to be a good idea. Adult advocacy could similarly begin during the investigation and substantiation stages for maltreatment reports, but it should certainly be utilized in all custody proceedings. Another step to ensure the rights of children is to allow them to testify in court (Parker, 1982). Strategies such as familiarizing children with court proceedings as well as having investigators, prosecutors, judges, and other court actors make special efforts to explain to children what is happening should be continued, along with further attempts to reduce the trauma related to court appearances. However, rather than letting a prosecutor or judge determine the quality of a child's testimony a priori, it is more appropriate to let the court evaluate the credibility and accuracy of such statements at trial, just as it does with adult witnesses.

Finally, there is a need for continued review and analysis of the procedures for terminating parental rights over children in both temporary and permanent proceedings. There appears to be considerable informality in many of these proceedings at present, whether during emergency placement, during investigations, or after a conviction is made. Yet the implication of these decisions for the welfare of both the child and the family are critical and far-reaching. Again, the use of a child advocate and raising the standards of proof and allowing for the court appointment of counsel to parents are potentially useful ways for improving this process.

References

American Humane Association. (1986). *Highlights of official child neglect and abuse reporting.* Denver: Author.

Bauer, H. (1983). Preparation of the sexually abused child for court testimony. *Bulletin of the American Academy of Psychiatry and the Law, 11,* 287–289.

Berliner, L., & Barbieri, M. K. (1984). The testimony of the child victim of sexual assault. *Journal of Social Issues, 40,* 125–137.

Bernstein, B. E., & Claman, L. (1986). Modern technology and the child witness. *Child Welfare, 65,* 155–163.

Bernstein, B. E., Claman, L., Harris, J. C., & Samson, J. (1982). The child witness: A model for evaluation and trial preparation. *Child Welfare, 61,* 95–104.

Besharov, D. J. (1977). The legal aspects of reporting known suspected child abusers and neglecters. *Villanova Law Review, 23,* 458–520.

Besharov, D. J. (1986). Child abuse: Arrest and prosecution decision making. *America Criminal Law Review, 24,* 315–377.

Bourne, R. (1985). Family violence: Legal and ethical issues. In E. Newburger & R. Bourne (Eds.), *Unhappy families* (pp. 39–46). Littleton, MA: PSG.

Claman, L., Harris, J. C., Bernstein, B., & Lovitt, R. (1986). The adolescent as a witness in a case of incest: Assessment and outcome. *Journal of the American Academy of Child Psychiatry, 25,* 457–461.

Cleveland Board of Education v. LeFleur, 414 U.S. 632 (1974).

Colby, I. C., & Colby, D. N. (1987). Videotaped interviews in child sexual abuse cases: The Texas example. *Child Welfare, 66,* 25–34.

Craft, J. L., & Clarkson, C. D. (1985). Case disposition recommendations of attorneys and social workers in child abuse investigations. *Child Abuse and Neglect, 9,* 165–174.

Cramer, R. (1986). A community approach to child sexual abuse: The role of the office of the district attorney. *Response to the Victimization of Women and Children, 9,* 10–13.

Davidson, H., & Bulkley, J. (1982). *Child sexual abuse: Legal issues and approaches.* Washington, DC: American Bar Association.

Duncan, E. C. (1973). Recognition and protection of the family's interest in child abuse proceedings. *Journal of Family Law, 13,* 803–817.

Duquette, D. N., & Ramsey, S. H. (1986). Using law volunteers to represent children in child protection court proceedings. *Child Abuse and Neglect, 10,* 293–308.

Farley, R. H. (1987). Drawing interviews: An alternative in technique. *Police Chief, 54,* 37–38.

Finkelhor, D. (1983). Removing the child and prosecuting the offender in cases of sexual abuse: Evidence from the National Reporting Department for Child Abuse and Neglect. *Child Abuse and Neglect, 7,* 195–205.

Gelles, R. J., & Straus, M. A. (1988). *Intimate violence.* New York: Simon & Schuster.

Globe Newspaper Co. v. Superior Court, 102 S. Ct. 2613 (1982).

Goodman, G. (1984). The child witness: Conclusions and future directions for research and legal practice. *Journal of Social Issues, 40,* 157–175.

Gothard, S. (1987). The admissibility of evidence in child sexual abuse cases. *Child Welfare, 66,* 13–24.

Kent, J. T. (1976). A follow-up study of abused children. *Journal of Pediatric Psychology, 1,* 25–31.

Libai, D. (1969). The protection of the child victim of a sexual offense in the criminal justice system. *Wayne Law Review, 15,* 979–986.

Littrell, W. B. (1979). *Bureaucratic justice: Police, prosecutors, and plea bargaining.* Beverly Hills, CA: Sage.

Mac Murray, B. K. (1988). The nonprosecution of sexual abuse and informal justice. *Journal of Interpersonal Violence, 3,* 197–202.

Mac Murray, B. K. (1989). Criminal determination for child sexual abuse: Prosecutor case screening judgments. *Journal of Interpersonal Violence, 4,* 233–244.

Melton, G. B. (1980). Psychological issues in child victim's interaction with the legal system. *Victimology, 5,* 274–284.

Melton, G. B. (1985). Sexually abused children and the legal system: Some policy recommendations. *American Journal of Family Therapy, 13,* 61–67.

Melton, G. B., & Corson, J. (1987). Psychological maltreatment and the schools: Problems of law and professional responsibility school. *Psychology Review, 16,* 188–194.

Melton, G. B., & Davidson, H. A. (1987). Child protection and society: When should the state intervene? *American Psychology, 42,* 172–175.

Melton, G. B., Bulkley, J., & Walkan, D. (1981). Competency of children as witnesses. *Child Sexual Abuse and the Law.* Washington, DC: American Bar Association.

Meyer v. Nebraska, 262 U.S. 390, 399 (1923).

Miller, R., & Weinstock, R. (1985). Conflict of interest between therapist-patient confidentiality: Duty to report sexual abuse of children. *Behavioral Science and the Law, 5,* 161–174.

Myers, J. B. (1985). The legal response to child abuse: In the best interest of children? *Journal of Family Law, 24,* 149–269.

Newburger, E. H. (1985). The helping hand strikes again: Unintended consequences of child abuse reporting. In E. Newburger & R. Bourne (Eds.), *Unhappy families* (pp. 171–178). Littleton, MA: PSG.

Nurcombe, B. (1986). The child as witness: Competence and credibility. *Journal of the American Academy of Child Psychiatry, 25,* 473–480.

Parker, J. (1982). The rights of child witnesses: Is the court a protector or perpetrator. *New England Law Review, 17,* 643–713.

Pynoos, R., & Eth, S. (1984). The child as witness to homicide. *Journal of Social Issues, 40,* 87–108.

Quinn, K. M. (1986). Competency to be a witness: A major child forensic issue. Special issue: Child forensic psychiatry. *Bulletin of the American Academy of Psychiatry and the Law, 14,* 311–321.

Rogers, C. M. (1982). Child sexual abuse and the courts: Preliminary findings. *Journal of Social Work and Human Sexuality, 1,* 145–153.

Saltzman, A. (1986). Reporting child abusers—Protecting substance abusers. *Social Work, 31,* 474–476.

Terr, L. C. (1986). The child psychiatrist and the child witness: Traveling companions by necessity, if not by design. *Journal of the American Academy of Child Psychiatry, 25,* 462–472.

Tyler, A. H., & Brassard, M. R. (1984). Abuse in the investigation and treatment of intrafamilial child sexual abuse. *Child Abuse and Neglect, 8,* 47–53.

Valentine, D. P., Stewart-Acuff, D., Freeman, M. L, & Andreas, T. (1984). Defining child maltreatment: A multidisciplinary overview. *Child Welfare, 63,* 497–509.

Weiner, B. A. (1985). Legal issues roused in treating sex offenders. *Behavioral Science and the Law, 3,* 325–340.

Wheeler v. United States, 159 U.S. 523 (1895).

Whitcomb, D. (1988). *Guardians ad lidem in criminal courts.* Washington, DC: U.S. Department of Justice.

Whitcomb, D., Shapiro, E. R., & Shellwagen, L. D. (1985). *When the victim is a child: Issues for judges and prosecutors.* Washington, DC: U.S. Department of Justice.

Wigmore, J. H. (1940). *On evidence.* Boston: Little, Brown.

Wolfe, V. V., Las, L., & Wilson, S. K. (1987). Some issues in preparing sexually abused children for courtroom testimony. *Behavior Therapist, 10,* 107–113.

Yates, A. (1987). Should young child testify in cases of sexual abuse? *American Journal of Psychiatry, 144,* 471–480.

5

Legal Issues in Violence toward Adults

Lisa G. Lerman and Naomi R. Cahn

Introduction

Until the 1970s, family violence was largely ignored by the police, lawyers, judges, and legislators. Law enforcement officials generally refused to intervene in domestic violence cases, viewing them as private matters to be handled within the family. A victim of spouse abuse[1] could get a divorce on the basis of her husband's cruelty, or she could get a piece of paper issued by a court warning her husband not to abuse her again. Mental health professionals responded in a similar fashion by treating the violence as a relational problem caused by both parties, rather than as a crime committed by one party against another.

In many places, the judges, prosecutors, and police remain reluctant to intervene in family matters. In most states, however, there are some legal tools that a victim of family violence can use to change her situation. Through the courts, she may get a civil protection order to compel the abuser to stop the violence; if the abuser violates the order, he can be jailed. These orders may require the abuser to participate in

---

[1]This chapter focuses on spouse abuse that includes battering of women by their male partners. The remedies are not gender-specific. The vast majority of victims, however, are female. Most remedies available for spouse abuse are also available for elder abuse and for child victims of family violence.

Lisa G. Lerman • Columbus School of Law, Catholic University of America, Washington, D.C. 20064.   **Naomi R. Cahn** • Sex Discrimination Clinic, Georgetown University Law Center, Washington, D.C. 20001.

counseling or to pay financial support to the victim, or they may evict the batterer from a residence. A victim of abuse may file criminal assault charges against the abuser; if the abuser is convicted, he may be put in jail, fined, or ordered into a counseling program.

The primary goal of these legal tools is to force abusers to take responsibility for stopping their violent conduct. Both criminal prosecution and civil protection orders are intended to punish or rehabilitate the abuser and protect the victim from further violence. Mediation and other informal legal intervention designed to conciliate is ineffective in accomplishing these goals.

Effective intervention in violent families requires a coordinated response of the law enforcement system and the mental health system. This partnership is essential. Mental health professionals have a critically important role to play in stopping family violence. The law enforcement system has the police power to enforce the criminal law, which provides that an adult may not commit an act of violence against another. The law enforcement system cannot monitor and rehabilitate criminal defendants without the assistance of the mental health system. The mental health system is needed to help implement the mandate of the law enforcement system that the violence must stop. It can do this by informing patients about legal remedies for domestic violence, and by offering treatment to perpetrators of family violence who are referred by the courts.

In working with the law enforcement system on stopping family violence, then, mental health professionals have a fairly specific role to play. They can help implement the legal mandate that violence must stop, and they can help the abuser to understand the boundaries imposed by law. The abuser must be made to understand that there is no excuse for battering, and that, while it is legal to get angry, yell, or to leave a situation, it is illegal to use violence, threats, and other forms of coercion.

This chapter examines the role of mental health professionals in assisting the law enforcement system in stopping domestic violence. It offers an overview of the legal remedies for domestic violence and discusses the points at which mental health professionals become actors in the law enforcement process. Mental health professionals who understand the legal system can be most effective both in responding to court-mandated cases and in referring family members for the appropriate legal action.

Legal Response

Each state has its own laws and its own court system. In every state, there are two types of laws—civil laws and criminal laws. Civil and criminal laws are usually enforced in different courts. In many states, an abused woman can choose to initiate both civil and criminal proceedings relating to the abuse she has suffered. Civil proceedings are generally quicker and less formal, but they may not be as effective as criminal penalties in deterring future violence. The following is a list of some important differences between civil and criminal cases.

Civil	Criminal
Purpose: To settle disputes between individuals and to compensate for injuries.	*Purpose*: To punish acts that are disruptive of social order and to deter other similar acts.
Remedies: Court may order payment of money to an injured party, or may order a defendant to stop doing certain acts. Court may order counseling.	*Penalties*: Conviction of a crime may result in a jail sentence, a fine, an order to pay money to the victim, or a term of probation during which certain conduct may be required or prohibited. Court may order counseling.
Proof: Violation of the law must be proven by a "preponderance of evidence." It must be shown to be more likely than not that the act in question occurred.	*Proof*: Violation of the law must be proven "beyond a reasonable doubt." This is a much higher standard than for a civil suit— more evidence is needed.
Lawyers: Plaintiff (victim) may hire a private attorney or a legal services lawyer. Defendant (abuser) also may hire a private attorney or go to a legal services lawyer. Either or both parties may proceed on their own, without a lawyer (pro se).	*Lawyers*: The state hires prosecutors (district attorneys) to enforce criminal law. The prosecutor represents the state; the prosecutor acts on behalf of both the victim and the community. (In some places, prosecution may occur even if the victim wants to drop charges, because the state has an interest in punishing a criminal even if the victim does not wish to do so.) Defendant has a right to counsel if conviction could result in a jail sentence, any may have a public defender appointed to represent him.

Civil Remedies

Before 1976, very few jurisdictions had legislation specifically providing civil remedies to victims of domestic violence (Note, 1982).

Since then, almost every state has enacted legislation creating new civil relief for domestic violence victims (Lerman, 1984a). Several forms of civil relief are available to battered women. These include protection orders, divorce or separation, child custody and visitation rights, alimony and child support, and money damages for personal injury.[2]

Protection Orders

A protection order (sometimes called a restraining order) is an order from a civil court to an abuser to require him to change his conduct. It can last for a period of up to 1 year. Depending on the state law, the court may order the respondent:

- To refrain from abuse of any household member.
- To stay away from the victim.
- To move out of a residence shared with the victim even if the title or lease is in the abuser's name.
- To make rent or mortgage payments even if he has been evicted.
- To provide alternate housing for the victim.
- To pay for the support of the victim and/or of minor children in her custody.
- To attend a counseling program aimed to stop violence and/or alcohol or drug abuse (both the abuser and the victim may be ordered to participate in counseling.
- To pay the victim a sum of money for medical expenses, lost wages, moving expenses, property damage, court costs, or attorneys' fees.

The court also may award temporary custody of children to the victim, and may order visitation with the abuser.

In many states, protection orders may be issued on behalf of anyone abused by a spouse, former spouse, family member, household member, or former household member. Some states limit relief to victims who are married to or living with their abusers. A protection order may be obtained by filing a petition in the court that has the authority to issue it. It is useful but not necessary for a victim to be represented by a lawyer when she files a petition. In most states, victims may represent themselves in the hearings. In some cities there are clinics that assist victims in writing their petitions.

When a petition is filed, the court schedules a hearing, usually within 2 weeks of the date of filing. The abuser is notified of the hearing and asked to appear. The abuser can be represented by a lawyer, but

---

[2]Standard domestic relations remedies also provide important relief to many battered women.

there is no requirement that he have legal counsel. The hearing is before a judge or magistrate; there is no jury. Both parties have an opportunity to testify as to why an order should or should not be issued.

In most states, a victim of abuse who is in immediate danger can get a temporary protection order. Temporary orders are emergency orders that may be issued within a few hours of the time requested. They are issued after a hearing at which only the victim is present.

To get a protection order, the victim must show that some type of "abuse" has occurred. "Abuse" for which a protection order is available may include (1) an act causing physical injury, such as hitting, shoving, or use of a weapon; (2) an attempt to cause physical injury, such as raising a fist, pointing a gun; (3) a threat to cause physical injury, such as saying, "I'm going to beat you up"; or (4) sexual abuse of a spouse or her children.

To get some of the types of relief available through a protection order, such as custody or support, a victim of abuse must show more than that violence has occurred. For example, to get temporary custody of children, the woman probably will need to show that this is in the "best interests of the child" (WLDF, 1986). Some states, such as Florida, require a court to consider spouse abuse as one factor in determining custody (Women's Legal Defense Fund, 1986).

In most states a protection order may last for up to 1 year. Once she gets an order, the victim must take steps to ensure that it is enforced, including making sure that the abuser and the police get copies of the order. If the victim is abused after the protection order is issued, many states allow police officers to make an arrest without obtaining a warrant. A majority of states allow warrantless arrest in domestic violence cases even if the officer did not witness the abuse and even if there are no visible injuries. The officer must have probable cause to believe that a protection order was violated or another crime committed by the person being arrested.

Violation of a protection order is either contempt of court or a misdemeanor offense, punishable by a jail sentence (in most states, up to 6 months), a fine (in most states, up to $500), or both, or a term of probation. (*Contempt of court* is the term used to describe any violation of a court order. Sometimes contempt is treated as a criminal offense, sometimes as a civil offense.) To prove that the protection order has been violated, the victim must go back to court for another hearing. She and the abuser will have the opportunity to present evidence. A judge or a commissioner will decide whether there has been a violation, and the appropriate remedy. If the abuser is released on probation, he may be required to attend counseling sessions, to avoid contact with the victim, to refrain from abuse, etc. The abuser must report to a probation officer, who is responsible for making sure that the abuser does what the order says.

Mediation

Some domestic violence cases are referred for mediation by responding police officers, court clerks, or prosecutors offices. In mediation, a neutral third party works with both parties to help them reach an agreement about their dispute. While mediation may be a cost-efficient way of handling *some* disputes, it is inappropriate in domestic violence cases and should not be used (Lerman, 1984b).

Mediation is useful to solve problems if the parties have equal bargaining power, and if both parties take responsibility for making concessions until they reach an agreement. In domestic violence situations, however, a battered woman does not have equal bargaining power with her abuser. Moreover, allowing an abuser to mediate about whether he will continue his battering implies that, in the absence of an agreement, he may continue his behavior. Other issues than violence, such as custody, visitation, or support, cannot be fairly mediated either if one party has been violent toward the other, because the implicit ongoing threat of violence creates an atmosphere of coercion in which real bargaining cannot occur. Another problem with mediation is that generally the resulting agreement is enforceable only as a contract. It does not become a court order, so it provides no real protection.

Cases in which domestic violence has occurred should not be mediated.

Other Civil Remedies

In addition to using civil protection order statutes, victims of family violence may be able to bring other types of lawsuits. In most states, a victim of domestic abuse can sue the abuser to obtain a court order requiring the abuser to pay for any injury to her or to her property. This remedy is not useful unless the abuser has significant financial resources. Some battered women have won awards of money damages.

In some cases in which the police have not responded appropriately, victims of domestic violence have successfully sued the police. They have claimed that the police respond differentially to domestic violence calls than to other requests for police help, or that the police have violated a duty of care toward victims of domestic violence (*Watson v. Kansas City*, 1988; *Thurman v. City of Torrington*, 1984). Battered women request money damages in these cases for injuries that occurred because of the police failure to act. In several cases, victims negotiated settlements with police departments to provide better response to domestic violence victims (e.g., *Bruno v. Codd*, 1979).

Criminal Prosecution

Assaulting another person is a crime. Every state has laws prohibiting physical assault and prohibiting threats of assault. These laws apply regardless of whether the assailant and the victim are strangers, friends, or family members. Some states have enacted laws that make spouse abuse a separate criminal offense.

Until the 1970s, and at present in many places, spouse abuse is treated as a family matter, and criminal law is rarely enforced against wife-beaters. Historically, prosecutors have been slow to respond to domestic violence cases. In many (perhaps most) jurisdictions, charges are filed against spouse abusers only in a few extreme cases. One writer estimated that of the cases in which charges are filed, as many as 50% of domestic violence cases are dropped before a disposition is reached (Comment, 1985). Prosecutors often blame battered women for the dropping of charges and use this as an excuse not to pursue domestic violence crimes. Some prosecutors' offices have established special domestic violence units to increase prosecution of domestic violence cases. These offices have developed procedures that ensure victim cooperation in the vast majority of cases (Lerman, 1980; Waits, 1985).

Many different types of conduct violate state criminal law and may be the basis of criminal complaints. These include hitting, slapping, shoving, or other physical assault; sexual assault, rape, or attempted rape; threat of physical assault; any act causing the death of another; destruction or theft of private property belonging to another; kidnapping or confining another against his or her will; and violation of the terms of a protection order.

There are two ways in which a criminal action against an abuser may be started. First, the police may make an arrest after being called for assistance. Second, the victim may go to a prosecutor's office or to an intake unit in criminal or family court to file a criminal complaint. In over half the states, new laws allow police to make arrests without warrants in domestic violence cases, even if no weapons are used and there are no serious injuries. Some of these laws allow warrantless arrest only if a protection order has been violated. In some states, there are mandatory arrest laws that may require police to make an arrest in certain situations in which domestic violence has occurred (Note, 1988).

Arrest of an abuser may be a deterrent to further violence, even if there are no other legal proceedings. In one study that set out to measure the effectiveness of different types of police response, researchers found that subsequent violence was more effectively prevented by police arrest than by attempting to counsel both parties or sending the abuser away from the home for a few hours (Sherman & Berk 1984).

After an arrest is made a criminal charge may be filed. In some places charges are filed by the police; in other places the police send a report to the prosecutor's office, and the prosecutor files charges.

A victim of domestic abuse may file a criminal complaint if the police were not called after the abuse occurred, of if they were called but failed to appear or did not make an arrest. After a complaint is filed, the prosecutor's office will conduct an investigation and decide whether criminal charges should be filed. If charges are filed, the court will issue a warrant for the arrest of the abuser or a summons directing him to appear in court on a certain date.

The arrest of the abuser and the filing of the criminal charge begins the process of prosecution. The next step is an arraignment or bail hearing, at which time the abuser may be required to submit a sum of money (bail or bond) to the court to ensure that he will reappear for his trial. Other conditions may be imposed on the abuser's pretrial release, such as participation in counseling, avoiding contact with the victim, or terminating the abuse. If the terms are violated, the abuser may be returned to custody until the prosecution is completed.

The filing of a criminal charge does not necessarily mean that there will be a trial. The charge may be disposed of in any of the following three ways. First, prosecution may be postponed after charges are filed in cases in which injuries are not severe and the abuser is a first offender. The abuser makes an agreement with the prosecutor that, for example, he will cease any violence, attend counseling, avoid contact with the victim, and/or move out of a shared residence. The prosecutor (or a probation officer) is responsible for making sure that the abuser complies with the agreement. If the abuser agrees to attend counseling, the prosecutor may request that the mental health professional provide reports on the abuser's attendance and progress. If the abuser complies with the agreement for the specified period, then the charges will be dropped. If he violates the order, prosecution will be resumed.

This type of disposition is called diversion. Many battered women's advocates oppose the use of diversion because the abuser may not be convicted of the crimes he has committed. On the other hand, diversion can offer more immediate intervention and closer supervision than traditional prosecution.

Second, there may be a plea bargain. In the vast majority of criminal cases, the prosecutor, the defense attorney, and the defendant (the person charged with a crime) make a deal in which the defendant agrees to plead guilty to charges and the prosecutor agrees to request a less severe penalty than would be imposed by a court after a trial. The process of making deals to avoid trial is called plea bargaining. A judge must approve this settlement before it goes into effect. Plea bargaining in spouse abuse cases usually results in a sentence of a period of probation. During probation, just as during diversion, the abuser may be required to refrain from abuse, to attend counseling, to move out of a shared residence, and/or stay away from the victim. If the abuser violates the terms of probation, he may be put in jail without a trial since he has already agreed to his conviction by admitting guilt during the plea bargaining.

Third, there may be a trial. If the abuser pleads innocent, he will be tried on the offenses charged. If convicted, he may be jailed, fined, or placed on probation. Jail sentences are rarely imposed in domestic assault cases and are seldom longer than 1 year. The possible terms of probation are the same as those available as a result of a plea bargain.

If a victim of abuse is required to testify at a trial, she may be able to get help either from the prosecutor's office or from another agency. She may need someone to go to hearings with her, or to explain the court system to her. She may need child care while she goes to court. She may need assistance in getting housing, public benefits, a divorce, or a protection order.

Sometimes, the battered woman may be the defendant in the criminal justice system. Battered women who kill their husbands usually face criminal charges and must defend their actions (Browne, 1987). If the prosecutor finds that a woman acted in self-defense, this may lead to a decision not to file charges. Those who are charged have the options, as discussed above, of diversion, a plea, or a trial.

Role of Mental Health Professionals

As the above discussion of the legal system indicates, there are many circumstances in which the legal and mental health systems should work together. In both civil and criminal cases, mental health professionals have an important role to play. Before, during, and after a case is adjudicated, the mental health system is involved in diverse ways with the legal system.

A fundamental issue for mental health professionals who work with the legal system is their attitude toward abuse. Therapists who respond by treating family violence as a crime can help end the violence. Therapists who attempt to reconcile the parties without addressing the issue of violence may only perpetuate the cycle of violence because, in most cases, if the relationship continues, the violence continues. To intervene and treat violent families effectively, mental health professionals need special training on the psychology of battering and the legal resources available within the community. With special training, they can make appropriate referrals for their patients, seek out involvement in court-mandated treatment programs, and play many other roles.

Referrals to the Legal System

Initially, mental health professionals need to recognize the occurrence of violence in the families of their patients. They should routinely ask their patients whether there is violence in their families, regardless of whether they observe signs of possible abuse. If they are aware that both victims and abusers tend to minimize the violence, then mental health professionals are more likely to understand the existence and the extent of the abuse. Early intervention by the mental health system can help prevent later violence (Goolkasian, 1986).

Therapists who learn of family violence can help family members stop the violence by referring them to the legal system. Mental health professionals who understand the differences between civil and criminal remedies can inform either the victim or the abuser of what the law requires or permits. Because patients may be unfamiliar with the legal system, the therapist may be an important source of information on what behavior is a crime, and how the abuse can be stopped. Just knowing what the law says may help the victim take action to stop the violence and may encourage the abuser to stop his criminal behavior.

When mental health professionals see patients who are involved in civil or criminal cases, they can provide counseling and support at each stage of the legal action. Mental health professionals can help victims with the trauma of testifying against their abusers. They also can provide referrals for shelter, medical services, or financial aid. Similarly, mental heath professionals who work in shelters or at other social service agencies that are concerned with domestic violence can provide victim assistance.

Court-Mandated Treatment

Once a criminal case has been adjudicated, the defendant's conduct must be followed outside the courthouse. He must be in a position of continuing accountability to the state to ensure continued nonviolence. Often, a probation officer is responsible for developing a comprehensive treatment plan and for monitoring the abuser's treatment and his compliance with any court orders. The probation officer may develop a plan requiring the abuser to attend individual or group counseling, such as a batterers' group, or an alcohol or drug treatment program.

The best treatment programs focus on stopping the violence and holding abusers responsible for their conduct. In conjunction with a probation officer, a court-mandated treatment program then becomes the eyes and ears of the law enforcement system. Communication between the different service providers and the courts is essential to ensure that the abuser is being treated effectively, and that the abuse is not recurring. Generally, the court must arrange for continued contact with victims to learn of any new incidents of violence.

If the abuser fails to appear, or if the violence recurs, the therapist must report back to the court so that law enforcement action can be taken against the abuser. Many court systems do not monitor cases effectively, so the therapist must take an active role to ensure that the information gets back to the appropriate official and is acted upon. Every professional who works with members of violent families must become an advocate.

In many other areas of mental health, it is generally agreed that patients respond most to treatment undertaken voluntarily. In treatment of spouse abusers, the opposite is usually true. Most abusers will not accept any form of treatment unless mandated by a court, and many respond well to compulsory treatment (Ganley, 1981).

Individual and group treatment of abusers is more likely to be effective in holding the abuser responsible for his conduct than couples counseling or family therapy, which tend to look at the responsibilities of all parties for their contribution to the problem. For the purpose of stopping the violence, it is necessary to require that the person committing the acts of violence stop using physical coercion to get what he wants. This requirement must be unconditional; any intervention that treats the victim as being partly responsible for the violence undercuts this message.

Mental health professionals who are specially trained in domestic violence issues should seek referrals from the court. They need to become familiar with how the legal system refers abusers for treatment. Once mental health professionals begin to treat abusers referred by the courts, they should work with the legal system to develop an effective monitoring program.

Other Roles

Another important role of mental health professionals is to testify in spouse abuse cases. Where child custody is an issue, the victim may need psychological evidence showing the detrimental effect of battering on children to help win her custody and to establish visitation rights of the abuser.

In cases in which a victim of abuse has been accused of killing the abuser, the victim may need testimony by a psychologist. Some battered women kill their mates in self-defense after being battered repeatedly. To prove self-defense, a woman must show that at the time of the homicide she reasonably believed that she was in danger of serious bodily harm and that she used reasonable force to prevent this harm. Many courts allow the women to use expert witnesses to support their arguments. Mental health expert witnesses can be very useful in informing the jury about the psychological impact of spouse abuse on a woman and explaining why a woman has been unable to leave the relationship.

Conclusion

In many states, a battered woman can use any of the legal remedies described, or she may want to use more than one. For example, a protection order is often useful to a woman who files criminal charges against her husband. The victim's decision about legal action should depend on her goals. Most victims want to end the violence. Some also may want to punish the abuser, to get help for him, to end the relationship, or all of these.

Mental health professionals have a critical role to play in the legal system. Through work with a mental health professional, the victim may be better able to understand her options and take legal action to stop the violence. Mental health professionals must seek out information from their patients about family violence, and inform victims of abuse about the remedies available through both the civil and criminal systems. When counseling abusers, a mental health professional can provide information about what behavior is criminal, and the potential penalties for that behavior. Abusers should learn that beating up family members is a crime that society takes seriously.

Mental health professionals and the legal system can work together to end the violence. But cooperation will be effective only if the legal and mental health systems have the same goals. The best responses of the mental health system are those that support the legal system in communicating that domestic violence is wrong, and that those who commit acts of violence may suffer severe consequences.

References

Browne, A. (1987). *When battered women kill.* New York: Free Press.
Bruno v. Codd, 47 N.Y.2d 582, 419 N.Y.S.2d 901, 393 N.E.2d 976 (1979).
Comment. (1985). Ex parte protection orders: Is due process locked out? *Temp. L.Q., 58,* 843–872.

Ganley, A. (1981). *Court-mandated counseling for men who batter: A three-day workshop for mental health professionals.* Washington, DC: Center for Women Policy Studies.

Goolkasian, G. (1986). *Confronting domestic violence: A guide for criminal justice agencies.* Washington, DC: U.S. Government Printing Office.

Lerman, L. (1980). *Prosecution of spouse abuse: Innovations in criminal justice response.* Washington DC: Center for Women Policy Studies.

Lerman, L. (1984a). A model state act: Remedies for domestic abuse. *Harvard Journal of Legislation, 21,* 61–143.

Lerman, L. (1984b). Mediation of wife abuse: The adverse impact of alternative dispute resolution on women. *Harvard Women's Law Jounal, 7,* 57–113.

Note. (1982). Restraining order legislation for battered women: A reassessment. *University of San Francisco Law Review, 16,* 703–741.

Note. (1988). Mandatory arrest for domestic violence. *Harvard Women's Law Journal, 11,* 213–226.

Sherman, L., & Berk, R. (1984). The Minneapolis Domestic Violence Experiment. *Police Foundation Reports, 1.*

Thurman v. City of Torrington, 595 F. Supp. 1521 (D. Conn. 1984).

Waits, K. (1985). The criminal justice system's response to battering: Understanding the problem, forging the solutions. *Washington Laws Review, 60,* 267–329.

Watson v. Kansas City, 857 F.2d 690 (10th Cir. 1988).

Women's Legal Defense Fund. (1986). *Representing battered women in custody disputes in the District of Columbia: Litigating custody as part of a civil protection order.* Washington, DC: Author.

6

Medical Issues with Child Victims of Family Violence

Susan E. Briggs

Introduction

Trauma, either accidental or nonaccidental injury, is the single most common cause of death in children between 1 and 15 years of age (see Briggs, 1989). Each year, about 20 million injuries occur in children. The consequences of the permanent disability, both physical and emotional, are incalculable. Injuries caused by child abuse, either from intentional or unintentional violence against children, unfortunately constitute an increasing percentage of the trauma statistics. One's concept of child abuse must include not only the well-described "battered child syndrome" but the many children who are the innocent victims of family violence arising from domestic quarrels, drugs, or alcohol intoxication. Each day, newspapers report cases of children shot to death accidentally in drug wars, the ultimate form of child abuse.

Although the exact incidence of child abuse is not known, it is estimated that over 1 million children are maltreated in the United States each year (American Humane Association, 1984). Violence against children may take many forms, and it is important for all members of the professional community working with such situations to recognize the unique manifestations of injury in children, from both physical and emotional abuse. Most children who die from abuse have had multiple recurring episodes of battering. Early recognition of family situations at

Susan E. Briggs • Harvard Medical School, Massachusetts General Hospital, Boston, Massachusetts 02114.

high risk for child abuse is critically important to prevent eventual death from either intentional or unintentional violence against children.

Violence against children, whether from emotional abuse and neglect or from unintentional injury to the child from violence between adults, is basically a disease of adults that finds expression in children, the innocent victims. The ultimate pathological expression of this disease is violence against children by other children seeking to emulate adult behavior for emotional or financial satisfaction. If optimal health care resources were available to all sectors of the community, the problem of child abuse, both intentional and unintentional, could be significantly ameliorated. Until that time, the key to prevention must be the ability to identify vulnerable children and parents in high-risk family and community situations that predispose to violent behavior against children.

Identification of Victims of Child Abuse

The spectrum of child abuse can take many different forms, such as physical or mental injury, nutritional or hygienic neglect, delayed or inadequate treatment of disease, sexual abuse or verbal abuse (Green, 1975). Unfortunately, in children (especially preschool children) the spectrum of injury from accidental to nonaccidental is often quite subtle, making the diagnosis of child abuse difficult for members of the professional team dealing with such situations. Careful history and physical examination of the child, combined with close communication with members of the community team dealing with the family unit, are the only way to ensure that the abused child will be identified and cared for appropriately. The severely battered child or the child that is dead on arrival from intentional or unintentional violence is not the diagnostic dilemma. It is the child who presents with subtle physical findings suggestive of abuse or neglect combined with any of the warning signs of abuse that is the most clinically demanding situation.

Above all, members of the professional team must maintain a high degree of suspicion in the face of any injury to a child and must remain alert to telltale signs of inappropriate behavior in the family members of the child if the true incidence of child abuse is to be appropriately identified and treated.

Clues to the diagnosis of child abuse include the following.

History

This shows (a) significant discrepancy between the stated history of the injury and the actual degree of physical injury observed in the child,

(b) prolonged interval between the stated time of the injury to the child and the time the child was brought to medical care, and (c) history of repetitive accidents to the child within a short period (Green, 1975).

Clinical Examination of the Child

The most common injuries to abused children are soft-tissue injuries, burns, fractures, and head trauma. The following clinical findings demonstrated by the child may alert one to the possibility of child abuse (see Green, 1975; Keen, Lendrum, & Wolman, 1975; Sobel, 1970): (a) poor hygiene or failure to thrive, (b) perioral injuries, (c) odor of alcohol, (d) fractures in children under 3 years of age, (e) evidence of frequent injuries (scars or old healed fractures), (f) bizarre injuries (bites, cigarette burns, branding burns such as with irons, grates, or rope marks), (g) untreated chronic diseases, (h) genital and perineal trauma, (i) second- and third-degree burns, especially in anatomical distributions, (j) subdural hematomas, (k) skull fractures, (l) ruptured viscus (internal organs), or (m) being dead on arrival.

Behavior Changes

Behavioral characteristics of the child on presentation to medical care may be important in identifying the abused child. Children who cry hopelessly or cry very little under examination or treatment, those who do not look to parents or guardians for reassurance, and children who are wary of any physical contact with adults or are constantly on the alert for danger should raise one's suspicion that the injury may not be accidental (Caffey, 1974; Feldman & Brewer, 1978; Green, 1975).

Parental or adult behavior may provide an important clue that the injury is a result of violence against the child. One should be suspicious of child abuse in the following instances:

1. Differences or changes upon repeated questioning between parent or guardians, or between the child and parents, in the history of the injury.
2. Failure of individuals with the child at the time of the injury to voluntarily provide information about the injury.
3. Failure to demonstrate concern about the injury, treatment, or prognosis of the child. Parents or guardians who respond inappropriately or do not comply with medical advice—i.e., refusing to admit the child to the hospital for observation if medically indicated—should alert one to the possibility of abuse.
4. Lack of physical or emotional support to the child, lack of physical contact with the injured child.
5. Inappropriate or no response to the crying child.

Anatomic Consideration in Injuries to Children

Size

The child's smaller size, as opposed to the adult size, yields a smaller target to which linear forces from the injuring agent are applied. The applied energy dissipates over the smaller mass of the child, resulting in a greater force to a smaller area and a high incidence of multiple organ injuries, especially internal (viscera) injuries. Children have less body fat, less elastic connective tissue, and closer proximity of multiple organs and, as a result, sustain significantly greater injuries than adults with the same applied force (American College of Physicians, 1988).

Skeleton

The child's skeletal structure is incompletely calcified, contains multiple active growth centers, and is more resilient than the adult's skeleton. This renders the child less able to absorb significant external trauma and results in internal organ damage without overlying bony fractures. For example, rib fractures in children are unusual, but lung contusions (bruises) are common injuries (Feldman & Brewer, 1978).

Surface Area

The ratio between a child's surface and body volume is the highest at birth and decreases throughout infancy and childhood. Loss of body heat thus becomes an important factor in a your child's sustaining trauma. Hypothermia (low body temperature) can be life-threatening in an injured child, especially the very young child.

Psychological Status

Caring for the injured child, especially the abused child, presents a significant challenge. The stress and pain of a traumatic injury frequently lead to marked emotional lability in the child and regressive psychological behavior. The child's ability to interact or communicate with unfamiliar individuals in strange environments is usually severely limited in violence-related injuries, especially if the child is experiencing pain. Thus, history taking and therapeutic manipulations may be extremely difficult.

Long-Term Effects

A major consideration for all members of the professional team dealing with injured children is the effect the injury may have on subsequent growth and development. Unlike the adult who has completed the growth and development processes, the child must not only recover from the traumatic event but continue the normal growth and development processes, and the physiological and psychological effects of injury on this process are significant. Children with even minor injuries may have prolonged cerebral function disabilities, psychological adjustments, or organ system deformities and disabilities.

Specific Injuries in Child Victims of Violence

All types of penetrating and blunt traumatic injuries have been demonstrated in victims of child abuse, intentional and unintentional. Recognition of patterns of injury suspicious for child abuse as well as characteristics of injury specific to children will alert professionals to the spectrum of child abuse.

Cutaneous Injuries

Cutaneous injuries represent one of the most common manifestations of child abuse (American College of Physicians, 1988; Caffey, 1974). The location of the injury, the pattern of the injury, the presence of multiple lesions of different ages, and the failure of new lesions to appear after the child is hospitalized or removed from the home environment help to distinguish accidental from nonaccidental injuries.

Bruises constitute the majority of intentional cutaneous injuries. Lacerations are more commonly associated with accidental injury. The most common areas of inflicted injuries in children are the upper arms and legs, trunk, sides of the face, neck, ears, genitalia, and buttocks. Bruises (especially facial and buttock bruises) seen in infants should be considered suspicious for child abuse until proven otherwise.

The injuring instrument, whether it be animate (e.g., human hand, foot, or teeth) or inanimate (e.g., shoe, belt, rope, electric cord, knife), will often leave a telltale mark, much like the steering wheel imprint on the chest wall of a victim who sustains a motor vehicle accident and is not wearing a seat belt. Thus, the pattern of the cutaneous injury may identify the inflicting instrument and the possible individual responsible for the violence against the child.

The typical lesion left by an electric cord is elliptical (Briggs, 1989); a belt or a buckle leaves a bruise conforming to its shape. Injuries inflicted by the human hand often leave characteristic parallel linear marks representing the spaces between the fingers. Rope burns may leave circular marks around the neck, suggesting strangulation. Human bite marks are characteristic lesions, and the size of the bites help identify the age of the biting person. Oval pressure marks in the arms or trunk suggest hard pressure from human hands.

Multiple bruises or other cutaneous lesions in varying stages of healing are indicative of repeated intentional injury. No new lesions appearing in the protective hospital environment or foster setting, combined with laboratory confirmation of normal bleeding studies, a history suspicious of child abuse, and cutaneous lesions indicative of inflicted injury raise the spectrum of intentional injury to the child in the family environment.

Burns

Burn injuries are a leading cause of accidental death in the pediatric population and the source of incalculable morbidity and long-term disability. Flame burns account for approximately 15% of pediatric thermal injuries and scald burns for approximately 85% of thermal injuries. The most disturbing cause of burns that has dramatically increased over the past decade is child abuse and neglect. Children are frequently abused with cigarettes as well as a variety of hot implements (grills, radiators, curling irons, flatirons, matches). As with all other types of child abuse, the location and pattern of the burn as well as the association of other social, psychological, and physical signs of child abuse are useful guides to the diagnosis of accidental versus nonaccidental thermal injury. Immersion burns are characterized by symmetrical anatomic region involvement (see Figure 1), such as the stocking glove distribution pattern of burn injury in which both feet are uniformly burned secondary to forceful immersion of a child in hot water.

Most accidental minor scald burns are characterized by a scatter distribution of thermal injury, as opposed to a burn with sharply demarcated edges, because the child will attempt to escape the burning agent unless forcibly restrained. Genital and perineal burns are suspicious areas for child abuse since these are unusual areas for accidental injury unless the child falls in a bathtub (American College of Surgeons, 1988).

The following characteristics help the examiner estimate the extent of burn. In general, in children under 5 years of age, scalding often inflicts third-degree burns because of the thin skin of the child.

Burns may be caused by heat from various sources, chemicals, electricity, and radiation. Extreme cold can also produce an injury similar to a burn. Burn depth significantly affects most subsequent pathophysiologic changes in the body.

A *first-degree* burn involves only the epidermis and is characterized by cutaneous erythema and mild pain. Tissue damage is minimal, and protective functions of the skin, located in the dermis, remain intact.

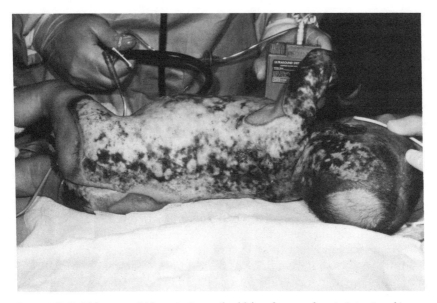

Figure 1. Full-thickness scald burn in 2-month-old female secondary to intentional immersion in hot water.

The chief symptom, pain, usually resolves in 48 to 72 hours. In 5 to 10 days, the damaged epithelium peels off, leaving no residual scarring. The most common causes of first-degree burns are overexposure to sunlight or brief scalding by hot liquids.

A *second-degree* burn involves injury to the entire epidermis and variable portions of the dermal layer. Vesicle (blister) formation is characteristic of second-degree burns. A superficial second-degree burn in extremely painful because the large number of remaining viable nerve endings are exposed. Superficial second-degree burns will heal in 7 to 14 days owing to regeneration of epithelium by the epithelial cells that line the hair follicles, sweat glands, and other skin appendages. A mid- to deep second-degree burn will heal spontaneously, but reepithelialization is extremely slow. Pain is present, but to a lesser degree than in more superficial burns because fewer intact nerve endings remain. Fluid losses and metabolic effects of deep dermal burns are essentially the same as those of third-degree burns.

A full-thickness or *third-degree* burn involves destruction of the entire epidermis and dermis, leaving no residual epidermal cells to regenerate. The wound will not epithelialize and can heal only by wound contraction or skin grafting. The lack of painful sensation in a third-degree burn is due to heat destruction of nerve endings.

Head Trauma

Children and adults differ significantly in their response to head trauma. In general, children recover better than adults from head trauma. Children less than 3 years of age have the worst prognosis from severe head injury. Head injury in abused children is often compounded by secondary brain injury from hypovolemia from associated internal injuries or hypoxemia (lack of oxygen) due to delay in appropriate treatment, especially institution of an adequate airway and ventilatory support. The young child with an open fontanel and mobile sutures is more tolerant of an expanding intracranial mass from head trauma. Vomiting is common in children after head injury and does not necessarily indicate significant increased intracranial pressure.

Seizures occur frequently in children following head trauma and are usually self-limiting. Elevated intracranial pressure without focal intracranial masses following head trauma is more common in children than in adults. A lucid interval prior to delayed neurological deterioration is sometimes seen in children with head injuries (American College of Surgeons, 1988).

Findings on clinical examination that may suggest child abuse and dictate a more extensive investigation include multiple subdural hematomas, especially without a fresh skull fracture, retinal hemorrhages, and old skull fractures on X-ray examination (Friedman & Morse, 1974). Hair pulling, a maneuver used for discipline as well as intentional injury, may cause alopecia (loss of hair) as well as scalp hematomas. Subdural hematomas are almost always traumatic in children. The signs and symptoms of head injury may be nonspecific, such as irritability, lethargy, or lack of desire to eat. More specific signs of head injury are signs of elevated intracranial pressure (e.g., vomiting, seizures, stupor, coma). The findings of retinal hemorrhages are suggested of whiplash origin of injury. Subdural hematoma associated with a skull fracture usually leaves external marks and is more easily diagnosed.

Chest Trauma

The child's chest wall is very compliant and allows energy to transfer to the intrathoracic structures more easily than the adult's thoracic cage (Green, 1975). Thus, children may sustain significant internal chest injuries without evidence of external trauma. Penetrating injuries to the chest in children are usually the result of unintentional injury to a child involved in the physical setting of violent conflict between adults. Blunt trauma to the chest in abused children often leaves telltale cutaneous marks from inflicting agents, such as a hand mark or a belt mark.

Abdominal Trauma

Abdominal examination of the child is extremely difficult, especially in abused children. Cutaneous manifestations of injury may be present. Most infants and children who are stressed and crying will swallow large amounts of air, which may mimic the findings of abdominal injury. Ability to elicit a history of abdominal pain is probably the most reliable sign of abdominal injury in the neurologically intact child and requires extreme patience and good communicative skills on the part of the examiner.

Visceral (internal injuries) are second only to head trauma as the most common cause of death from child abuse. Nonaccidental internal injuries usually involve structures below the diaphragm, and significant blood loss may be present without external signs of trauma. Many cases of significant intraabdominal injury from child abuse unfortunately are first diagnosed at autopsy examination.

Extremity Trauma

History is of vital importance in the diagnosis of nonaccidental extremity trauma in children. X-ray diagnosis of fractures and dislocations around joints is difficult in younger children because of the lack of mineralization of the bone and presence of a growth plate (physis). Bone in children grows in length as new bone is laid down by the growth plate near the end of the bone. Because of the nature of the immature bones, children may sustain a fracture of only one side (cortex) of the bone, the "greenstick fracture." Fractures in children under 3 years of age are unusual and raise the possibility of child abuse, as does the presence of old fractures in multiple sites seen on X-ray examination.

Summary

The question "Could this case of injury be the result of intentional or unintentional violence to the child?" should come to mind in all cases of traumatic injury to children.

No pattern of injury or psychological or socioeconomic background of the family unit will conclusively prove an instance of child abuse. A high degree of suspicion on the part of the professional team caring for the injured child, as well as close cooperation between community and medical resources involved in the care of the child, provides the best opportunity for early detection of child abuse and prevention of the ultimate complication of child abuse: death of the child.

References

American College of Surgeons Committee on Trauma. (1988). *Advanced trauma life support program for physicians, Instructor manual* (chap. 10, p. 217). Chicago: Author.

American Humane Association. (1984). *Highlights of official child neglect and abuse reporting 1982*. Denver: Author.

Briggs, S. E. (1989). First aid, transportation and immediate acute care of the burned patient. In J. A. J. Martyn (Ed.), *Anesthesia and critical care of the burned patient*. New York: Grune & Stratton.

Caffey, J. (1974). The whiplash shaken infant syndrome. *Pediatrics, 54,* 396–403.

Feldman. K. W., & Brewer, D. K. (1978). Child abuse, cardiopulmonary resuscitation and rib fractures. *Pediatrics, 62,* 1–7.

Friedman. S., & Morse, C. (1974). Child abuse: A five year follow-up of early case finding in the emergency department. *Pediatrics, 54,* 404–410.

Green, F. C. (1975). Child abuse and neglect: A priority problem for the private physician. *Pediatric Clinics of North America, 22.*

Keen, J. H., Lendrum, J., & Wolman, B. (1975). Inflicted burns and scalds in children. *British Medical Journal, 4,* 268–269.

Sobel R. (1970). The psychological implications of accidental poisoning in childhood. *Pediatric Clinics of North America, 17,* 653–685.

7

Medical Issues with Adult Victims of Family Violence

Richard L. Judd

Introduction

Interhuman violence is generally estimated to affect millions of persons in the United States. Violence in the context of this chapter refers to physical force that contravenes societal norms or penal codes. Abuse can generally be categorized as verbal abuse, battering, mobility restriction, communication restriction, or economic exploitation. A more inclusive categorization of abuse involves physical abuse (e.g., infliction of pain or injury), sexual abuse (e.g., rape, sexually transmitted diseases), emotional abuse (e.g., derogation, humiliation), neglect (e.g., abandonment, deliberate denial of food, medications), or financial exploitation (e.g., illegal or improper use of funds).

Violence has come to be an expected stranger in all echelons of our society. Within the adult population, while estimated figures vary widely from source to source, the number of reported abused persons is estimated to be in the range of 4 to 5 million (National Coalition Against Domestic Violence, 1988; *New York Times*, 1985; Plotkin, 1988). The wide variation in estimates of individuals who have suffered violence, particularly at the hands of family members or significant others, is thought to be related to several factors. These factors include the (1) fear of reporting the problem, (2) shame of having to acknowledge the person responsible for inflicting the abuse or violence, (3) unprecedented growth in

Richard L. Judd • Emergency Medical Sciences, Central Connecticut State University, and Allied Medical Staff, New Britain General Hospital, New Britain, Connecticut 06050.

the number of those over 65 years of age, and (4) lack of statutory provisions and definitive reporting systems.

The physical and emotional signs of abuse—those of rape, spouse beating, or nutritional deprivation in the elderly—are often overlooked or, perhaps, not accurately identified. Women, in particular, rarely report incidents of sexual assault to law enforcement agencies. It sometimes takes years for victims to work through their apparent loss of self-respect in order to confront the feelings of fear, grief, and rage. In the elderly population, sensory deficits, senility, and other forms of altered mental status (for example, drug-induced depression) may make it impossible or extremely arduous for them to report the maltreatment.

While the categories of emotional abuse and financial exploitation are of concern to clinicians in all health-related fields, physical abuse and neglect pose the greatest concern from the medical standpoint. Sometimes during periods of acute medical illness or trauma resulting from abuse, an individual may see a health care provider outside of the ordinary medical services system, and these providers may conduct an initial assessment. If the setting is one without medical services (e.g., a shelter for abused women), and victims attend such a facility prior to receiving prehospital or definitive medical care, the facility personnel should be competent in the assessment and recognition of life-threatening problems. They should also be prepared to provide basic life support as well as referral to an appropriate medical care facility.

Initial Assessment

Initial assessment of a patient involves evaluating those life support processes that, if not examined during a traumatic event or acute illness, may result in serious disability or death. These initial factors have been generally referred to as the *ABC's*—that is, airway, breathing, and circulation. It is not the intent, nor is it within the scope, of this chapter to provide training in the supportive or resuscitative measures required in such circumstances. Rather, major assessment regimens that are considered a standard in emergency medicine today will be presented. Indeed, any practitioner of the healing or helping medical arts who is involved with victims of adult violence should be competent in emergency medical care to a level appropriate to the environment in which the practitioner works. Human violence often involves trauma, and, therefore, lifesaving considerations must be part of any assessment.

The American College of Surgeons has developed a well-conceived protocol for assessing significant trauma in accident cases. These protocols are found in the College's *Advanced Trauma Life Support Program*

Table 1. Initial Assessment[a]

A. Airway and cervical spine

Is the airway patent, i.e., open and accessible?

Patency may be accomplished using the chin-lift or jaw-thrust maneuver.

Suction blood, secretions, remove foreign debris.

Insert an oral or nasal airway (BLS); intubation (ALS).

Remember: Assume cervical spine fracture in multisystem trauma, especially blunt injury above clavicle. Avoid hyperextension/hyperflexion

B. Breathing

Expose the chest: Is there adequate ventilatory exchange?

There are generally three major problems in the trauma case that impair adequate exchange of air; these are (1) tension pneumothorax, (2) open pneumothorax, and (3) large flail chest.

Determine rate and depth of respirations.

Inspect and palpate the chest for unilateral and bilateral chest movements.

Auscultate the chest bilaterally.

Ascertain the respiratory rate. A respiratory rate of greater than 20 per minute or less than 8 per minute indicates respiratory compromise.

C. Circulation

What is the blood volume and cardiac output?

What is the patient's state of consciousness?

When blood is reduced by half or more, cerebral perfusion is critically impaired, and unconsciousness results. Conversely, a conscious patient can be presumed to have at least enough blood volume to maintain cerebral perfusion.

Skin color: A patient with pink skin (or mucosa in dark-skinned persons), especially in the face and extremities, is rarely hypovolemic following injury. Conversely, the ashen, gray skin of the face and the white skin of blood-drained extremities are ominous signs of hypovolemia. These latter signs usually indicate a blood volume loss of at least 30% if hypovolemia is the cause.

Pulse: What is its quality, rate, and regularity? Full, slow, regular peripheral pulses are welcome signs in the injured patient. Check an easily accessible central pulse initially: femoral or carotid pulses signify coordinated cardiac action and at least 50% of the residual blood volume. Rapid, thready pulses are early signs of hypovolemia, but may have other causes as well. An irregular pulse is usually a warning of cardiac impairment. Absent central pulses at more than one site, without local injuries or other factors which preclude accurate palpation of pulses, signify the need for immediate resuscitative actions.

Bleeding: Initial step in managing shock is to recognize its presence. The majority of patients in shock are hypovolemic; cardiogenic shock may be the cause and must be considered in patients with specific injuries above the diaphragm. For all practical purposes, shock does not result from isolated head injuries. A significant number of patients in hypovolemic shock will require surgical intervention. Remember, compensatory mechanisms may have precluded a measurable fall in systolic pressure until the patient has lost 30% of blood volume. Direct attention to pulse rate, respiratory rate skin circulation, and pulse pressure. A narrowed pulse pressure suggests significant blood loss. Earliest signs are tachycardia and cutaneous vasoconstriction. In adults, tachycardia is indicated with pulse rates of greater than 100. It is important to note that the elderly may not exhibit tachycardia because of limited cardiac response to catecholamine stimulation or certain medications such as propanolol.

(continued)

Table 1. (*Continued*)

D. Disability

Rapid neurologic evaluation using the pneumonic AVPU, which translates to:

A = alert

V = responds to vocal

P = responds to painful stimuli

U = unresponsive

Assess pupils for size, equality, and reaction.

E. Exposure

Undress patient to facilitate thorough examination and assessment. The degree of undressing a patient must depend on the circumstances in which the patient is found and the current situation. If the patient is conscious and can competently advise on the nature of injuries, a full unclothing may not be necessary. In a sexual assault situation, undressing the patient may be contraindicated until appropriate personnel are available. And, in some circumstances, undressing the patient may not be appropriate due to psychologic factors. Emergency medical personnel have appropriate backgrounds to assist in this determination, as necessary. In the hospital emergency department setting, full exposure of the patient is required to conduct a competent assessment of injuries.

[a]Adapted from American College of Surgeons (1989).

(American College of Surgeons, 1989), consisting of a five-step process. The steps presented in Table 1 are frequently accomplished simultaneously. For example, the response to the question "What happened?" can provide immediate information about the patient's airway, breathing, and neurologic status. Simultaneously, the examiner can assess the patient's pulse, skin color, and capillary refilling time in 30 seconds of patient contact.

Characteristics of Abused Adults

Adult victims of violence most frequently are female, although males smaller than their spouses are victims as well. Likely victims are young pregnant women who are unable to resist the abuser (Goldberg & Carey, 1982). Women who have two or more children and few friends or relatives fall into the risk category (Geis, 1982). Those adults who are unhappy with their current existence, whose spouses (particularly husbands) have job security problems (out of work, part-time, or periodic employment), or who have a family violence history are potential victims of abuse. Families living in environments that are not conducive to normal, ordinary living or social customs (e.g., military reservations) may also be at high risk for maltreatment. Addiction to drugs, alcohol, or other substances is a major consideration of violence potential.

Accordingly, the medical history should seek to determine information in medical records of previous injuries or illnesses that may be related to violence incidents.

Characteristics that may assist the practitioner in identifying adult abuse include (1) repeated visits to the office, emergency department, or clinic, (2) a history of being "accident-prone," (3) soft-tissue injuries (see detail below), (4) implausible explanation of injuries, (5) simplistic, often vague, explanation of injuries, (6) psychosomatic complaints, (7) pain, especially chronic pain, (8) self-destructive behavior, (9) eating and sleep disorders, (10) lack of energy, (11) depression, (12) substance abuse, and/or (13) sexual abuse (Goldberg, 1982).

Medical Issues

Specific examination and inspection for bruises, burns, head injuries, abdominal injuries, fractures, and failure to thrive should be undertaken by the medical team. It is important that all personnel involved in violence cases, from prehospital (e.g., first responders, emergency medical technicians) to definitive care staff (e.g., nurses, physicians), perform exacting surveys and examination of the patient.

In the overall assessment of abuse, a key factor is pursuing the adequacy of explanation of the presenting incident. The astute clinician will look for those indicators that either conceal or avoid frank answers to questions that attempt to discover causation of the injury. Answers that are implausible or doubtful from anyone, including the patient who has sustained alleged abuse, the possible inflictor, or significant witnesses, require aggressive investigation. Questions raised by the examiner such as "Exactly where did this happen?" "What was she (the victim) doing, exactly?" "What time did it happen?" may provide valuable clues to the existence of maltreatment. A sense of clinical suspicion should develop when a practitioner reviews a medical history that raises such questions as "Does this make sense?" "Do I really believe this story?" When one sees burns, especially cigarette burns (one of the stigmata of abuse), or physical marks indicative that certain portions of the body systematically have been scalded, suspicion must be raised that abuse may be the cause. It is important to remember that many patients suffering abuse are terrorized into making false statements for fear of retribution. In the case of elder abuse by family members, fear of removal from the home environment may be the cause of lying about the origin of the abuse. In other cases of elder abuse, sensory deprivation or dementia may preclude adequate explanation (Judd, 1988; Kimsey, Tarbox, & Bragg, 1981; Schwartz, Bosker, & Grigsby, 1984).

The significance of these assessments is important in uncovering pathology as well as in identifying abuse that often is not reported by the patient for fear of reprisal or because of embarrassment or incapability of reporting. Some of these assessments will involve definitive diagnostic procedures by the physician, such as roentgenographic or magnetic resonance imagery. Others, such as malnutrition, can be observed by visual examination. Still others can be determined by palpation, as with the swelling of an extremity.

In addition to the implicit lifesaving care that must be administered during the assessment, one of the very significant concomitants of a thorough examination involves reducing further trauma from abuse through its very identification. It is well known that, in child abuse, the cycle of repeat abuse has a high mortality rate (McNeese & Hebeler, 1977). It can be inferred from the data on child abuse that one of the preventive measures in reducing additional maltreatment of adults is the knowledge of its occurrence, uncovered or identified by medical practitioners. This may allow for referral and protective services of human, social, and public safety agencies.

Clinical Signs of Physical Abuse or Neglect

The signs of physical abuse or neglect may be quite obvious (e.g., the imprint left by an item such as a fireplace poker) or subtle (e.g., undernutrition in the fragile elderly). A comprehensive and thorough physical examination, in which findings are recorded and documented, is mandatory in the clinical setting. Indeed, the medicolegal implications for not doing so are enormous. In general, the physical factors to be looked for, particularly when there is inadequate explanation, are (1) inflicted bruises, (2) burns, (3) head injuries, (4) chest injuries, (5) abdominal injuries, (6) bone injuries, (7) failure to thrive, and (8) sexual abuse injuries. Each of these will be discussed further in turn.

Inflicted Bruises

Typical sites of inflicted bruises are the buttocks and lower back, genitals and inner thighs, cheek (slap marks) or earlobe (pinch marks), upper lip and frenulum (from forced feeding of the elderly patient), and neck (choke marks). Pressure bruises, frequently the result of human hand marks, may be identified by oval grab marks (fingertips), pinch marks, handprints (e.g., on the face, buttocks), linear marks (fingers), or trunk encirclement bruises. Human bite marks are typically inflicted on the limbs and more likely involve the upper extremity. In addition to the trauma (lacerations, crushing) of the human bite, infection must also be a major medical concern since many diseases are transmitted from organisms located in the oral cavity.

Strap marks from belts, whips, and other similar devices may present as linear bruises and will carry characteristic marks indicative of the particular injuring agent. Loop marks from a doubled-over electric cord, rope, wire, or string may leave characteristic signs as well. Many of these may have resulted from ligatures used to restrain the patient. This is especially applicable to the elderly, who, for purposes of restricting movement, may have been tied in bed. Indeed, the author has been involved in one such case in which a demented elderly patient was tied to her bed and neglected to the point where the springs of the mattress physically invaded her skin. There are other reportable cases where, in order to prevent somnambulism, falling out of bed, or behavioral problems, elders are similarly restrained. In the nongeriatric adult population, restraint can be used to control aggressive behavior in retarded individuals or for other purposes of abuse (e.g., sexual).

Bizarre marks that are not easily identifiable may be the result of unusual causation. The specific instrument may leave telltale markings of blunt trauma (e.g., hammers, pliers, fireplace poker). Tattoos, fork mark punctures, or screwdriver indentations (Phillips-head) are also highly indicative of inflicted abuse.

Multiple bruises in various states of healing also require investigation. Some bruising may be normative (e.g., those resulting from physical activity involved in playing sports or banging into a kitchen counter). Again, careful questioning of the patient and a review of that individual's activities of daily living (ADL) are evaluative factors.

Serologic tests that include a bleeding disorder screen should be ordered in any unexplained bruising. Moreover, dating of bruising may also be helpful. Table 2 presents guidelines for judging the relative age of the bruising (Sussman, 1968).

Burns

Approximately 100,000 patients with burns require hospitalization each year; of these, 12,000 will die as a result of their injuries. It is estimated that a quarter of a million individuals sustain minor burns (e.g., second-degree burns of less than 15% of the body surface area) that are managed on an outpatient basis (Bunkis & Walton, 1986). Many burns considered less critical are not treated in any medical facility. Burns are a common form of maltreatment, and it is more than likely that most of the burns inflicted are not seen in any medical setting. For many reasons the elderly, including those not able to care for them-

**Table 2. Coloration of Bruises
According to Time**[a]

Age[b]	Color
24 hours	Swollen, tender; reddish with some blue or purple discoloration
1–5 days	Blue to bluish brown
5–7 days	Greenish coloration
7–10 days	Yellowish coloration
10–14 days	Brown
2–4 weeks	Clear

[a]Adapted from Sussman (1968).
[b]Adult values of these color changes are within these parameters.

selves, can suffer from this category of physical insult. Typical abuse from burns includes those caused by (1) cigarettes, (2) match tip or incense, (3) dry contact from forced contact with heating devices (e.g., heating grates, electric hot plate, radiators, irons), (4) branding by heated metals of various types, (5) scalds from forced immersion or direct pouring of hot liquids on body surfaces, (6) chemicals, such as acids or alkalis, and (7) electrical power sources.

In the initial assessment of burns, medical personnel must direct attention to any burns that may produce airway distress. Clinical indications include facial burns, carbonaceous sputum, singeing of eyebrows or nasal and other facial hair, and impaired mentation.

As in all abuse cases, obtaining a history of the presenting problem is imperative, but this is especially so in burn cases. The sequelae of burns and their attendant high mortality require vigorous attention to life support measures. The history given by the patient and others needs to be considered in terms of the plausibility of the injury.

Inspection of body parts should be observed for festering burn blisters (especially from cigarettes) and excavation marks from fresh burns (with particular attention to frequently traumatized areas such as the palms, soles, and buttocks). Imprints of items such as a hot poker or a household ironing device may be indicative of abuse. In managing circumferential burns of an extremity, removal of bracelets, watches, rings, and other such items is important to prevent constriction of parts distal to the circumferential item. Burns, particularly those classified as critical, are not well tolerated by the elderly for a number of complex reasons. In fact, a 70-year-old person with burns of 30% of the body surface area has a predicted mortality rate of 70% (Bunkis & Walton, 1986).

Head Injuries

Head injury in abuse cases is a serious concern from a traumatic standpoint. Injuries to the head inflicted by direct blows are generally a high cause of mortality in abuse cases. Overall, trauma as a mechanism of injury to the head causes more deaths and disability than any other neurologic cause in patients under age 50 (American College of Surgeons, 1989). The latter finding is related not only to abuse but to other mechanisms of injury (e.g., motor vehicle accidents, shootings). The following general injuries may occur from direct blows: (1) skull fractures, (2) scalp swelling and bruises, (3) retinal hemorrhage, (4) subdural hematomas, (5) subarachnoid hemorrhage, (6) subgaleal hematoma and/or traumatic alopecia, and (7) black eyes.

It is vitally important, owing to the high mortality of head injury and its sequelae, that patients who have suffered such violent abuse be seen by a physician in a proper medical facility capable of initial assessment and management. This requires appropriate triage and, in the initial medical management of the patient, attention to ventilation and hypovolemia. Thus is the potential for secondary brain damage obviated. Assuming that adequate and prudent initial stabilization of an abused head-injured patient has occurred, the matter of neurosurgical consultation may then be determined. At any rate, from the medical standpoint, the physician must determine what appropriate diagnostic studies (e.g., computed tomography [CT], skull roentgenograms) are needed. CT is considered to be a diagnostic procedure of choice for patients suspected of having sustained serious head injury. Other tests should be left to the discretion of the neurosurgeon.

The scalp is one of the more often affected areas in abuse cases. Injury can result from direct blows, lacerations, and pulling of the hair. Hemorrhage is not uncommon, and owing to the scalp's abundant blood supply, major blood loss is possible. The galea aponeurotica, one of the five layers of tissue covering the bone of the top of the skull, is separated by loose areolar tissue from the pericranium. It is in this area that hemorrhage can occur, resulting in subgaleal hematoma. Traumatic alopecia, or baldness, can occur from vigorous pulling of the hair, as well as its removal by force.

The skull is another vulnerable source of potential injury in abused adults. The skull anatomically is composed of the calvarium or cranial vault and the base. The cranial vault is particularly thin in the temporal regions. Injuries inflicted to this area of the abused patient must be regarded with a high index of concern.

Clinically, there are four major categories of skull fracture. These are classified as (1) linear, nondepressed, (2) depressed, (3) open, and (4) basal. Skull fractures are common in violent abuse cases but do not, by themselves, cause neurologic disability. Severe injury to the brain can occur without a fracture; the force alone transmitted by a blunt object to the skull can lead to damage. The significance of skull fractures from the trauma standpoint is that there is a high probability of intracranial hematoma. A victim of abuse who has sustained head injury should be admitted to a hospital for observation. Likewise, any abuse victim with a skull fracture should be seen by a neurosurgeon.

Blunt trauma, impalement injuries, and bullet wounds are the usual cause of intracranial hemorrhage. These may be classified as acute epidural hemorrhage, acute subdural hematoma, or subarachnoid hemorrhage. Acute subdural hematoma and subarachnoid hemorrhage require immediate surgical intervention because they are life-threatening. A hallmark of acute subdural hematoma is a fixed pupil on the same side as the impact area. Although alert, a patient with this type of injury typically complains of severe headache and is sleepy. It should be remembered in assessing head trauma that in cases of violent abuse, subdural hematomas are never spontaneous: Someone has caused the condition! Any neurologic deficit in an abuse case involving the head should be considered as critical. Alteration of consciousness is the hallmark of brain injury.

Nasal hemorrhaging, wounds or burns of the lips and tongue, missing or loose teeth, displaced nasal cartilages, fractures of the mandible, and bruises to the corners of the mouth should be evaluated in the context of the presenting patient's situation and history. Maxillofacial trauma, particularly that involving midfacial fractures, may indicate more serious skull fractures (e.g., cribiform plate).

Of particular concern for head-injured abused adults is damage to the eyes. General questions to consider in ocular trauma are these: Was there blunt trauma (e.g., fist insult)? Was there penetrating trauma (e.g., sharp object like a knife or pencil)? Were chemicals, particularly caustic, involved? The eyes should also be evaluated for pupillary size. Commonly encountered injuries consist of periorbital ecchymoses, subconjunctival hemorrhage, dislocated lens, detached retina, retinal hemorrhage, penetrating injuries, and traumatic cataracts.

Finally, the ears should be inspected for indications of (1) twisting, pulling, or pinching, (2) ruptured eardrums caused by blows to the head, (3) "cauliflower" ear caused by frequent blows to the pinna (projected part of the exterior ear), and (4) blood behind the tympanic membrane, a possible indicator of basilar skull fracture.

Chest Injuries

Blunt or penetrating trauma are the usual mechanisms of injury to the chest (e.g., hitting the chest with a baseball bat, or stabbing with an ice pick). The chest should be inspected for deformity and limitations of motion due to rib fractures. Blunt trauma from hitting with the fist or by object is a usual mechanism of injury. While marks from knuckles are sometimes discernable, often the perpetrator will use a hard bar of soap wrapped in a towel to hide telltale marks. Penetrating trauma from sharp instruments (e.g., knives, screwdrivers) must also be looked for in the examination. Observe the chest for contusions and hematomas that may be indicative of more occult or inexplicable trauma.

Careful assessment of the chest must be undertaken since the chest is often an area of assault for abuse victims. In females, the breasts are often a location for infliction of nonaccidental trauma (e.g., bites, lacerations, penetrating wounds, burns, and marks of disfigurement). In the elderly, restricting their movement by restraining them with various tie devices may result in rib fractures or more serious internal damage to the thoracic cage organs. Any impairment of respiratory effort must immediately be addressed. Definitive assessment of hemothorax, pneumothorax, and subcutaneous emphysema must be undertaken. Evaluation of the internal structures is necessary by stethoscope for auscultatory purposes followed by roentgenograms.

Abdominal Injuries

Abdominal injury has the potential for grave life threat, since there is the possibility of serious hemorrhage from the many visceral organs and vessels contained in the abdominal cavity. Blunt and penetrating trauma are the usual mechanisms, although other causes such as poisoning and forced ingestion of caustic substances may be involved. The internal organs can be damaged from blows inflicted to the back by the fist; lacerations to abdominal organs such as the small intestine sometimes occur from this mechanism.

The organs and tissues contained in the peritoneum, retroperitoneum, and pelvis most frequently injured are the (1) liver and spleen, (2) intestines, (3) duodenum or proximal jejunum, (4) major blood vessels (vena cava and aorta), (5) pancreas, and (6) kidneys.

The liver, spleen, and kidneys are the organs predominantly involved in blunt trauma, typically from blows administered by fists. The liver, spleen, and major vessels are prone to ruptures, the intestines to perforation, and the duodenum to hematoma from blunt trauma. Penetrating injuries from sharp objects (e.g., knives) and gunshot wounds result in varied exact organ or structural damage dependent upon the mechanism of injury. The circuitous trajectory of the bullet will determine that course. Stab wounds, depending on the length, width, and mechanism of entrance, will similarly determine which organs are involved.

An accurate physical examination diagnosis, diagnostic peritoneal lavage, and other adjunctive tests such as computerized tomography (CT) are the hallmarks of competent assessment of abdominal trauma by the physician. Unrecognized abdominal injury can lead to death. Note that although genitourinary injuries fall within the anatomical boundaries of the abdomen, they are included below in the section on sexual abuse.

Fractures

Visual examination should be made of the extremities for contusions or deformity. An assessment of neurovascular integrity should be undertaken as well. Definitive diagnosis of the existence of fractures, which are often concealed by other injuries, must be made by roentgenogram. A high index of suspicion of violent abuse must be maintained when repeated fractures to the same site are observed.

Ordinarily, fractures do not represent a grave threat to life in the adult patient. However, multiple fractures to major bony structures such as the femur or pelvis can lead to major hemodynamic instability and, therefore, may pose a life threat to the patient presenting with these injuries.

Failure to Thrive

In the adult abuse victim, failure to thrive (FTT) may not be as easily discernable as in children. The frail elderly patient who may already have reduced body volume and size is difficult to compare with others. Yet there are factors that may be considered in identifying FTT. Some of the diagnostic criteria and other factors are as follows: (1) Is the weight comparable to others in the age cohort? Is there undernutrition? (2) Is there a failure to gain weight in the current environment? Does this change when the environment is changed? (3) Is there a ravenous appetite? (4) Is the FTT due to withholding of medications? (5) Is the FTT due to withholding of the economic capability to purchase necessary food, medicine, and other biologic needs? (6) Are there signs of neglect, such as evidence of uncleanliness of body and personal clothing, unkempt hair, lack of shaving in males, poor dental hygiene, lack or deficiencies in cleanliness, temperature regulation, and reasonable amenities in the place of abode?

Sexual Abuse

Injuries to the genital, perianal areas or rectum, without direct evidence of antecedent trauma, must always be regarded as suspicious in any age group. In the elderly, where dementia, senility, or other causes of altered mental status (e.g., overmedication producing "chemical strightjacketing") are often observed, sexual abuse may never be reported by the abused party. In women, as previously noted, the shame and pressure to forget are common reactions, and therefore many cases go unreported for years. Owing to the difficulties many sexually abused persons have in reporting the violence, it is important that inadequate or implausible explanations be carefully scrutinized and reviewed.

Urogenital Injuries

Blunt trauma from direct blows to the flank or back that result in contusions, hematomas, or ecchymosis are the hallmarks of renal injury. A hematoma in the perianal area is indicative of bladder or urethral injury. Blood at the urethral meatus or inability to urinate also are signs of urethral injury.

Penetrating trauma from sharp instruments, and particularly from gunshot wounds, produces a number of internal injuries, including perforation of the ureter and bladder. Lacerations, bruises, or injuries to the external or internal genitalia, poor sphincter tone, and evidence of sexually transmitted disease (STD) or other infection must raise questions in the practitioner's mind as to cause. Finally, roentgenographic studies, including excretory urography utilizing intravenous pyelography, cystography, and computed tomographic (CT) scan, should be undertaken for definitive assessment of the genitourinary tract in violent abuse cases.

Summary

Abuse of any person presents the diagnostician with many challenges, not the least of which may be assessment and maintenance of basic life support functions. The clinical signs of abuse are often missed because the particular and usual mechanisms of trauma are not considered. It is abundantly and often distressingly clear, though, that the progress of the pathophysiologic insult is the same: high mortality and morbidity.

In developing the history of abuse the following key factors should be kept in mind:

1. If there are eyewitnesses, what was seen, who is accused, and who confesses?
2. Unexplained injuries are suspect first and ruled out only after careful analysis of all the evidence gathered, both personal and clinical.

3. Implausible histories need thorough investigation before being accepted as valid.
4. Alleged self-inflicted injuries must be carefully analyzed as to their origin; psychologic screening may be necessary to diagnose self-destructive behavior.
5. Delay in seeking medical care in the adult, except when altered mental status exists, is always questionable.

The management of abuse that results in physical violence is always fraught with many concerns. Detection of its existence by astute practitioners may be the single most important factor in its reduction by providing the proper medical care, referral, and protection afforded by social, human welfare, and public safety agencies. The high mortality involved when the vicious abuse circle closes is all too well known.

References

American College of Surgeons Committee on Trauma. (1989) *Advanced trauma life support program* (pp. 13–19; 133). Chicago: Author.

Bunkis, J., & Walton, R. L. (1986). Burns. In D. D. Trunkey & F. R. Lewis (Eds.), *Current therapy of trauma* (Vol. 2, pp. 367–373). Philadelphia: B. C. Decker.

Geis, G. (1982). The framework of violence. *Topics in Emergency Medicine, 3,* 2–3.

Goldberg, W. G. (1982). Behavioral assessment of the physically abused. In C. G. Warner & G. R. Braen (Eds.), *Management of the physically and emotionally abused* (pp. 111–125). Norwalk, CT: Appleton-Century-Crofts.

Goldberg, W., & Carey, A. L. (1982). Domestic violence victims in the emergency setting. *Topics in Emergency Medicine, 3,* 65–67.

Judd, R. L. (1988). Child, spousal, and elderly abuse: An overview. *Journal of Emergency Medical Services, 17,* 43–45.

Kimsey, L. R., Tarbox, A. R., & Bragg, D. (1981). Abuse of the elderly—The hidden agenda: The caretakers and categories of abuse. *Journal of the American Geriatrics Society, 29,* 465–472.

McNeese, M. C., & Hebeler, J. R. (1977). The abused child: A clinical approach to identification and management. *Clinical Symposia, 29,* 31–32.

National Coalition Against Domestic Violence. *NCADU Statistics* (May 1988). Washington, DC.

New York Times. (1985, May 23). Physicians alerted to risks of abuse (Sec. 3, p. 15).

Plotkin, M. R. (1988). *A time for dignity: Police and domestic abuse of the elderly* (p.8). Washington, DC: American Association of Retired Persons.

Schwartz, G., Bosker, G., & Grigsby, J. W. (Eds.). (1984). *Geriatrics emergencies.* Bowie, MD: Robert J. Brady Co.

Sussman, S. J. (1968). Skin manifestations of battered child syndrome. *Journal of Pediatrics, 72,* 99.

II

Violence toward Children

8

Child Physical Abuse

R. Kim Oates

Description of the Problem

Historical Background

Although child abuse did not become widely recognized by the medical and other professions until the late 1960s and early 1970s, the abuse of children has been a feature of most societies for many centuries. The Punch and Judy puppet play, which originated in the mid-17th century (Opie & Opie, 1951), tells how Judy gave Mr. Punch her baby. Despite being gently rocked by Mr. Punch, the baby begins to cry. This makes Mr. Punch rock the baby harder, becoming violent. Finally, when the crying persists Mr. Punch loses control, hits the baby, and kills him. A popular English nursery rhyme dated from the 18th century (Opie & Opie, 1951) describes "an old woman who lived in a shoe" who, because of her frustration at having to care for so many of her children, "whipped them all soundly and put them to bed." Even before this time, many cultures had used infanticide as an accepted method of family planning, it also being accepted practice to dispose of weak, premature, or deformed infants (Bakan, 1971).

One of the first medical descriptions of child abuse came from France, when Ambrose Tardieu (1860/1975), a forensic pathologist, published a medicolegal study of 32 children who had been battered to death. Little further was published about the condition until 1946 when

R. Kim Oates • Department of Pediatrics and Child Health, University of Sydney, and Division of Medicine and Child Protection Unit, The Children's Hospital, Camperdown, Sydney 2050, Australia.

an American radiologist, John Caffey, reported a new syndrome. Caffey (1946) reported 6 children with subdural hematomas who also had multiple fractures of the long bones. He noted other injuries, including bruising and retinal hemorrhages, and reported that some of these children were poorly nourished and delayed in their development. Caffey concluded that, in the absence of underlying skeletal disease, the fractures were most likely to be caused by trauma. He felt that negligence may have been a factor, but he was unable to obtain any history of trauma from the parents. Others recognized this condition, which became known as "Caffey's syndrome," but the true cause of these injuries was not clear to most practitioners. Such was the level of denial that parents could actually inflict serious injury on their own children. An important contribution to understanding these injuries was made in 1955 when Woolley and Evans took a fresh look at children with Caffey's syndrome. They emphasized the traumatic nature of these injuries and pointed out that the environments of these infants were often hazardous and undesirable.

The period of awareness of child abuse was ushered in by the landmark paper from the Denver group in 1962 (Kempe, Silverman, Steele, Droegemueller, & Silver, 1962). They coined the term *the battered child syndrome* as a way of directing attention to the seriousness of the problem and pointed out that physical abuse was a significant cause of death and injury to children. Since this time the extent of child abuse has been widely recognized and an extensive literature has developed. There now exists an International Society for the Prevention of Child Abuse and Neglect, formed in 1976, which publishes a quarterly journal, *Child Abuse and Neglect*.

Incidence

Kempe (1971) estimated the incidence of child physical abuse in the United States to be six cases per thousand live births. Because of difficulty and reluctance in making the diagnosis, the actual incidence is certain to be higher than the confirmed reported incidence. This has to be balanced by the fact that, while many cases go unreported, there also is the problem of overreporting. Besharov (1983) found that 60% of all reports are unable to be verified by the agencies that investigate them. Thus, there is the situation of simultaneous underreporting of many real cases and overreporting of cases where physical abuse may not have occurred. One of the best empirical studies on the incidence of violence toward children was done by Straus (1980), who, using a national probability survey of American children aged between 3 and 17 years, estimated that approximately 6.5 million children were physically abused each year. Although one can argue about the true incidence of child physical abuse, the important conclusion is that it is a relatively common problem. Indeed, it is far more prevelant than most single pediatric diseases to which considerable time and resources are allocated.

Types of Injuries

The clinical spectrum in physical abuse ranges from relatively mild trauma causing bruising through to florid cases with organ and skeletal damage. While bruises, head injuries, burns, and fractures are common, lacerations occur less often (Ryan, Davis, & Oates, 1977). Poisoning is thought to be an unusual feature of abuse. While it is not as common as bruising and fractures, it is now recognized as a distinct entity, often being surreptitiously used by the parent as a way of having prolonged hospitalization and investigation to find a cause for the child's unusual symptoms, a type of "Munchausen syndrome by proxy" (Meadow, 1977; Schnaps, Frond, Rand, & Tirosh, 1981).

The junction of the cartilage with the shaft of the long bone is one of the weakest areas in the skeleton of the growing child. These areas are very vulnerable to the torsion forces that occur when a child is pulled and shaken, so that epiphyseal separation and metaphyseal fractures are common injuries in abuse and unusual injuries in normal play or accidents. Spiral fractures or long bones also are unusual in childhood accidents and occur as a result of the twisting, shearing forces that an adult applies when violently twisting a child's arm or leg.

When an infant is shaken, the repeated acceleration-deceleration and rotation forces that are produced as the infant's head bounces back and forth can cause damage to the brain by direct contusion from the brain's hitting against the inside of the skull or by rupture of blood vessels within and around the brain. Shaking can also cause retinal injuries. These retinal hemorrhages usually undergo complete resolution but can be more serious and lead to permanent visual handicap (Mushin, 1971). A complete ophthalmic examination should always be included as part of the assessment of the abused child.

Burns are a relatively common manifestation of child abuse. Smith and Hanson (1974) reported serious burns or scalds in 20% of 124 abused children seen in England. These authors drew attention to burns of the buttocks or perineum inflicted by placing the child on a hot metal surface such as a stove. Other typical burns are marks caused by lighted cigarettes and glove and stocking burns of hands or feet suggesting that the child's limbs may have been forcibly held in hot water.

Other less usual injuries include (a) drowning, suggesting that abuse should be considered in the diagnosis of atypical immersion inci-

dents in infants (Pearn, Brown, Wong, & Bart, 1979), (b) subgaleal hematomas caused by hair pulling, (c) genital injuries, (d) tears to the floor
and roof of the mouth caused by trauma at feeding, and (e) traumatic
cysts of the pancreas and intramural hematoma of the bowel caused by a
direct blow to the abdomen and leading to symptoms and signs of
intestinal obstruction (Kempe, 1975). Sometimes skin lesions take the
shape of a recognizable object, such as a belt buckle, or a mark in the
shape of a loop caused by a loop of rope or electric cord.

Why Child Physical Abuse Is Important

The answer to the question "Why is child physical abuse important?" may seem obvious, but there is more to this condition than the
immediate physical injuries. It is true that child abuse is a major problem
resulting in many deaths and a far greater number of injuries, many of
them serious, each year. Perhaps just as important is that, with the
majority of abuse being caused by the child's parent or caretaker, the
actions that lead to the abuse deprive children of some of their basic
needs. Pringle (1975) has described the needs of children as the need for
love and security, the need for new experiences, the need for praise and
recognition, and the need for responsibility. These basic needs for security, recognition of one's worth, and praise are not met in children
who see their parents as people likely to injure them and who feel they
have to live in fear of a parental outburst. It is recognized that a proportion of parents who abuse their children were physically abused in their
own childhood, while recent long-term follow-up studies (Oates, 1986)
have shown that even though the abuse stops, many physically abused
children develop with poor self-esteem, inability to make adequate
friendships, lack of trust, and continuing behavior problems. This
makes it very difficult for many of these children to develop satisfactory
adult relationships, and even more difficult for them to cope with the
normal stresses associated with childrearing. Thus, child abuse is a condition that can be transmitted from one generation to the next. Breaking
this cycle is important both for the abused child and for that child's own
future children.

Case Description

Laura was the first child of Margaret and Danny, a young couple
living in an inner-city suburb. The pregnancy that produced Laura was
unplanned, and Margaret, aged 20, who had been a school clerical assistant, had given up her job in the last trimester, remaining at home after
the birth to care for Laura. Danny, aged 18, was a plumber and in regular
employment.

Laura was born at term weighting 3450 grams, the pregnancy being uneventful and the delivery accompanied by a lift-out forceps procedure. She was in good condition at birth, no resuscitation being necessary, and she was breast-fed.

Margaret had a regular Monday evening activity with friends from her old place of employment, and on these occasions Laura was left at home in Danny's care. When Laura was 3 weeks old, Margaret went back to her usual Monday evening outing, being away for just under 3 hours. Later that evening Laura was noted to be restless and crying in her sleep. During the small hours of the morning Margaret went to check on Laura and found her to be very pale and breathing irregularly. The parents then took Laura to the Children's Hospital, where her condition was serious enough to warrant immediate admission to the intensive care unit.

The medical findings when Laura was brought to the hospital were very serious. She was gasping irregularly and was unable to be roused although she was responsive to pain. The anterior fontanelle was raised and tense, a sign of increased intracranial pressure. Her right pupil was dilated and unresponsive to light. Examination of the right occular fundus showed extensive retinal hemorrhages. The left pupil reacted normally and there were no retinal hemorrhages. There were no bruises anywhere on the body.

Laura's condition continued to deteriorate quickly so that she was unable to breathe spontaneously and had to be artificially ventilated. A CT scan of the brain showed marked swelling in the right side of the brain and signs of bleeding within the brain substance. A radionucleide scan of the brain showed poor and delayed blood flow to the right side of the brain, thought to be a result of the marked swelling in this area. There was no skull fracture. These findings were consistent with an acute brain injury. A radiological survey of all Laura's other bones did not show any recent or old fractures.

The seriousness of Laura's condition was discussed with Danny and Margaret. They reported that Laura had always been an easy baby to care for, one who was fairly placid, slept well, and fed readily. On this evening, Laura was said to have settled down well after her usual 6:00 p.m. feeding, and when Margaret left her an hour later she was asleep. Danny said that while Margaret was out Laura had awakened crying and could not be comforted. He tried cuddling and feeding her but with little success. However, by the time Margaret returned home Laura appeared to be sleeping peacefully. Later that evening Laura woke crying and was very irritable, taking some time to settle. Much later that night she was noted to be pale and gasping, at which time her parents rushed her to the hospital. Both parents could offer no explanation for Laura's condition, Danny very early saying, "I didn't hit her or anything like that."

After the initial interview, which was conducted without any accusations, the parents said that they were planning to visit Laura again in 2 days' time, an unusual behavior in view of the seriousness of Laura's condition and the hospital's policy of encouraging parents to live in and visit as much as possible. Margaret and Danny were told of our responsibility to report injuries that had no explanation and where child abuse could be a possibility. In a later interview with the police, Danny said that he had placed Laura in a playpen that evening when she was crying and that he had then accidentally kicked the corner of the playpen, perhaps bumping Laura as well.

The medical opinion was that Laura had sustained an acute brain injury on the evening of her admission to the hospital, and that in the absence of any significant external head trauma, violent shaking was thought to be the most likely cause. Because Laura had been only with her parents during this time, it was felt that the injury must have been caused by one of the parents, the more likely one being Laura's father during the time Margaret was out of the house. It was felt that Laura probably did wake crying, and that in his frustration of not being able to settle her, Danny had shaken her, not realizing the serious damage that violent shaking can cause to a young infant.

A children's court order was obtained that placed Laura in her mother's care under supervision from the Department of Child Welfare, a condition of the placement being that Danny should live out of the home and not have access to Laura. In addition to the children's court order, criminal charges were laid against Danny by the police, and a number of court cases were heard over the subsequent 3 years. Despite the children's court order, there was very little in the way of Welfare Department supervision, and after the first few months Danny moved back into the family home. A second, healthy child was born to Danny and Margaret 14 months after Laura's injury. This child developed normally and is not known to have had any injuries. The paternal and maternal grandparents have been very supportive of the family.

At the end of 3 years the final court hearing was held, the police aiming for a conviction of Danny for attempted manslaughter. The defense case was based on the possibility that the forceps delivery may have been responsible for the injury, and this, coupled with some degree of conflict in opinion by the various hospital specialists who had seen the child, was enough for the prosecution's case to be lost.

Laura's condition remained unstable and critical for the first few days of her admission to the hospital. She was eventually able to come off the ventilator but was left with permanent, severe cerebral damage. She has been followed regularly over several years and is extremely handicapped. She is severely intellectually retarded, has spastic quadriplegia, is blind, and is very irritable. She developed infantile spasms and now has epilepsy, which is difficult to control. She has been linked with a variety of community resources, which include physiotherapy, respite care, and the state blind society's infant stimulation program, and she receives special schooling. Margaret has coped admirably with her, always keeping appointments and being fully involved in her various therapies.

Medical Issues

Establishing the Diagnosis

Those involved in treating children need to be aware that child physical abuse is relatively common. If a condition is common, the practitioner needs to be aware of it, and physical abuse should be considered a possibility, even if only to be dismissed, in any child who presents with an injury, particularly if that injury is not adequately explained. Kempe and Helfer (1972) estimated that 15% of children under 5 years of age who attend hospital casualty departments are likely to have inflicted injuries. Springthorpe, Oates, and Hayes (1977), in a study of children coming to an emergency room at a children's hospital, found that 40% of children under 5 years of age with burns or injuries had features strongly suggestive of abuse. These studies suggest that it is important for those working in emergency rooms to gain expertise in child abuse detection and management and to have an appropriate level of suspicion when seeing children with injuries. Similarly, when an infant is brought unconscious to an intensive care unit, child abuse, particularly from a shaking injury, should be considered along with the other diagnostic possibilities.

The danger of shaking infants was pointed out by Caffey in 1974. Caffey's paper drew attention to the high vulnerability of the infant head, brain, and eyes to the stress of shaking, and pointed out that the shaking of infants can be an important cause of mental retardation and permanent brain damage. It is likely that many of the so-called spontaneous subdural hematomas of infancy described in older pediatric texts were actually cases of child abuse resulting from violent shaking. It is interesting that while older pediatric textbooks discussed the spontaneous subdural hematoma of infancy—a not uncommon diagnosis in that period—they did not mention child abuse. More recent texts now discuss child abuse, but the so-called spontaneous subdural hematoma of infancy is no longer mentioned. The concept of these brain injuries being solely due to shaking, however, has been recently called into question (Duhaime, Gennarelli, Thibault, Bruce, Morgulies, & Wiser, 1987). These researchers feel that direct physical injury also usually occurs and showed that in more than half the cases they studied, although no evidence of external trauma was noted on the initial physical examination, careful autopsy did show evidence of scalp contusion and skull fractures. Although there may still be some doubt about the mechanism, it is clear that abuse must be considered as a possible cause when a child presents with evidence of acute brain injury.

Clinical signs from a shaking injury may not be immediate and can take several hours to appear. This is particularly likely when the bridging veins within the skull are torn. Bridging veins cross the potential surface between the dura, a tough, thick membrane that is the outer membrane covering the brain, and the arachnoid, a much thinner membrane lying beneath the dura. Bleeding from these veins is under low pressure, and symptoms may not appear until a significant volume of blood starts to expand and accumulate in the space between the dura and the arachnoid.

One problem in a child with a skull fracture is to decide the likelihood of the injury's being nonaccidental. While the diagnosis is based largely on the presence of any associated injuries and on the "fit" between the parents' story and the physical findings, Hobbs (1984) has provided some useful information on skull fractures in children under 2 years. He found that accidents were more likely to result in single, narrow, linear fractures, usually involving the parietal bone with no associated intracranial injury. In contrast, fractures associated with abuse were more likely to be multiple, complex, depressed, or wide, to involve areas other than the parietal bone, to involve more than one bone, and to be associated with intracranial injury.

Modern imaging techniques can help the diagnosis of intracranial injury (Frank, Zimmerman, & Leeds, 1985). The CT findings can include contusion and hemorrhages in single or multiple sites in the brain substance as well as evidence of bleeding between the brain and the skull. In severe cases, the CT scan later shows hypodense areas as much of the damaged brain tissue becomes resorbed, leaving markedly enlarged ventricles and atrophy of brain substance. The advent of magnetic resonance imaging has been shown to be superior to CT scanning in detecting brain injury, particularly subdural hematomas (Alexander, Schor, & Smith, 1986).

What few studies there are on the outcome of children who sustain severe head injuries suggest that, as in the case of Laura, there are usually permanent handicaps (Dykes, 1986), with a high incidence of death, visual loss, seizures, and developmental delay.

The diagnosis of physical abuse is not based solely on the injuries. It is also based on the history, particularly if the explanation is inadequate or inappropriate. Other features that may raise the level of suspicion include inconsistent explanations for the injury given by each parent, a long delay between the injury and presenting the child for treatment, and inappropriate affect on the part of the parents. Other physical findings in favor of this diagnosis include unusual patterns of bruising, especially "grab marks" in the shape of finger marks where the limbs of the child may have been forcefully gripped, bruises suggesting the pattern of an object, bruises in areas usually not injured accidentally, two black eyes, unusual fractures such as spiral fractures in long bones or chip fractures at metaphyseal regions suggesting a twisting injury, and evidence of old and recent fractures showing different stages of healing on the skeletal survey. The diagnosis of abuse is sometimes clear-cut, but often there are gray areas where clinical experience, careful family assessment, and consultation with more experienced colleagues will all help in establishing the diagnosis.

Rather than trying to reach a "whodunnit" diagnosis in every case, it is far more fruitful to look at the strengths and weaknesses in the family where abuse is suspected, and to take steps to relieve some of the stresses by providing realistic support services. What is most important is the future protection and mental health of the child. Most families have the same concern for the child as the child protection worker—that is, for their child to grow up well and healthy. Many families do not have the skills to achieve this, reverting to violence in the face of stress and frustration. Supporting these families in parenting and recognizing that there must be a long-term commitment to them is for most families a more realistic approach than seeing detection and prosecution as the beginning and end of involvement with the family.

Accepting the Diagnosis

One problem in making the diagnosis of child abuse may be the professional's own denial about being faced with this condition. In the past, many medical professionals have been poorly trained to deal with child abuse. They often are reluctant to become involved in court action and may be uncomfortable working cooperatively with other professionals. There is then the danger of accepting at face value a most unlikely explanation for the injury rather than seeking its real cause (Oates, 1979; Sanders, 1972). Sanders (1972) reports that, in his experience, it can be more difficult to tell parents he is reporting them, than it is for them to accept his action.

A review of 52 situations in which physicians had difficulty in making a diagnosis of child abuse was undertaken by Silver, Dubbin, and Lourie (1969). These researchers found that in each case the prime difficulty was the physician's own subjective feelings or his misunderstandings of his responsibility under the child abuse reporting laws. Gregg and Elmer (1969) studied 146 accidents, 30 of which were due to abuse. They found it was difficult to separate the two groups on the history of the accident alone and stressed that assessment of the family, particularly its child care practices, was the most useful differentiating factor. With widespread acceptance that child abuse is a major problem, and with the availability of child protection teams in most centers, these difficulties in reporting have become less, although the individual practitioner still needs to be aware of the unconscious tendency to overlook this diagnosis.

The Child Protection Team

The management of child abuse usually requires a team approach. However, child protection teams don't just happen. A team of individuals who work in parallel without mutual trust and respect for each other and without close cooperation as a team in name only. Considerable effort has to go into creating a child protection team with complementary skills where the members can work comfortably with each other. In Laura's case, the initial interview with Danny and Margaret was conducted jointly by the social worker and the pediatrician. Some of the subsequent interviews were held jointly or separately but always with discussion between the social worker and the pediatrician at their conclusion. The case conference is an important process in creating a management plan. In Laura's case, there was an early case conference attended by the pediatrician and the social worker, the child welfare agency (which has the statutory authority for child protection), the intensive care ward staff, and the police. At the case conference, minutes are taken and a management plan is made. It is essential that the recommendations made at the case conference are realistic and able to be carried out with named members of the team being recorded as being responsible for particular aspects of the management. If the management plans have to be varied, subsequent case conferences or reviews are needed to ensure that any altered circumstances are taken into account and that the management plan remains viable.

It is also important for the child protection team to be involved early. Asking the team to see a child for the first time when the child is about to be discharged after 2 weeks in the hospital devalues the role of the team and makes working with the family extremely difficult. With Laura, the child protection team was notified within an hour of Laura's arrival at the hospital so that early involvement with the family was possible. This early, initial interview often is very helpful in establishing a relationship with the parents. Child protection teams based in hospitals should try to have a high profile in terms of teaching and in offering a high-quality, quickly responding 24-hour-per-day service. This credibility will encourage early consultation.

The members of the team have to be careful not to confuse their responsibility to the family with their responsibility to the child. They need to be aware of a natural tendency not to want to become involved in some cases, and also of the temptation that sometimes occurs to empathize so closely with the parents that the child's needs are overlooked. While being able to have some sympathy with and understanding for the parents' problems, it is important to be able to look closely at the needs and rights of the child. This includes the provision of a treatment program made specifically for the child's needs. This is particularly important in view of the follow-up studies showing high incidence of developmental delay in these children (Oates, 1986).

Those involved in child protection often experience anger and frustration. Each team member needs to try to help the others in the team as well as those involved in the hospital, such as nursing staff on the child's ward, to contain this anger or to express it constructively. Many members often find it helpful to look beyond the team for personal support, and many teams find it helpful to have an advisor not directly involved with the family with whom they can discuss the problems of the child abuse as well as their own feelings about it.

Legal Issues

In Laura's case, the legal issues were taken on two fronts. The child welfare department's interest was to protect Laura. They had her case heard in the children's court, where decisions were made "on the balance of probability," a much less stringent criterion than that of "beyond reasonable doubt," which is used in the criminal court (of course, legal procedures will vary from country to country and by jurisdiction). The children's court readily accepted the need to offer Laura protection, and, since the maternal grandparents were nearby and supportive, and since it seemed that the injury was caused when Margaret was out of the house, a decision was made for Laura to be placed in Margaret's custody but with Danny being required to live apart from them. Supervision was not adequate, and before long Danny and Margaret were together again.

In retrospect it can be seen that no harm came to Laura from the breakdown of supervision, but it does point out the need for court orders to be realistic and for supervision to be provided in a specified way rather than just ordered without any formal review process to ensure that it is actually happening. As it turned out, a variety of supporting services were provided for Margaret and Laura, and Margaret cooperated fully in all of these arrangements. However, if the hospital team had not worked to obtain long-term hospital and community-based support for this family, this support might not have been forthcoming. A more realistic court order might have been for Laura to live away from her parents while the assessment of their strengths and weaknesses continued, and then, if Laura was returned either to her mother or to her grandparents, or put in foster care, for an audit to be made to ensure continuing treatment for Laura.

The other legal avenue used was the criminal court. Because Laura was close to death, the police proceeded with an attempted manslaughter charge. Delays in the justice system, with frequent deferrals of the case and frequent adjournments, meant that it was 3 years before the case was concluded. By this time, memories were hazy, although fortunately careful documentation of the injuries and treatment had been made at the time, an essential procedure in all child protection cases.

The child protection team was convinced that the injury was not accidental, although there was a real possibility that Danny was unaware of the extent of the injury he would cause by violently shaking Laura. The evidence presented by the hospital could have been more carefully prepared. The neurosurgeon, a key witness, was very reluctant to appear in court and, as a result of several emergency neurosurgical procedures that coincided with the court hearings, did not give evidence apart from a written statement describing the injuries but failing to express an opinion as to the cause.

The neurologist who had been involved in Laura's care gave evidence but was reluctant to be definite about the cause of the injury and, under pressure from cross-examination for the defense, conceded that it was possible for trauma occurring at the time of the forceps delivery to be responsible for Laura's sudden illness and present condition. The child protection team had made an error in not ensuring that the neurologist was fully conversant with the obstetric details before giving evidence. The record from the obstetric hospital and discussion with the obstetrician soon after Laura's initial presentation showed that the birth was uncomplicated, that forceps were applied only lightly at the "lift-out" stage of the delivery, and that Laura was in good condition at birth. The cross-examination of the neurologist by the defense had not revealed this, the implication being that the delivery was far more hazardous than it actually was.

Another difficulty was that the neurologist was unfamiliar with child abuse literature, including studies on head injuries, and so was not able to be definite in his conclusions and was persuaded that birth trauma could have been a possible cause. This evidence was in conflict with that of the pediatrician from the child protection team, who stated that the injuries were consistent with violent shaking and not at all consistent with birth trauma. However, the conflict in evidence meant that there was "reasonable doubt," and so the prosecution's case was lost.

It can be seen now that things have probably worked out better from Laura's point of view as a result of this decision. Danny and Margaret matured considerably over the 3 years between the injury and the final court case. Danny has been able to remain in employment and the family has been materially much better off than if he had been in prison. There has been good support from the grandparents on both sides, with little in the way of recrimination, allowing continuing support from both sides of the family. Hospital and community support have also been provided. Danny and Margaret have a continuing tragedy in their lives, that of having to care for a child born potentially normal but now with severe intellectual impairments and major physical disabilities. However, in other cases the result might have been different, and the results in this case do not diminish the need for those involved in this area to develop expertise in preparing cases for court and in teaching other professionals who may be involved about some of the techniques needed to be able to present effectively in court.

Some useful papers have been written on giving evidence in court (Knight, 1978) and developing courtroom skills (Carson, 1984). It is essential for the expert witness to prepare for the case and to have a careful mastery of the facts. Doctors should not retreat into the security of complex technical jargon. This makes their evidence incomprehensible to a jury and may make it open to misinterpretation. There is no substitute for plain, everyday language. Thus, "two black eyes" is a much more understandable term than "bilateral periorbital hematomas."

Attention to other techniques, such as appropriately conservative dress, avoiding constantly shuffling papers, using eye contact when answering questions, and avoiding fidgeting, will all help the expert witness's credibility. It is often very helpful for those starting work in a child protection team to have several visits to court to observe more experienced members of the team giving evidence in preparation for the time when they will also be called as witnesses.

It is important to remain calm and controlled. Becoming angry or sarcastic does nothing to enhance the expert witness's credibility. It also is important to be impartial and honest. Being honest may mean acknowledging when a question is outside your area of expertise. The expert witness should never be tempted to step beyond the bounds of his own skill and competence. Doing so may cause embarrassment to the witness if his lack of expertise in the area into which he has strayed is revealed. It also lessens the credibility of the evidence given in an area of expertise.

Finally, the testimony of the expert witness should be regarded as a scholarly endeavor (Brent, 1982). The expert witness is there to help arrive at a decision about the truth, not to try to win a case for one side or the other. It is essential to be well informed, to be nonpartisan, and not to step beyond the bounds of one's own expertise, tempting as that may be.

Social and Family Issues

Family Strengths and Weaknesses

Margaret

Laura's family had a number of positive features. Margaret was of good intelligence, had a stable background, and had a good relationship with her own parents, who lived nearby. She had made firm friends in her work as a school clerical assistant and also maintained contact with some of her old school friends. She was able to seek help when needed and was able to telephone her family doctor or her pediatrician whenever problems relating to Laura, such as seizures, occurred. She participated in the physiotherapy and infant stimulation programs and did all that was asked of her with regard to Laura's care, which was complex and, at times, stressful.

She could not be described as an "open" person, appearing calmly efficient on the outside but unwilling to discuss positive or negative features of her family life. She readily responded to all practical suggestions to assist Laura but was unable to be engaged by the social worker in any therapeutic work. This raises the question of how much one should probe or try to become involved in deeper family issues when it is resisted. In this case, it was decided to be available but not to exert any pressure that might have lost cooperation with the various community support and medical treatments in which Laura and Margaret were involved.

Danny

Danny was only 18 when Laura was born. He is a large young man who had been involved in junior wrestling. He had undertaken a successful apprenticeship as a plumber and had remained in full employment during a time when unemployment was high. His parents also lived nearby and were supportive of him, Margaret, and the marriage. He had a close relationship with his mother, frequently telephoning her for advice on a wide variety of subjects, including childrearing. He was reported to have a quick temper and had been known to have been involved in fights with minimal provocation. He was proud of his physical strength.

While his parents were supportive and readily available, the early years of his childhood had been unhappy. There had been a great deal of stress between his parents, often resulting in his father's being violent toward his mother. He was unable to recall any abuse to himself, but his memory of his father, who separated from his mother when he was 6 years of age, was generally negative. His mother remarried when he was 11. He had no contact with his natural father but had formed a cordial but not affectionate relationship with his stepfather.

The Community

Margaret and Danny were fortunate to live in a suburb with strong community supports. While not being aware of any need for these supports before Laura's injury, the ready availability of an extremely supportive and understanding family doctor and a visiting community nurse, and easy access to physiotherapy and other services for Laura were all important factors in reducing some of the stresses on the parents after the injury and in allowing a realistic management plan to be implemented.

The Future

This family has a long way to go. Laura will become an increasing physical and financial burden as she becomes older and heavier. She will never be independently mobile and requires almost constant supervision. Their second child has remained well and free from injury, the community support services being involved to ensure that her needs are not overlooked. Although involvement by the same professional group has continued with this family for over 4 years, many more years will be required. This is one of the major challenges in child protection work where in many families the problems and stresses remain much longer than the involvement of any particular worker. While helping these families to develop skills in coping and in parenting, it is important that, when professionals move on to other positions, they carefully prepare the family for this loss and adequately hand the case over to their successors.

Assessment of Psychopathology

Neither Danny nor Margaret had a formal psychiatric assessment. Margaret was cooperative but self-contained, a concrete thinker, and possibly not readily available for a therapeutic approach involving introspection. It was felt most appropriate to continue at a practical level, providing ready access and supportive services. On the surface this appears to have been effective, her management of Laura having been exemplary and her subsequent child developing normally and free from abuse.

Danny appeared to be somewhat less intelligent than Laura. He enjoyed physical activity and the company of other males, and he had a hot temper. He did not communicate easily with professionals and had an unhappy childhood, witnessing violence toward his mother, to whom he was closely attached, but not suffering physical abuse himself. He felt that, as a result of the early example of his natural father, most conflicts could be resolved by force, and he demonstrated this by getting into occasional physical fights. Having married at 17 years of age, he had missed out on some aspects of normal adolescent development. It has never been established exactly what happened to Laura, but it appears likely that Danny did lose control with her, probably during Margaret's absence, resulting in violent shaking that did far more harm than he probably intended.

Many abusive parents do not have clear-cut psychiatric disorders, but they do display psychopathology. Steele and Pollock (1972), in a study of 60 abusive families, commented that "with few exceptions these parents had emotional problems of sufficient severity to be accepted for psychiatric treatment had they presented." These and other studies have come from groups of patients referred to psychiatrists for assessment, do not have controls, and would be expected to show a high incidence of psychopathology by the very nature of their referrals. However, a random community survey (Bland & Orn, 1986) has convincingly shown that child abuse as well as family violence correlates strongly with psychiatric disorder in the parents.

Recent attempts to categorize psychiatric disorders in abusive parents have led to the concept of borderline personality disorder being a feature of many of these parents. Five factors considered to be the major characteristics of child abusing parents have been described by Prodgers (1984) as arrested emotional development, poor self-image, emotional isolation, depressive loneliness, and poorly suppressed anger. These features were not found in Margaret, but Danny could be considered to have arrested emotional development, poor self-image, and poorly suppressed anger. The concept of borderline personality as it relates to abusive parents has been thoughtfully reviewed by Brennan (1986).

Treatment Options

The management options in this case included the following:

1. Psychotherapy. This approach was not chosen.
2. A practical approach providing supportive services and regular contact with the family. This was the option chosen, although, if supportive services had not been so readily available, this would have been a difficult option to organize successfully.
3. Removal of Laura to foster care on either a short-term or a long-term basis. This was one option available to the children's court, although the decision was made for Laura to remain with her mother.

4. Group work with the parents. This can be an effective form of treatment, although it requires some motivation on the part of the parents and was not chosen in this case.

The evaluation of the effectiveness of treatment programs for physically abused children is difficult, and there is much more written about how to treat these children than about results of treatment, suggesting that there are many problems in this area (Oates, 1982). A collection of 43 major papers on child abuse (Cook & Bowles, 1980) did not include any that described the results of treatment to either the parents or the children. More recent efforts in this area (Kelly, 1983), however, show promise for interventions with abusive parents.

Three prerequisites for optimal long-term management have been suggested by Schmitt and Beezley (1976): (1) a comprehensive diagnostic assessment of the family, (2) a multidisciplinary team to make decisions and to plan treatment, and (3) the availability of diversified treatment options for periodic assessment of treatment plans. Those involved in child abuse treatment should be clearly aware of their short- and long-term responsibilities to the families. Because the situation is complex, it is essential to have a treatment plan that is flexible, is reviewed periodically, and is realistic and practical. The multidisciplinary team that produces an ideal but totally unrealistic plan does little for these children.

Although it has been argued by some (Bishop & Moore, 1978) that the majority of parents would benefit from psychiatric intervention, treating the parent can be hazardous. It has been reported that stressful psychotherapy sessions for abusive parents are likely to precipitate future episodes of abuse (Winkler, Ginn, & Miletic, 1979). Even if the answer did lie in simply providing psychotherapy, there would never be enough skilled therapists available for the size of this problem. In contrast, Rosen and Stein (1980) suggested that rather than psychotherapy, the parents require educative and supportive treatment aimed at enhancing their own self-esteem and lowering their unrealistic expectations for the child.

The advantages of nonprofessional volunteers, who can give abusive parents some of the parenting they missed in their own childhood, and thus prevent the parents from depending on the child for their emotional needs, have been described by Gray and Kaplan (1980). Because of the size of the abuse problem in relation to the number of professionals available, and because volunteers can provide a type of caring that professionals cannot give, this seems to be a particularly valuable form of treatment.

The form of treatment offered to parents depends on the degree of problem found in the family. While some parents will respond to relatively simple and supportive measures, these are less likely to work for a hard core of parents (variously estimated at between 20 and 40% of cases) who have serious personality disturbances (Besharov, 1983). These parents will require intense skilled and sustained intervention, while serious consideration should be given to alternate care of the child in some of these cases.

Where there is severe family pathology it may be in the child's best interests to be removed from the parents and placed in foster care. It would be naive, however, to believe that this solves the problem. A review of over 5000 children in foster care (Bolton, Laner, & Gai, 1981) showed that the risk of maltreatment at the hands of a foster parent was over three times greater than in a natural family. Being placed in foster care is a confusing and unsettling experience for a child. Children need to be prepared for this sort of separation and should have a specific treatment program provided for them during the period of fostering. Without this, the potential adverse emotional sequelae for the child may be even more harmful.

In some cases, short- to medium-term fostering with eventual return to the parents may be less in the child's interests than permanent placement. A 4-year follow-up of 50 abused children from Liverpool (Hensey, Williams, & Rosenbloom, 1983) found that those children for whom an early decision had been made to sever all family contacts fared significantly better than those who were returned to their parents.

Since most abused children remain in their homes, it is in this context that most treatment should be planned. Ruth Kempe (1981) has pointed out that treatment starts with a complete evaluation of the child's strengths and weaknesses. She noted that treatment of the infant involved working with the mother, that preschool children often respond to a therapeutic day care center, and that a more traditional psychotherapeutic approach may be suitable for the school-aged child. Carter (1982) showed the value of therapeutic day care by interviewing a random sample of parents whose children were receiving this treatment. The majority of parents reported that their child's behavior had become easier to manage and that they themselves had benefited from meeting other parents.

Other forms of treatment include residential programs for the parent and child (Brazier, Davis, & Shier, 1982; Coote, 1981; Lynch, Steinberg, & Ounsted, 1975). These programs appear to be successful, although they are expensive facilities that are available only to a small number of carefully selected families. Perhaps more practical is the type of program that provides a therapeutic preschool environment for abused children in conjunction with a supportive program for parents (Petheram & Thomson, 1981).

Conclusions

As in many child abuse cases, the cause of Laura's injury was never completely determined, although it is virtually certain that it was caused by an adult, Danny being the most obvious perpetrator. Could this injury have been prevented? The family was not known to any agencies prior to this episode, and apart from Danny's youth, there was nothing to single this family out from any other. If a prenatal detection program (Geddes, Monaghan, Muir, & Jones, 1979; Gray, Cutler, Dean, & Kempe, 1977) aimed at looking for families where there was a potential for abuse had been available, this family might have been detected as having risk factors, such as low paternal age and a past history of aggression. Supportive services could then have been provided from birth, thus possibly resulting in, but by no means ensuring, prevention of Laura's injury.

Helfer and Kempe (1980) have described a number of preventive measures aimed at parents and children at different stages of their lives that, taken together, are thought likely to prevent many cases of child abuse. These are the following:

1. Perinatal coaching to provide new parents with the skills necessary to communicate with their new child.
2. Home care assistance where parents are provided with visitors to help them with practical child care problems and to improve their communication skills with their infants.
3. Expanded baby care.
4. Teaching preschool and primary school children interpersonal, cognitive-problem-solving skills to help them with resolving everyday problems.
5. The teaching of interpersonal skills for high school children, with emphasis on how to get on with people of all ages and at all levels in society.
6. A crash course in "childhood" for adults and some young adults who need a second chance to learn skills that should have been learned during their childhood.
7. A pre-parent refresher course for "soon-to-be" parents to revise previously taught concepts of appropriate ways to interact with their partners and children.

In Laura's case, supportive and preventive services could be provided only after the injury. This family has a continuing tragedy caused by Laura's severe handicap, but it seems to be managing well with a supportive approach. A long-term commitment to this family needs to be maintained, as it does to the majority of families where child physical abuse has occurred.

References

Alexander, R. C., Schor, D. P., & Smith, W. L. (1986). Magnetic resonance imaging of intracranial injuries from child abuse. *Journal of Pediatrics, 109*, 975–979.

Bakan, D. (1971). *Slaughter of the innocents: A study of the battered child phenomenon.* San Francisco: Jossey-Bass.

Besharov, D. J. (1983). Child protection: Past progress, present problems, and future directions. *Family Law Quarterly, 17*, 151–172.

Bishop, F. I., & Moore, B. G. (1978). *Maltreating families.* Victoria, Australia: Ministry of Health.

Bland, J., & Orn, H. (1986). Family violence and psychiatric disorder. *Canadian Journal of Psychiatry, 31*, 129–137.

Bolton, F. G., Laner, R. H., & Gai, D. S. (1981). For better or worse? Foster parents and foster children in an officially reported child maltreatment population. *Children and Youth Services Review, 13*, 127–129.

Brazier, J., Davis, A. A., & Shier, J. (1982). "Montrose" Child Life Protection Unit: A treatment and assessment model in child abuse intervention. *Child Abuse and Neglect, 6*, 389–394.

Brennan, J. (1986). The borderline parent-child relationship (Abstracts). Sixth International Congress on Child Abuse and Neglect, Sydney. Abstract No. 24, p. 128.

Brent, R. L. (1982). The irresponsible expert witness: A failure of biomedical graduate education and professional accountability. *Pediatrics, 70*, 754–762.

Caffey, J. (1946). Multiple fractures in the long bones of infants suffering from chronic subdural hematoma. *American Journal of Roentgenology, 56*, 163–173.

Caffey, J. (1974). The whiplash shaken infant syndrome. *Pediatrics, 54*, 396–403.

Carson, D. (1984). Developing courtroom skills. *Journal of Social Welfare Law, 110*, 29–38.

Carter, J. (1982). Family day centres and child abuse. In R. K. Oates (Ed.), *Child abuse—A community concern.* Sydney: Butterworths.

Cook, J. V., & Bowles, R. T. (1980). *Child abuse: Commission and omission.* Toronto: Butterworths.

Coote, S. (1981). Beryl Booth Court—An innovative residential program in child maltreatment in Victoria. In *Second Australasian conference on child abuse, conference proceedings.* Queensland, Australia: Government Printer.

Duhaime, A., Gennarelli, T. A., Thibault, L. E., Bruce, D. A., Margulies, S. S., & Wiser, R. (1987). The shaken-baby syndrome. *Journal of Neurosurgery, 66*, 409–415.

Dykes, L. J. (1986). The whiplash shaken infant syndrome: What has been learned? *Child Abuse and Neglect, 10*, 211–221.

Frank, Y., Zimmerman, R., & Leeds, N. M. D. (1985). Neurological manifestations in abused children who have been shaken. *Developmental Medicine and Child Neurology, 27*, 312–316.

Geddes, D. C., Monaghan, S. M., Muir, R. C., & Jones, C. J. (1979). Early prediction in the maternity hospital. *Child Abuse and Neglect, 3*, 757–766.

Gray, J. D., & Kaplan, B. (1980). The lay health visitor programme: An eighteen-month experience. In C. H. Kempe & R. E. Helfer (Eds.), *The battered child* (3rd ed.). Chicago: University of Chicago Press.

Gray, J. D., Cutler, C. A., Dean, J. G., & Kempe, C. H. (1977). Prediction and prevention of child abuse and neglect. *Child Abuse and Neglect, 1*, 45–53.

Gregg, G. S., & Elmer, E. (1969). Infant injuries: Accident or abuse. *Pediatrics, 44*, 434–439.

Helfer, R. E., & Kempe, C. H. (1980). An overview of prevention. In C. H. Kempe & R. E. Helfer (Eds.), *The battered child* (3rd ed.). Chicago: University of Chicago Press.

Hensey, O. J., Williams, J. K., & Rosenbloom, L. (1983). Intervention in child abuse: Experience in Liverpool. *Developmental Medicine and Child Neurology, 25*, 606–611.

Hobbs, C. J. (1984). Skull fracture and the diagnosis of abuse. *Archives of Disease in Childhood, 59,* 246–252.

Kelly, J. A. (1983). *Treating child abusive families: Intervention based on skills-training principles.* New York: Plenum.

Kempe, C. H. (1971). Paediatric implication of the battered baby syndrome. *Archives of Disease in Childhood, 46,* 28–37.

Kempe, C. H. (1975). Uncommon manifestations of the battered child syndrome. *America Journal of Diseases in Children, 129,* 1265–1266.

Kempe, R. S. (1981). Individual treatment planning for the child. *Child Abuse and Neglect, 5,* 317–323.

Kempe, C. H., & Helfer, R. E. (1972). *Helping the battered child and his family.* Philadelphia: J. B. Lippincott.

Kempe, C. H., Silverman, F. N., Steele, B. F., Droegemueller, P. W., & Silver, H. K. (1962). The battered child syndrome. *Journal of the American Medical Association, 181,* 17–24.

Knight, B. (1978). How to give evidence. *British Medical Journal, 2,* 1414–1415.

Lynch, M., Steinberg, D., & Ounsted, C. (1975). Family unit in a children's psychiatric hospital. *British Medical Journal, 2,* 127–129.

Meadow, R. (1977). Munchausen syndrome by proxy: The hinterland of child abuse. *Lancet, 2,* 343–345.

Mushin, A. S. (1971). Ocular damage in the battered baby syndrome. *British Medical Journal, 3,* 402–404.

Oates, R. K. (1979). Battered children and their families. *New Doctor, 14,* 15–18.

Oates, R. K. (1982). Management—The myth and the reality. In R. K. Oates (Ed.), *Child abuse—A community concern* (pp. 287–297). Sydney: Butterworths.

Oates, R. K. (1986). *Child abuse and neglect: What happens eventually?* New York: Brunner/Mazel.

Opie, I., & Opie, P. (1951). *The Oxford dictionary of nursery rhymes.* London: Oxford University Press.

Pearn, J. H., Brown, J., Wong, R., & Bart, R. (1979). Bathtub drownings: Report of seven cases. *Pediatrics, 64,* 68–70.

Petheram, R., & Thomson, J. (1981). Child abuse—The search for an effective service model. *Second Australasian conference on child abuse, conference proceedings.* Queensland, Australia: Government Printer.

Pringle, M. K. (1975). *The needs of children.* London: Hutchinson.

Prodgers, A. (1984). Psychopathology of the physically abusing parent: A comparison with the borderline syndrome. *Child Abuse and Neglect, 8,* 411–424.

Rosen, B., & Stein, M. T. (1980). Women who abuse their children. *American Journal of Diseases of Children, 134,* 947–950.

Ryan, M. G., Davis, A. A., & Oates, R. K. (1977). One hundred and eighty-seven cases of child abuse and neglect. *Medical Journal of Australia, 2,* 623–628.

Sanders, R. W. (1972). Resistance to dealing with parents of battered children. *Pediatrics, 50,* 853–857.

Schmitt, B. D., & Beezley, P. (1976). The long-term management of the child and family in child abuse and neglect. *Pediatric Annals, 5,* 165–176.

Schnaps, Y., Frond, M., Rand, Y., & Tirosh, M. (1981). The chemically abused child. *Pediatrics, 68,* 119–121.

Silver, C. B., Dubbin, C. C., & Lourie, R. S. (1969). Child abuse syndrome: The "grey areas" in establishing a diagnosis. *Pediatrics, 44,* 594–600.

Smith, S. M., & Hanson, R. (1974). One hundred and thirty-four battered children: A medical and psychological study. *British Medical Journal, 3,* 666–670.

Springthorpe, B. J., Oates, R. K., & Hayes, S. C. (1977). Non-accidental childhood injury presenting at a hospital casualty department. *Medical Journal of Australia, 2,* 629–632.

Steele, B., & Pollock, C. (1972). A psychiatric study of parents who abuse infants and small children. In R. Helfer & C. H. Kempe (Eds.), *The battered child* (3rd ed.). Chicago: University of Chicago Press.

Straus, M. A. (1980). Stress and physical abuse. *Child Abuse and Neglect, 4,* 75–88.

Tardieu, A. (1975). *Etude medico-légale sur les services et mauvais traitements exercés sur des enfants.* In S. M. Smith (Ed.), *The battered child syndrome.* London: Butterworths 1975. (Original work published 1860)

Winkler, R. C., Ginn, D., & Miletic, R. (1979). Child abuse in the 24 hours after psychotherapy sessions. *Medical Journal of Australia, 1,* 239–240.

Woolley, P. V., & Evans, W. A. (1955). Significance of skeletal lesions in infants resembling those of traumatic origin. *Journal of the American Medical Association, 158,* 539–543.

9

Child Neglect

Arthur H. Green

Description of the Problem

Neglect is by far the most common form of maltreatment. The reported cases of neglect outnumbered those of physical abuse by 11 to 1 in New York City in 1987. Despite the fact that neglect is so much more prevalent than physical abuse in our country, it has received much less attention from child care professionals, child psychiatrists and psychologists, researchers, and social agencies. Neglect is often less obvious and less dramatic than physical or sexual abuse, and it is more difficult to measure and define. According to the New York State Child Protective Services Act of 1973, neglect is legally defined as the failure of the parent or guardian to supply the child with adequate food, clothing, shelter, medical care, and supervision (see section on legal issues). In many cases, neglect appears to be unintentional and closely associated with substandard living conditions in impoverished inner-city slum areas. Polansky, Hally, and Polansky (1975) defined child neglect as "a condition in which a care-taker responsible for the child either deliberately or by extraordinary inattentiveness permits the child to experience avoidable present suffering and/or fails to provide one or more of the ingredients generally deemed essential for developing a person's physical, intellectual, and emotional capacities." In broader terms, neglect might refer to the failure to provide the child with adequate parenting to ensure the realization of his potential for normal physical and psychological growth and development. Neglectful practices might include inadequate par-

Arthur H. Green • Department of Psychiatry, Columbia University College of Physicians and Surgeons, Columbia Presbyterian Medical Center, New York, New York 10032.

enting, interruption of maternal care, affective and social deprivation, inappropriate or premature expectations of the child, parental detachment, indifference, overstimulation, and failure to anticipate or respond to the child's needs at specific changes of development (Green, 1980). Neglect frequently involves "sins of omission," while abuse entails "sins of commission." It is clear that neglect, more than physical abuse, is subject to wide interpretation and is more influenced by community standards of child care.

According to the New York State Central Registry for Child Abuse, 54,250 reports of neglect were made in 1988, compared with 4262 reports of physical abuse. In 1978, a decade earlier, there were 19,865 reports of neglect and 6442 reports of physical abuse. The almost threefold increase in neglect during this period is striking and might reflect better reporting and a heightened public awareness of child maltreatment. However, there is an apparent real increase in neglect in New York City due to larger numbers of homeless families and those living in substandard welfare hotels. At the same time, the volume of neglect reporting has been swelled by increasing numbers of mothers testing positive for drugs at the time of the birth of their infants. These women are deemed neglectful because their infants are often addicted in utero and their substance abuse places them at risk for maltreatment of the children.

This increase in the reporting of maltreatment has also been documented on the national level. The American Association for Protecting Children (AAPC, 1986) noted that 1,726,649 children were reported as maltreated in 1984, an increase of 158% since 1976. Approximately 55% of the cases reported in 1984 involved physical neglect, 25% involved physical abuse, 13% involved sexual abuse, and 11% involved emotional maltreatment. The discrepancy between reported cases of maltreatment and the actual incidence of abuse and neglect was documented by a federally funded National Incidence Study (Westat, 1981), which revealed that only a third of the identified cases were reported.

Characteristics of Neglecting Parents

A wide variety of psychological and social deviancy has been attributed to neglecting parents. Pavenstedt (1967) described typical personality characteristics of neglecting parents encountered in disorganized lower-class families during a community intervention project. Many of these parents were psychotic, alcoholic, or antisocial. Most of them had a previous history of deprivation and neglect during their own childhood, and they tended to repeat these patterns of deprivation in their own families. They were often too overwhelmed to recognize the needs of their children, and they were unable to provide them with adequate adult role models. These parents displayed poor object relationships, owing to a basic mistrust of others, and exhibited an impaired self-concept. They also were limited in language development and abstract thinking and were, therefore, action-oriented and impulsive. They failed to provide their children with sufficient physical and verbal stimulation and rarely played with them. They often left their children alone or with the nearest available neighbor and neglected their health care. They were frequently aggressive with the children in an unpredictable manner. Giovannoni and Billingsley (1970) studied neglecting mothers in a poverty-level population, using a control group of adequate mothers. The neglecting mothers had more children, were less often married, experienced greater stress, had poorer relationships with their extended families, and were poorer than their adequate counterparts. Polansky, De Saix, Wing, and Patton (1968) studied child neglect in a rural setting. They described five types of neglecting mothers: the apathetic-futile, the impulse-ridden, the mentally retarded, the reactively depressed, and the psychotic. Polansky, Chambers, Buttenwieser, and Williams (1981) replicated these findings in a subsequent study of neglect in an urban setting. Most of the neglecting mothers fit into the "apathy-futility syndrome," characterized by a pervasive feeling of futility, emotional numbness, clinging and loneliness in interpersonal relationships, incompetence in many areas of living, passive-aggressive personality traits, stubborn negativism, verbal inaccessibility, and the tendency to generate the same sense of futility in others. Green (1976) compared neglecting, abusing, and normal control mothers from a similar poverty background on the basis of their responses to a structured interview. The neglecting mothers reported the highest incidence of unplanned pregnancies and the absence of a husband or boyfriend at home. They also demonstrated the highest rates of alcoholism, psychosis, and chronic physical illness. Galdston (1968) differentiated two types of neglecting parents on the basis of their defensive organization. The first type uses projection as a major defense and perceives the child as a symbol of their own undesirable attributes. This type is similar to child abusers, who also use projection, but instead of striking out at the children, they withdraw or delegate the care of the child to someone else. The second type uses denial as the preferred defense, and they do not regard the child as belonging to them. These parents do not bond with their children and are unable to empathize with them. They have great difficulty in caring for and feeding their children.

In summary, neglect is associated with prominent psychiatric, physical, social, and cognitive impairment in the parents, which often are embedded in poverty and substandard living conditions. It is likely that neglect is the end result of a combination of these interacting factors, which interfere with the normal processes of parenting. Family disorganization and the lack of material resources further undermine parental functioning by diminishing the availability of childrearing support systems.

Characteristics of Neglected Children

The harmful sequelae of neglect and maternal deprivation in infants and young children living in institutions have been described in the pioneering studies of Bowlby (1951), Goldfarb (1945), Spitz (1945), and many others. These children exhibited physical and developmental retardation and cognitive impairment, especially in the area of speech and language. They also were impaired in their ability to form human attachments. The unavailability of a consistent caretaker in the institutional setting was felt to be the cause of these symptoms.

Subsequent studies by Coleman and Provence (1957) and Prugh and Harlow (1962) demonstrated that similar types of deprivation leading to impaired development might be encountered in children living at home as a result of inadequate maternal care. The most common sequelae of neglect in these children, as described by Marans and Lourie (1967), Malone (1967), Rutter, (1972), and Green (1980) are pathological object relationships and difficulties in attachment. These result from maternal unavailability and multiple substitute caretakers, diminished initiative and enjoyment in play due to a lack of maternal support and of play materials, speech and language delays caused by inadequate verbal stimulation, poor self-care, and accident-proneness due to physical neglect, depression, apathy, and withdrawal. Some of these children are malnourished, dirty, and inadequately clothed. Many neglected children exhibit poor impulse control and conduct disorders, which may ultimately lead to delinquency and antisocial behavior (Polansky et al., 1981).

Recent studies have documented intellectual impairment in neglected youngsters. Polansky et al. (1981) reported significantly lower IQ scores in neglected children compared with normal controls. The IQs of these children were positively correlated with the mother's Childhood Level of Living Scale (CLL), which measures the quality of child care in the family. Sandgrund et al. (1974) found that the mean IQs of neglected children (79.97) were 11 points below the normal controls and were not significantly different from those of a comparison group of abused children. Twenty percent of the neglected children were retarded, with IQs below 70. Green, Voeller, Gaines, and Kubie (1981) reported significant neurological impairment in these same neglected children on the basis of pediatric neurological examination including EEGs and perceptual motor testing designed to elicit soft signs of CNS impairment. The neurological deficits were attributed to poor prenatal and infant care, abnormal (insufficient or excessive) sensory stimulation, poor nutrition, and inadequate medical care. Neglected children, like their parents, are physically and cognitively comprised and exhibit developmental and neurological impairment. These deficits may be attributed to insufficient or inappropriate parenting during the critical periods of infancy and early childhood.

Case Description

Alan B., currently 13 years old, was referred to the Family Center (a treatment program for maltreated children and their families) when he was 5 years 10 months old and in the first grade. The school guidance counselor, who made the referral, noted that Alan was disruptive in the classroom and bothered other children. He stole from these children and appeared to be restless and hyperactive. His physical appearance was often dirty and unkempt. Alan would not follow the classroom routines and rarely did schoolwork. Most striking was Alan's tendency to eat garbage and nonedible substances. Alan's mother, Miss Mary B., noticed that the child was often accident-prone (e.g., he stepped on nails in the house and was often bruised when returning from play). He once hit himself on the head while playing with a broomstick. Mary informed the social worker that her refrigerator had not been working for the past 4 months, and she kept some food on the windowsill, but Alan had to go to his grandparent's apartment for such items as milk and juice.

Mary was abandoned by Alan's father 1 week before he was born. They had known one another for a year and a half. Mary said that she wanted to have a baby, but when her boyfriend deserted, she had thought about giving Alan up for adoption, but then she changed her mind and decided to keep him. Alan was born after an uncomplicated pregnancy and delivery. The gestation was 36 weeks and he weighed 6 pounds, 6 ounces at birth. He developed pneumonia shortly after birth and remained in the hospital for 2 weeks. Mary was 34 years old when Alan was born. She described Alan as an active baby who sat up at 5 months and walked at 13 months. He spoke his first words at 15 months and began to use sentences between 18 and 24 months. He was toilet-trained at 2½ years.

When Alan was 2, he was hospitalized for 3 days with asthma. After his discharge from the hospital, Mary was provided with homemaking services because her difficulties in caring for Alan and managing the household became obvious. Alan was hospitalized once again for asthma at age 4.

Following acceptance in the program, Alan was seen on a weekly basis for play therapy, and Mary was provided with child guidance sessions and psychotherapy. During this intervention, Alan frequently ran away from his mother. After a year, treatment was discontinued because Mary failed to keep her appointments and did not bring Alan for his therapy sessions.

Two years later, when Alan was 8½ years old, Mary returned to the program to get help for Alan and herself. The presenting problems included Alan's leaving the house without permission and staying out late, his refusal to eat food cooked by his mother, oppositional behavior at home, and Mary's perception that she had little or no control over the child. Alan was also stealing money from his mother.

Alan was attending a class for emotionally disturbed children at this time. The guidance counselor noted problems with lateness and absenteeism, as well as Alan's arriving at school dirty and without his homework. Alan's oppositional behavior intensified to the point where he would talk back to his mother, curse her, and even hit her when he did not get his way. He often ran away from his mother when they were walking on the street together, and he would roam the streets at night. Additional problems surfaced, such as frequent nightmares depicting violence, sporadic nighttime enuresis, anxiety around sexual issues, poor grooming, and academic and behavioral difficulties in school, where Alan was noted to be very distractible. Alan also experimented with lighting matches but denied any firesetting. Attendance at the program improved, although Mary was still chronically late for her appointments.

Mary B. is the third oldest of five children and was 39 years old when she was referred to our program for the first time. Her parents are still living. Her father (age 80) is a retired bookkeeper, and her mother (age 71) sells cosmetics on a part-time basis. Mary and Alan live in an apartment in the same building as her parents, who often help to care for Alan. Mary's sister Janet is 4 years her senior. She is married with two children and lives in the neighborhood. Mary's brother Don is 2 years older and is a successful accountant. He is married with four children, and Alan often stays with him on holidays. Another brother, Bill, is married with one child and lives nearby, and the youngest brother died in Vietnam. Despite their proximity, Mary has little contact with her siblings.

Mary presents as an anxious, highly disorganized person who often speaks in a tangential confusing manner, so that it is often difficult to follow her train of thought. She had been a quiet, rather timid young woman who lived with her parents and was employed as a secretary until she was 24. At that time she began to exhibit some psychiatric difficulties, which appeared to be associated with breaking up with a boyfriend because her parents disapproved of him. She developed delusional ideas concerning people reading her thoughts and trying to influence her. She threatened to kill her father and talked about suicide. She was admitted to a psychiatric hospital at that time and was given the diagnosis of acute paranoid schizophrenia. Following this hospitalization, she had a series of part-time jobs, but her primary source of income has been from public assistance. Mary has taken part-time housecleaning and laundry jobs while having trouble managing these tasks in her own home. Mary's social contacts are very limited. She relates primarily to Alan and her elderly parents. She does not socialize with men, and she has a few female acquaintances.

Mary demonstrates love and concern toward Alan, as well as a desire to improve her parenting skills; however, she has had chronic difficulty with understanding his needs and relating to him in an appropriate manner. She has been both neglectful and overly intrusive, and her expectations are often so high that she has difficult rewarding Alan's progress and good behavior without simultaneously criticizing other behaviors. Mary needs constant guidance in setting limits with Alan, reinforcing and praising good behaviors, meeting his basic needs, and keeping appropriate boundaries. For years, Alan and Mary slept in the same bed or on separate floor pads next to one another, and Mary has resisted suggestions to provide Alan with his own room.

Mary has major difficulties with her finances. Her public assistance has often been suspended for unclear reasons, and she has needed constant help in having this reinstated. She also requires assistance with budgeting, home management, and negotiating with her landlord about housing problems and the constant need for repairs in her apartment. Mary tends to be chronically late for her appointments and frequently misses them completely. Her attendance improves when she experiences crises or unusual stresses.

Medical Issues

Medical issues play an important role in child neglect, in that physical and psychiatric illness in the parent is often a crucial factor in the initiation and sustaining of neglectful childrearing practices, which in turn pose a danger to the child's health and normal development. Parents with chronic medical illness are often depleted in energy and are unable to assume the burdens of child care. They are likely to become depressed or self-absorbed, which make it difficult for them to respond adequately to the needs of their children. Their failure to provide effective supervision increases the risk of accidental injury to the child, who may sustain burns or injuries due to falls. Unsupervised children are also prone to ingesting household poisons or medications. Children who are inadequately clothed or fed are at risk for illness and impaired physical development. Neglected children who become ill are unlikely to receive prompt medical attention, or the recommended medical treatment is not likely to be implemented. Neglectful parents also fail to provide routine pediatric care for their children and rely on emergency rooms in case of illness. Neglected children often fail to obtain the required immunizations. Some neglected children who are not adequately nourished may develop the nonorganic failure-to-thrive syndrome. It is therefore imperative that all family members in a neglectful household receive medical examinations if these were not recently obtained. The adults and children should be provided with their own internist and pediatrician, respectively.

Medical services were provided to the B. family immediately after their acceptance into our treatment program. Alan was referred to the pediatric outpatient clinic at Presbyterian Hospital, in which the Family Center is located. We were initially concerned with Alan's ingestion of nonedible substances, such as garbage and crayons, which placed him at risk for lead poisoning. The B.'s apartment was inspected for evidence of toxic substances, such as lead, which might have been ingested by Alan. Lead levels in Alan's blood were determined and found to be within normal limits. Alan's pica subsided rapidly after he and his mother entered the program, and he was assigned to a pediatrician who would follow him regularly. Alan was provided with an inhaler and medication for his asthma. Mary was referred to an internist, who acted as her family physician. Even more important for Mary was the regular monitoring of her psychiatric status by the clinical director of the Family Center, who is a psychiatrist. This was the first time that Alan and Mary had regular medical care. During his participation in the program. Alan was treated for such conditions as impetigo, shingles, poison ivy, strabismus, and an abscessed tooth, which had to be extracted.

Legal Issues

According to the New York State Child Protective Services Act of 1973, the legal definition of child neglect is the following: A "neglected" child is a child under 18 years of age, impaired as a result of the failure of his parent or other person legally responsible for his care to exercise a minimum degree of care (1) in supplying the child with adequate food, clothing, shelter, education, medical or surgical care, though financially able to do so or offered financial or other reasonable means to do so, (2) in providing the child with proper supervision or guardianship, (3) by reasonably inflicting or allowing to be inflicted harm or a substantial risk thereof, including the infliction of excessive corporal punishment, (4) by using a drug or drugs, (5) by using alcoholic beverages to the extent that he loses self-control of his actions, or (6) by any other acts of a similarly serious nature requiring the aid of the family court. A child is also to be considered maltreated when, under 18 years of age, he has been abandoned by his parents (or whoever else is legally responsible for his care).

Reporting Child Neglect

From 1964 to 1968, all 50 states, the District of Columbia, the Virgin Islands, and Guam enacted child maltreatment reporting laws. Physicians are specifically designated as mandated reporters in most states, along with other professionals, such as osteopaths, dentists, chiropractors, nurses, hospital administrators, psychologists, social workers, pharmacists, nurses, and religious healers. All reporting laws provide immunity from criminal and civil liability for mandated reporters. Most states have laws that include penalties for nonreporting. Friends, relatives, and neighbors are also encouraged to report suspected cases of maltreatment, but these nonmandated reporters are not required to identify themselves.

Most states have reporting systems that use one toll-free telephone number for reports from anywhere in the state. These reports are then transmitted to the local child protective agency, which is obliged to initiate an investigation within 24 hours.

The psychiatrist or mental health professional treating a member of a family in which physical abuse or neglect takes place is required by law to report such maltreatment, as is any other professional. Recurrence of abuse or neglect by parents who are receiving help for previous maltreatment must also be reported by the therapist. The reporting laws take precedence over the privileged doctor–patient relationship so that confidentiality cannot be maintained. When maltreatment takes place, the legal rights of the child take precedence over those of the parents. The potential negative impact of the reporting laws on the therapeutic relationship can be minimized if the therapist discusses his obligation to report maltreatment at the beginning of any intervention with abusing or neglecting parents.

Investigation

The child protective agency, usually located in the county or state department of social services, is authorized by law to investigate reported cases of abuse or neglect to determine the validity of the allegations. The protective services caseworker carries out an intake procedure in order to obtain information about the suspected maltreatment. The worker checks the central registry for previous reports of abuse or neglect involving the child and his family. The worker may also interview neighbors, relatives, schools, and other agencies to gather relevant information about the family.

If the presence of maltreatment is confirmed by the investigation, the child may be protected in one of several ways. Depending on the severity of the case, the child may be hospitalized, may remain at home under the supervision of the child protective agency, which may provide the family with supportive services, or can be placed in a shelter or foster home on an emergency basis. If the report of maltreatment cannot be validated, the case is closed and the report is expunged from the central registry.

Legal Rights of the Child

The allegedly maltreated child is entitled to representation in all legal proceedings. Many states require that a special guardian, or guardian ad litem, be appointed by the court to protect the child's interest. He acts as the child's advocate and ensures that the court receives all relevant data. He also gathers relevant information concerning the causes, nature, and extent of the maltreatment, and ensures that the child's interests are protected by law.

Legal Rights of the Parents

The parents or any other alleged perpetrator of maltreatment against a child must be informed of their legal rights by the local authority. These include the right to receive written notice of one's record in the child abuse registry and of court orders and petitions filed, the right to obtain legal counsel, the right to a court hearing prior to removal of the child, the right to appeal child protective case determinations, and the right to refuse agency services unless mandated by a court. The files in the central registry pertaining to the alleged maltreatment should be kept in strictest confidence to prevent unauthorized disclosure of identifying information concerning the parents.

The Judicial Process in the Juvenile or Family Court

A pretrial conference may be held prior to any hearing in order to decide which reports and evidence will be admissible. The judge and the attorneys for all parties participate in this conference, which is usually successful in settling the majority of cases by some form of consent decree, in which the parent agrees to cooperate with the child protective agency.

If the pretrial conference is unsuccessful in settling a case, an adjudicatory or "fact-finding" hearing takes place. This is the "trial" stage of the proceedings, in which the allegations of abuse and neglect are examined and argued. The judge makes his final decision about whether or not the allegations are confirmed. If the allegations are proven, the judge makes a "finding" of abuse or neglect.

A dispositional hearing follows the adjudication. At this hearing, the child protective agency managing the case presents a plan of intervention to the court and the parents, outlining the conditions and arrangements designed to protect the child and a time schedule within which the plan is to be implemented. The dispositional order may require counseling, psychiatric treatment, or provision of social services for the parents. In case of placement of the child outside of the home, a visitation schedule should be included in the case plan. Once the plan is agreed upon, the court should ensure parental compliance by periodically reviewing their participation in the rehabilitative process.

Social and Family Issues

The concrete aspects of poverty (i.e., lack of money, substandard and overcrowded living conditions, high crime rate, family disorganization) exert a stressful impact on families and parental functioning. While they might trigger the onset of abuse, it is likely that a background of poverty is more intimately related to neglect. Many of the substandard living conditions encountered in our decaying inner cities are considered neglectful by middle-class standards and might be used by child protection caseworkers to confirm otherwise equivocal allegations of neglect. When these impoverished parents are unable to provide adequate food, clothing, and shelter for their children, it might not be under their voluntary control. Many of these "involuntarily" neglectful families are headed by overwhelmed and depleted single mothers without adequate support systems. They cannot rely on spouses or family members for childrearing assistance or emotional support. Homeless families and families living in shelters are also exposing their children to neglectful and noxious environments through no fault of their own.

The current epidemic of drug addiction in the inner cities is more directly related to neglect of children. Substance-abusing parents are not likely to consistently recognize and respond to the needs of their children. In addition, the children are at risk for exposure to other drug-taking adults. Women who abuse substances during pregnancy inflict medical damage on the fetus. They are automatically charged with neglect if they test positive for drugs at the time of childbirth. Infants born to these addicted mothers become addicted themselves in utero and may be born with withdrawal symptoms. Similarly, an actively alcoholic mother may give birth to a child with fetal alcohol syndrome.

Assessment of Psychopathology

Since a high incidence of psychopathology and cognitive impairment has been demonstrated in neglecting families, the children and their parents should receive in-depth psychiatric evaluations designed to assess their psychopathology and document the presence of a psychiatric disorder. Exploration of the child's play, fantasy life, conflicts, and defenses will provide information about psychodynamic issues and behavioral symptoms that will assist in designing an intervention strategy for the child. Careful assessment of the parent's psychopathology, coping skills, and parenting ability will provide clues for treating and supporting the parent. The psychiatric evaluation of the neglected child should be supplemented by psychological testing, which will yield additional information about how the child perceives himself, his family, and the environment, and will identify the extent of any cognitive impairment.

Assessment of Alan

Psychiatric Evaluation

Alan is an appealing, "waiflike" 5-year-11-month-old boy with a dirty face and unkempt appearance. He is fully oriented and makes good contact with the examiner. Speech is coherent and goal-directed but is somewhat pressured. There is no evidence of a thinking disorder, delusions, or hallucinations. Alan is very distractible and frequently breaks off contact as the interview progresses, in order to explore the various games and toys in the examiner's office. He requires periodic refocusing during the evaluation. When asked about school, where he is a first-grader, he reports that the teacher says that he is a "bad boy" because he talks too much and gets out of his seat. He admits to punching kids in the classroom "if they get rough with me." Alan reluctantly acknowledges eating crayons and food from the garbage can in school because "I'm hungry and there isn't enough food at home." When asked about running away from home, Alan states that he wants to play with a friend in the neighborhood and runs off to see this boy because his mother won't let him out of the house. Alan realizes that this makes his mother "sad," and this makes him feel like a "bad boy." When he is away from home a long time, he thinks of his mother looking for him; then he is afraid to return home because he might get a "spanking."

Alan is unable to sustain interest in any of the play materials for more than a few minutes. He puts the family dolls on the roof of the play-house, leaves them there, and is apparently unable to engage in symbolic play. His figure drawings are primitive undifferentiated stick figures. His mood is labile and ranges from overexcitement to boredom and moderate depression. His affect is constricted and shallow. He goes to open the door from time to time to peer out into the corridor to see if his mother is around. In the cognitive sphere, Alan is unable to read. He appears to be of at least low average to average in intelligence.

DSM-III-R Diagnosis

Axis I	Attention-Deficit Hyperactivity Disorder
	Pica
	Oppositional-Defiant Disorder
Axis II	None
Axis III	Asthma
Axis IV	Psychosocial Stressors: Mother with chronic psychiatric illness
	Disorganized and neglectful home
	Severity: 4—Severe
Axis V	Current GAF 65
	Highest GAF past year 70

Psychological Assessment

Alan was initially tested at the age of 6 years 2 months, shortly after being admitted to our program. On the WISC-R, his verbal IQ was 95, his performance IQ was 105, with a full scale IQ of 100. On the Wide Range Achievement Test he achieved a grade level of 1.7. In academic achievement he received a 1.9 grade equivalent in word recognition, 1.7 in spelling, and 0.9 in arithmitic. He scored less than 1.1 in accuracy, less than 1.0 in comprehension on the Gilmore Oral Reading Test, and 99 (age equivalent 6 years 1 month) on the Peabody Picture Vocabulary Test. In general, this rather hyperactive and distractible youngster fell within the average range of intellectual functioning.

When Alan returned to the program 2 years later at age 8½, he showed a deterioration in intellectual functioning. On the WISC-R he received a verbal IQ score of 86, a performance IQ of 84, and a full scale IQ score of 84. The WISC-R scaled scores were as follows:

Verbal tests		Performance tests	
Information	6	Picture Completion	13
Similarities	3	Picture Arrangement	4
Arithmetic	7	Block Design	5
Vocabulary	11	Object Assembly	8
Comprehension Span	14		
Digit Span	8		

Alan was in the low average range of intellectual functioning and his responses in various areas varied widely. He was above the norms in his ability to distinguish essential from unessential visual details, in his ability to find solutions to problematic social situations, and in his vocabulary and verbal fluency. Alan did very poorly on tasks involving factual information, verbal conceptual thinking, the sequential analysis and understanding of social events, and the analysis and synthesis of visual patterns in terms of their parts. His academic achievement was at a second-grade level, commensurate with his intellectual functioning. Reading was at a 1.9 grade level, spelling at 2.4, and arithmetic at 2.6.

On the Bender-Gestalt Test of perceptual motor development, Alan's reproduction of designs contained numerous errors, including errors in integration and angulation, as well as rotations of designs. His human figure drawings were oversimplified and had peculiar characteristics. Overall graphomotor response was suggestive of both neurological and emotional difficulties.

Alan achieved a social age equivalent of 7 years on the Vineland. Overall social adaptation fell into the borderline to low-average range.

The projective material revealed a very confused, impulse-ridden, extremely anxious youngster who feels unstable, inadequate, and incapable of dealing with the world in an effective manner. Alan is preoccupied with his inner promptings and may perseverate on them, yet he lacks any insight; he is likely to misinterpret situations and respond inappropriately. He also has little understanding of interpersonal relationships, especially with his father, though he associates such relationships with bad feelings, including anger and sadness. There are also some indications of premature sexual feelings and preoccupations. Finally, Alan seems to feel both physically and emotionally deprived. His anxious, impulse-ridden behavior may stem from feelings of internal emptiness, hunger, and vulnerability.

Alan's most recent psychological testing at the age of 11 revealed an increase in his performance IQ to 98, a 14-point gain, while his verbal IQ remained virtually the same, at 85. His full scale IQ was 90. However, Alan failed to make any progress in academic skill since the previous testing. He was in the lowest percentile of the population in word recognition, spelling, and arithmetic, and he displayed multiple areas of moderate learning weakness with no strong compensatory strengths. He was weak in abstract thinking and acquired learning, with poor visual memory. In writing and reading he manifested rotational, directional, and sequential reversals of letters. His visual perception remained impaired and immature. Decoding was so laborious that the easiest reading comprehension passage could be accomplished only with great help. At the time of this evaluation Alan still retained the characteristics of an attention deficit disorder.

Assessment of Mary

Psychiatric Evaluation

Mary is a shabbily dressed 40-year-old woman who appears anxious and disorganized and considerably older than her stated age. She is fully oriented and relates to the examiner in a cooperative but rather distant manner. Her speech is coherent but is occasionally tangential and rambling. While there is no evidence of an organized delusional system, Mary displays paranoid ideas of reference pertaining to people on the street who do not like her or who talk about her behind her back. As a result, she usually stays by herself. Mary occasionally hears voices when no one is present; however, the content of these auditory hallucinations is benign. When asked about her work history, Mary admitted that she did not feel capable of having a regular job since her "nervous breakdown" several years ago. Since that time she obtained sporadic employment as a part-time clerical worker or housecleaner. She fears that the pressures of a full-time job would be too stressful for her. Mary has no real friends; she has a few acquaintances but spends most of her time with her parents, who live in her building. Mary's affect is constricted but not grossly inappropriate. Her mood is moderately depressed. Her memory is intact, and her intellectual functioning appears to be in the low normal range. Her thinking is very concrete.

DSM-III-R Diagnosis
Axis I   Schizophrenic Disorder, Residual Type
Axis II   None
Axis III   None
Axis IV   Psychosocial Stressors: Problems with collecting welfare
                               payments
                               Problems handling her child

Severity: 3—Moderate
Axis V   Current GAF 60
Highest GAF past year 65

Treatment Options

Intervention in cases of child neglect should be based on the psychopathology of the neglected child and his parent(s), on an assessment
of their unfulfilled needs, and on the determination of the neglectful
and pathological caretaking practices compromising the child's development.

In the case of Alan and Mary, Alan required individual counsel-
ing/psychotherapy to deal with his feelings of deprivation and damage,
his symptoms of pica and hyperactivity, and his oppositional tendencies. In addition, he required psychoeducational assistance to help him
cope with his numerous learning difficulties. It is clear that such intervention would be minimally effective without modifying Mary's neglectful and ineffective parenting. This, in turn, would require a combination of counseling and individual psychotherapy for Mary, vigorous
casework intervention to help Mary negotiate the welfare system and
improve the home environment, and parenting education to help Mary
respond more effectively to Alan's physical and emotional needs. Both
child and mother were also candidates for psychopharmacological intervention. Alan might have benefited from Ritalin, but Mary would not
agree to this plan. Mary did, however, consent to our recommendation
that she receive a tranquilizer, Haldol, in order to stabilize her psychological functioning and to minimize the impact of her anxiety and
disorganization.

Mary was able to benefit from our interventions and made some
progress in managing the household and improving her parenting of
Alan. However, renewed conflicts with her landlord and an abrupt termination of her Medicaid payments intensified her anxiety and disorganization. Furthermore, Alan's entering adolescence created additional
stress for Mary, since it became more difficult for her to adequately
supervise him and monitor his school attendance. Mary began to miss
many of her therapy appointments, and Alan's tendency to wander
away from home and to stay away from school increased. At this point,
Alan was referred to a residential treatment center that could provide
him with structure, supervision, therapy, special education, and socialization experiences. The latter, of course, was less available in his
home environment. The residential setting would also provide Alan
with positive adult role models. The final treatment goals with Mary

were designed to help her to accept Alan's entry into residential treatment and to assist her in working through the separation from her son.

More intact neglecting families manifesting marked disturbances in family interactions might benefit from a family systems approach, with the use of family therapy.

Summary and Conclusions

Neglect is by far the most common form of maltreatment, having a more severe impact on the child's cognitive and psychological functioning than physical or sexual abuse. Neglectful parents are likely to be psychologically or physically compromised. The psychological deviancy and psychopathology associated with neglect is clearly described in the case presentation. Environmental factors may have a more profound effect on neglect than on the other forms of maltreatment.

Intervention with neglecting families should be based upon a careful assessment of environmental stressors, individual psychopathology, and the deficiencies in the family system. The intervention should be designed to strengthen the family functioning by (a) reducing the environmental stress through provision of concrete services and outreach and consolidating support systems, (b) dealing with the individual psychopathology of the parents and children by means of individual psychotherapy and psychopharmacological agents when necessary, (c) correcting deviations in the family system through a family therapy approach, and (d) strengthening parenting skills by providing parenting education. While the general thrust of intervention is aimed at preserving and strengthening the family unit, in some cases temporary or permanent placement of the children might be necessary.

Acknowledgment

The author is indebted to Pat Coupe, M.S., for her valuable assistance in the preparation of the case description.

References

American Association for Protecting Children. (1986). *Highlights of official child neglect and abuse reporting 1984.* Denver: American Humane Society.

Bowlby, J. (1951). Maternal care and mental health. *Bulletin of the World Health Organization, 31,* 355–533.

Coleman, R., & Provence, S. A. (1957). Developmental retardation (hospitalism) in infants living in families. *Pediatrics, 19,* 285–292.

Galdston, R. (1968). Dysfunctions of parenting: The battered child, the neglected child, the exploited child. In J. G. Howells (Ed.), *Modern perspectives of international child psychiatry* 571–586. Edinburgh: Oliver and Boyd.

Giovannoni, J., & Billingsley, A. (1970). Child neglect among the poor: A study of parental adequacy in families of three ethnic groups. *Child Welfare, 49,* 196–204.

Goldfarb, W. (1945). Psychological privation in infancy and subsequent adjustment. *American Journal of Orthopsychiatry, 102,* 247–255.

Green, A. (1976). A psychodynamic approach to the study and treatment of abusing parents. *Journal of the American Academy of Child Psychiatry, 15,* 414–429.

Green, A. (1980). *Child maltreatment.* New York: Jason Aronson.

Green, A., Voeller, K., Gaines, R., & Kubie, J. (1981). Neurological impairment in battered children. *Child Abuse and Neglect, 5,* 129–134.

Malone, C. (1967). Developmental deviations considered in the light of environmental forces. In E. Pavenstedt (Ed.), *The drifters: Children of disorganized lower class families* (pp. 125–161). Boston: Little, Brown.

Marans, A., & Lourie, R. (1967). Hypotheses regarding the effects of child-rearing patterns on the disadvantaged child. In J. Hellmuth (Ed.), *The disadvantaged child* (pp. 19–41). New York: Brunner/Mazel.

New York State Central Registry for Child Abuse. (1988).

Pavenstedt, E. (Ed.). (1967). *The drifters: Children of disorganized lower class families.* Boston: Little, Brown.

Polansky, N. A., De Saix, C., Wing, M., & Patton, J. D. (1968). Child neglect in a rural community. *Social Casework,* October, 467–474.

Polansky, N. A., Hally, C., & Polansky, N. F. (1975). *Profile of neglect.* Washington, DC: Department of H.E.W., Public Services Administration.

Polansky, N. A., Chambers, M., Buttenwieser, E., & Williams, D. P. (1981). *Damaged parents: An anatomy of child neglect.* Chicago: University of Chicago Press.

Prugh, D., & Harlow, R. (1962). "Masked deprivation" in infants and young children. In *Deprivation of maternal care: A reassessment of its effects.* Geneva: World Health Organization.

Rutter, M. (1972). Maternal deprivation reconsidered. *Journal of Psychosomatic Research, 16,* 241–250.

Sandgrund, A., Gaines, R., & Green, A. (1974). Child abuse and mental retardation: A problem of cause and effect. *American Journal of Mental Deficiency, 79,* 327–330.

Spitz, R. (1945). Hospitalism: An inquiry into the genesis of psychiatric conditions of early childhood. *Psychoanalytic Study of the Child, 1,* 53–74.

Westat and Developmental Associates. (1981). *National study of the incidence and severity of child abuse and neglect.* Prepared for the National Center on Child Abuse and Neglect under Contract No. 105-76-1137.

10

Child Sexual Abuse

David J. Kolko and Janet Stauffer

Description of the Problem

Child sexual abuse (CSA) has received considerable national attention, owing, in part, to accumulating evidence as to its prevalence, patterns, severity, and long-term effects (see Finkelhor, 1984). Studies of the incidence of CSA have estimated that more than 80% of the victims are female and that perpetrators are generally known to their victims (Alter-Reid, Gibbs, Lachenmeyer, Sigal, & Massoth, 1986). The short-term and long-term effects of CSA have been documented with increasing regularity (Browne & Finkelhor, 1986; Finkelhor & Browne, 1985; Lusk & Waterman, 1986; Mrazek, 1983). Browne and Finkelhor (1986) have conceptualized the traumatic impact of CSA in terms of a broad range of physical and psychopathological symptoms that reflect traumatic sexualization, betrayal, stigmatization, and powerlessness.

Although females are more commonly victimized and have been studied in greater detail, male children remain vulnerable not only to involvement in sexually abusive experiences but also to its serious sequelae. Indeed, sex differences have been examined in an effort to better understand the patterns, precipitants, and consequences of CSA. Farber, Showers, Johnson, Joseph, and Oshins (1984) found greater physical evidence of sexual abuse among girls and a higher incidence of oral-genital contact among boys, but there were no other differences in other factors (e.g., abuser relationship, referral source, number of

David J. Kolko and Janet Stauffer • Department of Psychiatry, Western Psychiatric Institute and Clinic, University of Pittsburgh School of Medicine, Pittsburgh, Pennsylvania 15213.

abusers, incidence of abuse of others, abuse chronicity, use of bribes/coercion, concurrent physical abuse). In contrast, Finkelhor (1984) found that boys tended to be younger, to come more often from poorer and broken families, and to have experienced physical abuse. Pierce and Pierce (1985) also found sex differences in family composition, perpetrator characteristics, variables that heightened the repetition of abuse, and the services offered to the child and family. For example, offenders of males received harsher treatment and were more likely to be perceived as emotionally ill. Male victims were younger, more likely to reside with their mothers and to have no father at home, and more likely to be offered shorter treatment and to complete treatment, while mothers of male victims were regarded as more emotionally disturbed. Finally, boys were more likely to be abused by nonfamily members, especially stepfathers, to reside in families where more than one child was sexually abused, and to have received threats and coercive force from their perpetrators, but less likely to have been removed from home.

Although the specific impact of these characteristics on the adjustment of male victims remains to be more sufficiently documented, findings suggest that males, like females, are adversely affected by the experience. Reported effects include feelings of shame and self-blame, a fear of becoming homosexual, drug and alcohol abuse, self-injury, and involvement in pornography and sexual molestation of other children (see Vander Mey, 1988). Clinical experience suggests that male CSA victims are at risk for becoming offenders in adulthood (Freeman-Longo, 1986).

Such findings highlight the occurrence and negative impact of male CSA, as well as relative differences between males and females in risks for and response to the abuse. This chapter presents a case study of a young male victim of CSA who was referred for psychiatric hospitalization. As poignantly articulated by Vander Mey (1988), questions regarding the way in which the child was abused, the expected psychosocial impact of the experience, and follow-up outcomes on child and family adjustment will be addressed. In addition, issues are raised regarding the validity of allegations and relationship between the investigation and therapeutic processes (Benedek & Schetky, 1987a, 1987b; Newberger, 1985).

Case Description

Neil was a a 7-year-old white male who attended the second grade of a regular school. He lived with his 35-year-old mother, a 10-year-old brother, and, for much of the time, the mother's 41-year-old boyfriend. He had three prior admissions to a local psychiatric hospital in the past 9 months.

Reasons for Referral

Neil was referred by the hospital to which he had been admitted three times previously owing to long-standing problems with impulsivity and aggressiveness. Various medications had been tried at this hospital with little improvement. Requests of hospitalization were to verify a diagnosis, evaluate medication needs, and increase family involvement in inpatient and follow-up services.

In terms of sexual behavior, Neil admitted to pulling up girls' skirts or pinching buttocks in the past, though this was not confirmed. Although he was precocious in his discussion of sexual activities, the mother and her boyfriend denied any knowledge of sexual abuse. However, they acknowledged his involvement the previous summer with a 9-year-old neighborhood boy who offered Neil his friendship in return for fondling his genitals.

His peer relations were described as poor. Neil seldom kept friends for any length of time and was unable to share a friend. He frequently fought both at school and in the community, which became a chronic problem resulting in a school suspension. At the same time, he appeared to compete for his mother's attention at home and frequently complained of vague aches and pains in an effort to get her attention. Since the mother's car accident in February 1987, he had been more jealous of her affection and voiced concerns that she might die. He also became more clingy and demanding of her attention at this time.

History of Presenting Problems and Prior Treatment

The mother reported hyperactivity, inattentiveness, aggressiveness, and intrusiveness at school since age 3. This corresponded to the time of Neil's father's death, at which time his mother became depressed and began to abuse solvents. He was expelled from preschool at age 4, owing to inappropriate sexual acts with the girls at the school. The expulsion prompted referral to a partial hospitalization program.

Neil's first hospitalization was initiated for treatment of these chronic conduct problems and a possible attention deficit disorder. The latter disorder was adequately controlled with medication for several months until his behavior began to deteriorate, as evidenced by a loss of weight, insomnia, and frequent temper tantrums. Alternative medications only worsened his behavior, which was further compounded by the family's failure to comply with outpatient sessions. Readmission was sought to address Neil's increasingly destructive, agitated, and belligerent behaviors. Additional medications had resulted in some symptomatic relief. However, Neil returned home after mother's separation from her boyfriend (because of his abuse of alcohol) and then grew increasingly more unmanageable, aggressive, and destructive. A third hospitalization was initiated during which he received additional medications and a recommendation to seek treatment elsewhere.

Medical History

Prenatal history was positive for several complications (e.g., smoking, alcohol, marijuana use). Labor and delivery were uncomplicated. However, he was hospitalized four times at an early age after suffering from gastrointestinal problems and intolerance to formulas. He also had a history of asthma that required approximately 15 hospitalizations since birth. Developmental milestones were reached within normal limits, and physical growth parameters were at least average. He was Tanner I. Family history was positive for cardiovascular disease, substance abuse, seizure disorder, hypothyroidism, obesity, and leukemia.

Social and Family History

Neil's biological father died suddenly of a heart attack in 1983 at age 36. Family psychiatric history was positive for maternal depression and substance abuse, and for paternal substance abuse and posttraumatic stress disorder (PTSD). There was also a family history of drug abuse, alcoholism, suicidal behavior, and possible bipolar disorder. It was also learned that Neil's maternal uncle had sexually abused his mother.

The mother's boyfriend attempted to serve as a parental figure for Neil, although the mother frequently undermined his efforts. He, too, was a veteran with a history of both PTSD and depression, and he suffered from a drinking and drug use problem, though he provided few details regarding the nature of these problems.

Mental Status

The patient was well groomed and neat in appearance, and he displayed appropriate and pleasant affect. He indicated that the primary reason for hospitalization was because he was "hyper," which was consistent with his behavior throughout the interview. That is, he displayed a high activity level, fidgeted, and was distractible by irrelevant noise. Attention span was short, and he needed prompting or restatement of a question when his focus shifted to an irrelevant object in the room or some other topic. Speech rate and rhythm were a bit pressured at times but never unintelligible. There was no evidence of a formal thought disorder, and he denied depressive affect, sleep and appetite disturbance, anhedonia, and other affective symptomatology. However, he admitted to sometimes being easily annoyed or unhappy that he lacked friends. When asked why he lacked friends, he stated, "Because I fight with them," and excitedly bragged about a recent run-in with a neighborhood boy. He denied fears/phobias or other anxiety-related symptoms with a similar degree of certainty.

Problem List

Neil's initial problem list included the following psychiatric and behavioral symptoms: (1) impulsivity, distractibility, and other ADD/H symptoms, (2) verbal and physical aggressiveness, (3) precocious sexual play, and (4) lack of friends. Family problems included marital conflict, a weak parental coalition, and parental psychiatric problems.

Disclosure and Circumstances of Abuse

It was during this final hospitalization that concerns about sexual abuse and permissiveness were raised. A brief inquiry into the possibility of sexual abuse conducted on admission was negative. Upon reviewing Neil's sexual activities and family history, however, the treatment team became increasingly concerned about the possibility of abuse and requested an interview by a specialist in the area of child sexual abuse to further explore his sexual behavior.

At the outset of the interview, Neil willingly discussed some concerns regarding his sexual feelings toward a 13-year-old female on the unit. He acknowledged sending her notes and feeling in love with her, and also cautiously reported that he had thought of raping the girl. His verbal and nonverbal behavior, along with picture drawings, graphically depicted his knowledge of and desire for sexual activity.

Although appearing anxious upon being asked if anyone had touched or abused him sexually, he then proceeded to describe an incident 3 years earlier when the mother had left her boyfriend and him in bed together one night after she had moved to the sofa downstairs. He alleged that the boyfriend then initiated anal intercourse ("He bopped me up the butt") but denied any subsequent occurrences. At this point, the interview was terminated because of a concern about Neil's jumping on tables and chairs in the room.

In subsequent interviews with his psychiatrist, Neil verified his allegation and addressed some of his anxieties around the disclosure. He was very concerned about his family's reaction and the impact of his allegation on his relationship with his mother's boyfriend, denying any threats made by the boyfriend for disclosing this information.

Medical Issues

Neil's medical status and general physical health were generally normal. An admission physical suggested the possibility of an inquinal hernia. There was no evidence of sexually transmitted disease, hickeys or facial bruises, or related findings that would suggest oral sex or anal penetration. However, precocious sex play was reported by the mother, and there was a question about possible sexual abuse in the past. Overall, there was no medical information to suspect the possibility of sexual abuse.

Legal Issues

Involvement in the legal or judicial system is often prompted by the need to protect children, even though such involvement may elicit or exacerbate other adjustment difficulties. Although not necessarily new concerns, the family's sexual permissiveness, Neil's history of sexualized behavior, and his recent allegation of sexual abuse committed by an adult nearly 3 years before implicated the mother's boyfriend, who had continued to live in the home. In light of the disclosure and Neil's appearance as a credible source, we responded to the legal mandate as professionals to file a SCAN documenting the incident to the child abuse hotline for further investigation by the local Children and Youth Service (CYS) agency. Neil's credibility was upheld on the basis of their interview findings that included both his report and several sexually explicit drawings of the incident. The local CYS agency forwarded a report to Neil's home county CYS that included details of our findings.

Our report of the incident and the discussion with his mother that ensued regarding the need for a prompt investigation diverted the focus of intervention away from the family system and toward the determination of whether this man was guilty and should remain with the family. One consequence of filing the report was the family's preoccupation with understanding why Neil would say this, whether he was credible, and how their family life and the boyfriend's future would be harmed if the investigating agency found the allegations to be true. We chose to discontinue our efforts at clarifying the family's boundaries and structure, Neil's sexual knowledge and acting-out, existing community supports, and the impact of the mother's boyfriend's alcoholism on family life and his sexual behavior. Instead, it appeared more important to prevent Neil's involvement in further episodes of abuse, though it was equally clear that this could be accomplished only by a comprehensive intervention with the family that extended beyond his involvement in an incident that occurred 3 years before.

The mother, in particular, responded to Neil's allegations with considerable apprehension. She was asked to describe any information that could aid in understanding the basis of the allegation. Of course, she was quite surprised by this development and denied any such knowledge. Initially, she vacillated between being suspicious of and angry toward her boyfriend, on the one hand, and defending the boyfriend by maintaining his innocence and then attributing Neil's lack of credibility to his apparent psychological problems, on the other.

During the preceding family session, she had vigorously attempted to find inconsistencies in Neil's statements. Soon thereafter, she began to question him repeatedly during phone conversations, conveying in subtle but meaningful ways both her disbelief of this report and her anxiety over the implications of his statements. Sensing her disbelief and anxiety, he seemed to change his story as a way of showing his loyalty to his mother. Specifically, Neil was reported by his mother to have admitted to some confusion and acknowledged that it had actually been his now deceased father who had molested him. Upon recounting this information to the treatment team, the mother and the rest of the family were greatly relieved to hear this alternative allegation and to receive confirmation of the boyfriend's innocence. Because of the traveling distance, Neil's home county CYS agency waited to interview him until he was discharged from the hospital several weeks later. In the meantime, the mother's boyfriend was ordered out of the home until the SCAN could be evaluated in order to ensure Neil's safety. Eventually, Neil maintained the accuracy of his revised claim upon subsequent interview by a representative of his home county CYS agency, who then unfounded the SCAN on that basis.

Aside from this reversal in Neil's allegation, of clinical import was the fact that he had still alleged to have been sexually abused, though neither his family nor the children's agency seemed interested in addressing this experience. As long as there was no one to prosecute, it was as if the event had never happened. No legal recourse seemed available to initiate comprehensive family therapy and therapeutic involvement designed to address the sequelae following his victimization. In retrospect, the family's focus on our filing of the SCAN and its eventual status as unfounded may have impeded any therapeutic efforts to address family issues regarding loyalty, protection, and sexual intrusiveness. The family had attended three sessions with the sexual abuse outpatient treatment center to which we had referred them, but terminated as soon as the SCAN was unfounded.

Ultimately, the appropriate legal response was made by filing the SCAN and reporting Neil's allegations to the Children's Service to assure Neil's protection. Despite the SCAN's professional appropriateness, however, the investigation itself may have placed him at greater risk for reabuse or family rejection, if not both (Newberger, 1985). This investigation process appeared to contribute to further family disruption since the mother's boyfriend was restricted from residing in the home until the investigation was completed. Potentially, the family's general anger toward Neil placed him at risk for emotional and psychological abuse. Furthermore, Neil's relationship to the boyfriend, who provided emotional support and structural stability in the family as a primary disciplinarian, could have been weakened. One has to wonder, then, to what extent Neil, or his family, will confide and trust in other mental health professionals as they recall the distress associated with the investigation of these allegations.

Social and Family Issues

Cases of child sexual abuse require an analysis from a systems perspective since these events are often related to factors that interact to weaken the natural protective elements of the family. Understandably, abusive experiences do not occur in a vacuum but instead are abetted by dysfunction in the family and social system. As argued by Tierney and Corwin (1983), life stressors can precipitate involvement in incestuous relationships, which, in this case, reflected a vulnerability the family had experienced after a tragic death. The goal of conceptualization from a systems perspective should go beyond "blaming the victim" or the family, especially since this often increases the tendency to ignore the perpetrator's culpability. Rather, it provides the framework from which to address a continuum of issues that influence the initiation and maintenance of abusive environments, beginning with prevention, proceeding to assessment of allegations of abuse, and then designating treatment services.

There were many weakened social and familial factors in Neil's case. First, there was inappropriate sexual permissiveness in the family. The mother was unable to establish boundaries designed to protect her children from overstimulation and sexual exposure. During periods of the mother's extended absence from the home, substitute adult caretakers exhibited sexually inappropriate behavior and used sexually provocative language in front of the children. The boys were permitted to watch pornographic movies and read explicitly sexual adult books. For 9 months following their father's death, mother and both sons slept together in the family living room, where his cremated ashes lay in a vase. She was unable to return to the bedroom in which he had died. This lack of privacy may have encouraged the display of sexual activity in front of or actually with the boys during those months. Discussions of Neil's sexual behavior simply resulted in frequent denial of its existence, as evidenced by the fact that repeated contacts with the mental health system were initiated for complaints regarding related problems, such as aggression, hyperactivity, or peer conflicts.

Neil's mother was also overwhelmed by her own psychological problems as she continued to experience unresolved grief over her husband's death. Apart from living without a partner, the mother had to assume several new responsibilities with which she was unprepared to cope. Although she had entered a drug rehabilitation program because of her addiction to solvents, she was unable to complete the treatment and signed herself out prematurely. She then continued actively to abuse drugs and was occasionally "high" at home. A serious motor accident left her in a condition of chronic and disabling back pain that limited her mobility to the first floor of the house. She had difficulty setting limits or disciplining the children on a consistent basis, which often seemed to relate to her own feelings of guilt and inadequacy as a parent. This apparent overprotectiveness or uninvolvement shielded the boys from the structure and boundaries they needed, heightening their vulnerability to physical or sexual misconduct. The mother also expressed an ambivalence regarding her relationship with her boyfriend that was exacerbated during conflicts around discipline. During these angry incidents, her successful efforts to elicit the children's loyalty in siding against the boyfriend compromised any efforts the couple made to achieve consistency in their exercise of control strategies.

In terms of her own vulnerability, the mother had been sexually abused as a child by her uncle on one occasion while he was intoxicated, though this had never been revealed prior to her making this disclosure to a member of her hospital treatment team. She was unable to tell her own mother because of the mother's close relationship to the uncle. Thus, she appeared to minimize the importance of the event in her own life, saying that "we don't talk about those kinds of things." In spite of, or because of, her own experience of abuse, Neil's mother was unable to believe her son's allegation of abuse, and, not surprisingly, he had never reported the incident to her. Being unable to acknowledge and confront effectively her own victimization, in all likelihood, contributed to the mother's unavailability in providing support for her own son at the time of his disclosure. On a more practical level, she had minimal energy to nurture and care for her sons as a consequence of her unresolved grief over the husband's death, abuse of solvents, physical disability, and relational conflicts.

Other sources of existing family stress were evident. Two other children, Neil's 12-year-old brother and 17-year-old adopted sister, stayed at home with the boyfriend when the mother was out of the home. The 12-year-old brother was physically aggressive toward Neil and had repeatedly used him as a scapegoat for his own predicaments. During one altercation 2 months prior to admission, the brother had forced a rope around Neil's neck and caused an asthma attack. The two boys frequently fought about isolated minor matters. The boyfriend's alcoholism and the seriousness of his medical problems also had an impact on the family in that he was frequently unemployed and spent much of his time in the house. Owing to the conflictual nature of his relationship to the mother, there were occasional fights at home and brief, but disruptive, separations.

A comprehensive assessment of family functioning would be incomplete without recognizing and validating a family's strengths. Throughout these proceedings, the family managed to maintain its many important functions. There was much genuine care and concern for each family member, despite some limitations in focusing their attention in productive ways. The mother's requests for mental health services on several occasions were based, albeit circuitously, on a sincere desire to address Neil's behavioral difficulties. The boyfriend continued to reaffirm the need for added structure and more effective behavior management with the children. He and Neil had established several common recreational pursuits and hobbies, such as water sports and fishing. The family also looked to the boyfriend for emotional support and stability throughout the SCAN process. At certain times, the family appeared to share several positive experiences and several humorous moments.

Outside of the family, however, Neil was socially unable to maintain friendships, and even his peer relationships often had a sexual quality to them. As noted earlier, Neil had been coerced by a neighborhood boy to engage in mutual fondling and other sexual activities during the past year, though few details were recalled regarding this relationship. In yet another incident that occurred just before admission, Neil was observed fondling a young girl in his neighborhood. The family as a whole lacked a strong support system with extended family or regular contacts with the neighborhood, church, or social community. These indigenous supports might have been helpful in altering the family's reluctance to participate in treatment at the mental health or drug and alcohol centers.

It seems quite unfortunate that family intervention was not initiated earlier in Neil's childhood, since many of the vulnerabilities inherent in his family were evident even then. Instead of expulsion from the preschool program because of what the school perceived as sexualized behaviors toward classmates, school personnel who were better trained to identify families who are susceptive to violence and sexual exploitation could have performed a more extensive assessment and/or engaged the family in a preventive, community-based program. This involvement could have enhanced the family's supports in a way that might have reduced the continuation of inappropriate family routines and relationships. Of course, no such family intervention was implemented at that time. Even later, upon Neil's referral for mental health treatment for aggression or attention deficit problems, the family's sexualized routines that affected his own behavior remained unexplored. Eventually, Neil was brought to our tertiary care facility for inpatient psychiatric hospitalization on the children's unit in light of these and other concerns.

Assessment of Psychopathology

The case manager and the attending physician conducted a comprehensive psychiatric interview with Neil and his mother on admission. An interdisciplinary team conference that was conducted 2 weeks later evaluated the admission data base (e.g., clinical findings, unit observations, academic reports, social history) and yielded Axis I diagnoses of conduct disorder: undersocialized/aggressive and other specified family circumstances. The diagnosis of attention deficit disorder with hyperactivity had been ruled out using teacher ratings on the Connor's Teacher Questionnaire and unit observations. On the WISC-R, he obtained a verbal IQ of 105, a performance IQ of 104, and a full scale IQ of 104. In terms of parent self-report and interview measures, mother's completion of the Interview for Antisocial Behavior yielded a high score on the overt behavior factor (82) and low scores on the covert behavior (19) and self-injury factors. His overall score on the Matson Evaluation of Social Skills of Youngsters (-22) indicated greater involvement in inappropriate than appropriate behaviors.

The frequency with which Neil engaged in the eight symptom categories of the Hospital Chart Review was determined in order to compare his behavior to those of sexually abused, hospitalized children (Kolko, Moser, & Weldy, 1988). Children with a history of sexual abuse have been found to exhibit a greater frequency of specific categories (e.g., sexual behavior, fear/anxiety) than nonabused children. During his 8 weeks of hospitalization, Neil exhibited 23 separate incidents of sexual behavior, primarily involving sexual gestures and play with other peers. He also appeared to be sad/depressed on 15 occasions and engaged in physical aggression 5 times.

In terms of family characteristics, the Family Environment Scale revealed low cohesion, high conflict, and high organization and control. On the Dyadic Adjustment Scale, the couple was rated as somewhat low in satisfaction, cohesion, and affectional expression. The mother's score on the Beck Depression Inventory was 27. It should be recalled that Neil's mother and father, and the mother's boyfriend, all suffered from problems with depression, anxiety, and substance abuse. The impact of these problems was most clearly felt by increasing their dependency on Neil for assistance and limiting their availability to both provide for his own needs and promote his interests. In addition, these problems diminished their general involvement in family activities. The relationship between these vulnerabilities and the occurrence of abuse, however, can be only roughly approximated at this point.

Treatment Options

Short-Term Outcome

Brief treatment was initiated with Neil and his family during hospitalization, but it was impeded by the limitations of a short hospital stay and a driving distance of 3 hours for the family. Therefore, greater attention was paid to adequately assessing the nature of any psychiatric dysfunction and Neil's experience of victimization in order to facilitate referral for the most appropriate type of treatment in his home area. To provide a context for his experience, Neil met on an individual basis during hospitalization with his attending child psychiatrist for supportive work around his disclosure regarding the abuse and to help him understand the impact of the events that had just occurred to him. One of Neil's concerns directly related to the incident dealt with his fear of having AIDS and of being homosexual. The psychiatrist also helped him to express his anxiety following the disclosure and his apprehension as to the family's reaction and the future of the mother's boyfriend.

Neil participated in a group therapy program designed to encourage the use of appropriate social skills with peers in an effort to address his difficulty in maintaining friendships. A special behavior program was also implemented to reduce nighttime noncompliance and encourage going to bed both on time and without disruption. Briefly, compliance with these expectations was reinforced by extra social time the next day or bonus points in the milieu program. Both of these therapeutic efforts appeared to result in expected improvements.

Prior to Neil's disclosure, meetings with the family attempted to address the family's permissive attitude toward the viewing of sexually explicit materials, the need for appropriate structure and boundaries for the boys, and the frequent conflicts between mother and boyfriend. Following the disclosure, an effort was made to help them understand Neil's experience and better respond to his needs, though this was met with minimal success. The family's own lack of interest in discussing the allegation made it especially important for the treatment team to avoid perpetuating a denial of the family's sexual problems and adopting the system's idiosyncratic perception of reality. After all, these events were unpleasant and painful realities for all involved. Still, the support of the treatment team in processing these issues together and planning interventions was crucial.

In cases such as this one, the development of plans for intervention that have utility on a long-term basis is often suspended. A decision first must be made as to whether the family's strengths are sufficient to support a child's return home or if family resistance to change or any ensuing rejection are likely to complicate the child's reintegration and later adjustment. It was certainly possible that Neil might sustain greater impairment in his emotional and sexual development by continuing to reside in an environment of sexual stimulation fostered in his family and community. We were very concerned that Neil was at great risk to become a sexual perpetrator himself should he remain in his environment without receiving follow-up treatment. Out-of-home treatment in a group facility was an alternative option that would have fostered intensive individual work under controlled living circumstances. However, the goal of group home facilities is often to eventually return the client to his family. It was felt that Neil's family ties could be utilized constructively to facilitate change and to maintain more appropriate interactional patterns among family members. To remove Neil permanently from the family at this point did not seem wise. He was emotionally very close to family members, and such an action might simply compound the unresolved losses that had already incapacitated the family.

A decision was then made to have Neil return home to his family. Ideally, treatment was encouraged to focus on each of the weakened aspects of the family system noted previously to ensure future protection for Neil and his siblings. This approach would have attempted to strengthen individual family relationships that would reduce a given member's vulnerability to mistreatment of any kind. A complementary strategy would also involve teaching Neil to better manage both his own and others' behavior. Of course, there was a clear need for Neil to participate in counseling designed to address the sequelae of victimization and his concerns regarding sexuality and appropriate sexual expression. It was also assumed that the mother would benefit from the resolution of her grief over the loss of her spouse, as well as her own childhood sexual victimization. Relatedly, a commitment to protecting the children by providing more consistency in the setting of boundaries and use of structure was seen as crucial. The mother was encouraged to engage in more active problem solving to mediate individual conflicts with her boyfriend and free the children from loyalty struggles that prevented them from trusting either parent figure. Finally, the mother and her boyfriend needed to confront their respective problems with drug use and alcoholism, and to minimize their impact on their limited availability to the family. Throughout the case, the couple's fragile relationship was seen as a primary therapeutic target.

The reality, however, was that the family was not ready to undertake these challenges and confront these issues. We referred them to an excellent agency in their area that specialized in the treatment of sexually misused and abused persons. Concerned with the possibility of sexual abuse, the agency was prepared to help Neil understand his own sexuality and to understand and express his feelings about being taken advantage of sexually. Agency staff expressed an additional concern regarding Neil's risk of becoming a sexual perpetrator should he not find more healthy expression of his sexual feelings, and they were willing to work toward ensuring Neil's protection within the family system. Neil participated in three sessions until the allegations against the mother's boyfriend were considered unfounded by his home county Children and Youth Agency. The family promptly terminated at that point under the assumption that it would be confusing to seek treatment when it appeared that the entire incident had never occurred in the first place. Although sexual expression issues were still of real concern, the family was reluctant to pursue this threatening topic further. Instead, the family took Neil and his brother to a former counselor who had never addressed sexual issues with them, but that too only lasted a few sessions. Since the Children and Youth Agency's focus was limited to finding the SCAN valid or invalid, they were unable to mandate that the family continue with treatment.

Long-Term Outcome

A 1-year follow-up phone call revealed that Neil was attending a specialized child behavior management class in the school district and had brought his school marks up to A's and B's. At the same time, a Child Behavior Checklist completed by the mother indicated that Neil continued to exhibit clinically significant levels of both externalizing and internalizing symptoms. Specifically, he engaged in hyperactive (e.g., can't concentrate, hyperactive), aggressive (fights, unliked), and delinquent (destroys property, steals) behaviors, was quite withdrawn (poor peer relations, teased), and showed obsessive-compulsive (e.g., obsessive, can't sleep) and depressive (e.g., lonely, cries) symptoms. In terms of social competence, he was perceived as doing well in social activities and school performance, but as showing significant problems in social skill and peer relations. There were no difficulties reported on individual items representing sexual behavior and preferences.

The situation of the mother and the family had improved significantly. The mother was now employed full time, and her health was much improved. No further episodes of abuse by the boyfriend or neighborhood children had been acknowledged, which she suggested was an indication that the crisis of the previous year had passed. She was successful in imposing additional structure in the home for the boys and had curtailed their exposure to pornographic movies in the house after realizing that prior attempts to protect them arose out of her own guilt about the experience and were, in retrospect, countertherapeutic. She also acknowledged her boyfriend's assistance in providing this needed structure and a more cohesive relationship with him due, in part, to the threat of his removal from the home as a result of the allegations. In turn, the boyfriend has been able to relate positively to Neil.

Summary and Conclusions

Admittedly, a more complete assessment of current family functioning by a mental health professional would have been preferred to assess outcome. Nevertheless, it seems that the family was no longer in crisis and had become more stable, even though other family issues were yet unresolved. Because other aspects of the family's protective structure and functions were not fully addressed, there is still the potential for heightened vulnerability to abuse during periods when the mother is out of the home.

The knowledge that violence may have been directed toward children, especially in the form of sexual abuse, creates its own distress among practitioners working with the family and the impulse to terminate the abuse at all costs. Generally, the focus of treatment is directed toward identifying the perpetrator and removing him from the home. The structures of our legal system and child agencies reinforce that approach. As advocated by many practitioners, however, a broadened perspective of families in which they are viewed more systemically is needed. Clearly, child protection is a priority. Of course, concern regarding the acts of the perpetrator must be balanced by a concern for maximizing the family's protective functions. The difficulty for legal and mental health practitioners is, in some cases, judging the relative benefit of removing a perpetrator from the home for an isolated event or preserving the family constellation when that person serves as a supportive and strengthening family function. The judicial process is currently based on the "offender guilty–offender goes" principle, which may have specific benefits in terms of protection and deterrence but which may not directly serve the family's present interests. Assuming for the moment that the boyfriend had been the perpetrator in the past, he still maintained a pivotal family position by providing day-to-day assistance to the mother in several important roles, such as financial, emotional, disciplinary, and personal. Plausibly, any ensuing legal battle and removal from the home may prove to be more costly and disruptive to the family than the initial abusive act. To expand its therapeutic benefit, the legal system in such cases might be used to motivate families to participate in treatment and to monitor progress or compliance. At present, the risk–benefit ratio associated with this decision has yet to be carefully articulated (see Newberger, 1985).

Critical assessment, then, of family strengths or assets and limitations or pathology, within the context of their social situation and community supports, needs to occur before an adequate decision about intervention can be made. Specific targets to be evaluated include perceptions of the event by individual family members, the role these individuals played in initiating, disclosing, or concealing the event, and the impact of the event on family relationships and operations (cf. Conte & Schuerman, 1987). As also suggested by this case, therapeutic efforts aimed at increasing the understanding and support of parents should be initiated as early in the case as possible, beginning with the preliminary investigation phase (MacFarlane, 1986).

This case also highlights the need for more cohesive, consistent, and timely interagency work, particularly in evaluating child allegations of abuse. The SCAN investigation appeared to be too fragmented given that our hospital staff provided information for diagnostic purposes, though it was difficult to convey this information to the child's community agencies. Such cases are especially frustrating when the family's denial is so extensive as to result in alternative impressions of the child's allegations.

The usual questions about how to ascertain credibility in children apply to Neil as well. In general, recanting is the exception, not the rule, and can be investigated more fully (Benedek & Schetky, 1987a,b). Still, a child's changing conception of the implications of an allegation and the family's initial reactions may contribute to variations in the child's description or recollection of this experience (Coppens, 1986). Perhaps a more definitive accounting of the facts of this case will come to light as Neil and the family reach maturity.

Even less is known about how best to help and treat children who are sexually overstimulated or exploited. Existing evidence suggests that various modalities may prove helpful, particularly, individual, group, and family therapies (Kolko, 1986). Major treatment issues for consideration in this case include trust, protection, divided loyalties, and limit setting. Progress in the resolution of such issues may be expedited through involvement in a well-integrated set of services designed to prevent or at least alleviate the long-term sequelae of child sexual abuse. While protection of individual family members from reabuse can never be assured, efforts can be taken to bolster the family's protective network as a means of greatly minimizing the risk.

Acknowledgments

The authors acknowledge the contribution of Ana Rivera-Tovar, Ph.D., Janet Borden, Ph.D., and Craig Coleman, M.D., to the preparation of case materials. Janet Stauffer is now affiliated with the Fredericksburg Family Therapy and Counseling Center, P.O. Box 452, Tan and Chestnut Streets, Fredericksburg, Pennsylvania 17026.

References

Alter-Reid, K., Gibbs, M. S., Lachenmeyer, J. R., Sigal, J., & Massoth, N. A. (1986). Sexual abuse of children: A review of the empirical findings. *Clinical Psychology Review, 6,* 249–266.

Benedek, E. P., & Schetky, D. H. (1987a). Problems in validating allegations of sexual abuse. Part 1: Factors affecting perception and recall of events. *Journal of the American Academy of Child and Adolescent Psychiatry, 26,* 912–915.

Benedek, E. P., & Schetky, D. H. (1987b). Problems in validating allegations of sexual abuse. Part 2: Clinical evaluation. *Journal of the American Academy of Child and Adolescent Psychiatry, 26,* 916–921.

Browne, A., & Finkelhor, D. (1986). Impact of child sexual abuse: A review of the research. *Psychological Bulletin, 99,* 66–77.

Conte, J. R., & Schuerman, J. R. (1987). Factors associated with an increased impact of child sexual abuse. *Child Abuse and Neglect, 11,* 210–211.

Coppens, N. M. (1986). Cognitive characteristics as predictors of children's understanding of safety and prevention. *Journal of Pediatric Psychology, 11,* 189–195.

Farber, E. D., Showers, J., Johnson, C. F., Joseph, J. A., & Oshins, L. (1984).The sexual abuse of children: A comparison of male and female victims. *Journal of Clinical Child Psychology, 13,* 294–297.

Finkelhor, D. (1984). *Child sexual abuse: New theory and research.* New York: Free Press.

Finkelhor, D., & Browne, A. (1985). The traumatic impact of child sexual abuse: A conceptualization. *American Journal of Orthopsychiatry, 55,* 530–541.

Freeman-Longo, R. E. (1986). The impact of sexual abuse on males. *Child Abuse and Neglect, 10,* 411–414.

Kolko, D. J. (1986). Treatment of child sexual abuse: Programs, progress, and prospects. *Journal of Family Violence, 2,* 303–318.

Kolko, D. J., Moser, J. T., & Weldy, S. R. (1988). Behavioral/emotional indicators of child sexual abuse among child psychiatric inpatients: A comparison with physical abuse. *Child Abuse and Neglect, 12,* 529–541.

Lusk, R., & Waterman, J. (1986). Effects of sexual abuse on children. In K. MacFarlane, J. Waterman, S. Conerly, L. Damon, M. Durfee, & S. Long (Eds.), *Sexual abuse of young children: Evaluation and treatment* (pp. 101–118). New York: Guilford Press.

MacFarlane, K. (1986). Helping parents cope with extrafamilial molestation. In K. Mac-

Farlane & J. Waterman (Eds.), *Sexual abuse of young children: Evaluation and treatment* (pp. 299–311). New York: Guilford Press.

Mrazek, P. B. (1983). Sexual abuse in children. In B. B. Lahey & A. E. Kazdin (Eds.), *Advances in clinical child psychology* (Vol. 6, pp. 199–215). New York: Plenum.

Newberger, E. H. (1985). The helping hand strikes again: Unintended consequences of child abuse reporting. In E. H. Newberger & R. Bourne (Eds.), *Unhappy families: Clinical and research perspectives on family violence* (pp. 171–178). Littleton, MA: PSG.

Pierce, R., & Pierce, L. H. (1985). The sexually abused child: A comparison of male and female victims. *Child Abuse and Neglect, 9,* 191–199.

Tierney, K. J., & Corwin, D. L. (1983). Exploring intrafamilial child sexual abuse: A systems approach. In D. Finkelhor, R. J. Gelles, G. T. Hotaling, & M. A. Straus (Eds.), *The dark side of families: Current family violence research* (pp. 102–116). Beverly Hills, CA: Sage.

Vander Mey, B. J. (1988). The sexual victimization of male children: A review of previous research. *Child Abuse and Neglect, 12,* 61–72.

11

Incest

Judith A. Cohen and Anthony P. Mannarino

Description of the Problem

Incest is a particular type of child sexual abuse that often has severe consequences for the child, the perpetrator, and the family as a whole. Webster's dictionary defines incest as "sexual intercourse between persons too closely related to marry legally." However, in the field of child sexual abuse, it more commonly refers to any sexual activity between a child and a close relative. This obviously includes many diverse behaviors, which vary, for example, in frequency, duration, or type of contact.

There is no "typical" psychological outcome of incest. As with other forms of child sexual abuse, children exhibit a wide variety of psychological symptoms in response to incest. In two different studies, the authors found no significant group differences in symptomatology between children abused by relatives, and children abused by nonfamilial perpetrators (Cohen & Mannarino, 1988; Mannarino, Cohen, & Gregor, 1989). This supports the notion that the child's relationship to the perpetrator per se does not determine the degree of trauma he or she experiences. However, there are several other aspects of intrafamilial sexual abuse that may make it particularly difficult for victims to recover.

The first is the frequency of the sexual abuse. There is some evidence to indicate that with a greater number of abusive episodes, there is a higher rate of self-reported symptomatology, such as depression, anxiety, and poor self-esteem (Mannarino *et al.*, 1989). Although some

Judith A. Cohen and Anthony P. Mannarino • Department of Psychiatry, Western Psychiatric Institute and Clinic, University of Pittsburgh School of Medicine, Pittsburgh, Pennsylvania 15213.

cases of incest involve only one abusive episode, many incest victims have experienced ongoing sexual abuse. Some of these children have been abused for months or years on a regular basis. In these cases, the frequency of abuse may result in an increase in psychological symptoms.

The family's reaction to the abuse and its disclosure may also be a very important determinant in how the child functions. Although this issue has not been adequately examined in an empirical way, most clinicians suggest that familial support is a very important factor in the child's recovery (Friedrich, Luecke, Beilke, & Place, 1988; Wyatt & Mickey, 1987). It is important to note that the stereotypical incestuous family, where the "collusive mother" knows all along about the sexual abuse of her child and tolerates or even promotes it, is not representative of the families that we have seen. Other researchers report this also (Faller, 1988). Many of these children report the first episode of abuse to their mothers, who often take immediate appropriate action to protect the child and remove the perpetrator from the home (Mannarino & Cohen, 1986). There are many other mothers who express a great deal of ambivalence and have difficulty in "choosing sides," but who still take steps to prevent ongoing abuse. (One such family is presented in the case that follows.) There are, unfortunately, some families that tolerate the abuse or persistently disbelieve the victim despite overwhelming evidence that incest is occurring. (It should be noted that much variability in response to the victim occurs in extrafamilial sexual abuse cases as well; these victims' families are also not uniformly supportive, protective, or readily willing to believe the child.)

Legal involvement is often more complex in an incest case than with extrafamilial sexual abuse. Frequently the perpetrator represents the main source of family income. Pressing charges that may entail a subsequent prison sentence and loss of job could significantly decrease the family's standard of living, resulting not only in financial hardship but also in resentment of the victim by other family members. Removal of the perpetrator (with or without criminal charges being pursued) frequently deprives other family members of an emotionally important figure in the home, which may also cause ambivalence, anger, or resentment toward the victim. Custody issues frequently have an impact not only on the abused child but on other siblings as well. In addition, public knowledge about the sexual abuse may cause significant shame or embarrassment to the family members owing to their relationship to the perpetrator. All of these factors may significantly add to the stress experienced by the family and the abused child.

In the case of incest, the victimized child usually has a relationship with the perpetrator that also has had positive aspects. Although the perpetrator objectively has betrayed the child's trust, the latter may not perceive it this way. The emotional attachment that the child has to the perpetrator may make it much harder for her or him to reach some resolution regarding the abuse, because the perpetrator is still, and may always be, a member of the family. This may add complications and conflicts that a victim of extrafamilial abuse would not have to address.

The following case demonstrates many of the issues discussed above, which are potential problems that may be encountered in cases of incest. However, it is important to recognize that each sexual abuse case has its own characteristics, and there are no "absolute" dimensions that distinguish incest from extrafamilial child sexual abuse. Each situation must be assessed individually to determine relevant clinical, familial, and legal issues.

Case Description

Ann and Marie were sisters, aged 14 and 13, respectively, who were brought for an evaluation by their mother because of the girls' disclosure of sexual abuse by their natural father. The girls were living with their mother (a college-educated housewife) and their 18-year-old sister, Michele. The father, a Protestant minister, had lived with them until his arrest a few weeks prior to evaluation.

Ann had first attempted to tell her mother about the sexual abuse 2 years previously. She did this by asking her mother, "Do you know what sexual abuse is?" The mother apparently did not make anything of Ann's question and did not pursue the subject at that time. Ann let the matter drop. The following year, Marie disclosed the sexual abuse to a counselor at a church camp. Child protective services were called to investigate, but Ann was very angry at Marie for telling someone at camp (partly because it was affiliated with the father's church). Consequently, Ann refused to talk to the caseworker. In an attempt to lessen Ann's anger at her, Marie also refused to talk to the worker. Because the girls would not speak to the investigator, the report was unfounded. Apparently, the mother did not question the girls as to whether they had been abused or why Marie had reported it. She did, however, confront the father, who was already in individual therapy for treatment of work-related stress. The mother went with the father to see the father's therapist, and he did admit to "inappropriate love and affection" for both girls. (It should be noted that this was the first time his therapist learned about this, after 5 years of ongoing psychotherapy.) Shortly thereafter, the father called the children into his room and, in his wife's presence, praised Marie for her disclosure and apologized for his behavior. He promised it would never happen again, and the mother assumed that it would not.

However, in the last several months, the mother had noted that Marie was frequently fighting with her father and seemed to feel a great deal of hostility toward him. For this reason, the mother brought Marie to a private therapist for individual treatment. During the evaluation by this therapist, Marie again disclosed ongoing sexual abuse by her father. Child protective services were called, and this time Marie described the abuse to the investigators. The father was arrested, and both Ann and Marie were referred to our clinic for treatment.

Apparently, abuse of both girls began at about the same time, when Ann was 5 years old and Marie was 4 years old. Each girl was evaluated individually. Ann presented as an attractive, well-developed, articulate adolescent. She felt very ambivalent about Marie's disclosure, expressing both relief that her father would get some help and anger that Marie had gotten him into trouble by disclosing the abuse.

Ann reported that, most commonly, her father would fondle her in the breast area and between her legs. At different stages of her life, he would perform different sexual acts on her, which she and Marie would discuss on occasion. The most extensive abuse Ann experienced was what the girls called the "full treatment." This consisted of the father's undressing her, fondling her, and lying down in bed with her back to his chest. He would roll her around his genital area and touch her on her breasts and vaginal area. During the course of the interview, Ann related many incidents of this type being perpetrated against her, almost on a weekly basis during certain periods of her life. She could remember one of many trips out of town with the family, when the mother slept with Michele in one room, and the father slept with Ann and Marie in another room. She stated that while they were sleeping together in the same bed, he attempted to fondle her once again. She asked him to stop and he did. He asked her if she wanted to go in with her mother and she replied yes. Ann related that she felt guilty that she went into the other room with her mother and left Marie alone with her father. She stated that she always knew that the abuse was wrong but did not know how to stop it at the time.

The abuse continued on a regular basis, with Ann stating that frequently she would see her father entering Marie's bedroom and would know the abuse was occurring. On several occasions, she attempted to stop her father from abusing Marie by entering the room and beginning a conversation. In her estimation, she was never able to ask him to stop abusing Marie or herself until the first disclosure. Ann stated that she felt in her mind that she had given her mother many hints that the abuse was occurring. When she went to her mother and asked her, "Do you know what sexual abuse is?" Ann felt that this should have been a sufficient hint for her mother, but it was not. After the first disclosure, with her father apologizing to her and Marie, she felt that the abuse would no longer continue. Even when he would still attempt to enter her bedroom and give her back rubs, which resulted in his hands moving to her chest, she was able to say no, but she knew in her heart that the abuse was continuing with Marie. She was very angry at Marie for disclosing at camp and felt that it threatened the family. She was "trying to be so good for Mom" so as not to add any additional emotional burdens on her mother. She was unsure that her mother would be able to handle the family without her husband and felt quite guilty about having "wrecked" their marriage. She was able to state that she felt that she needed help to discuss feeling "dirty" about what had happened and what effect this would have on future relationships with the opposite sex. She was also able to express some anger at Marie for acting-out emotionally when she herself was trying to be so good and hold the family together.

Ann expressed fear that Michele would be angry at her, although Michele had expressed support for her. Ann stated that what she dreaded the most was having to go to court and face everyone and discuss what had happened to her. She stated that she felt everyone would be looking at her, thinking about the abuse that had been perpetrated against her, and that this made her feel "dirty." She was somewhat angry at father but expressed more sorrow for him, stating that he "must have problems" and that "he is a sick man." Ann denied any suicidal thoughts or ideation. She reported being sad, angry, and confused, and believed very strongly that she needed to talk to somebody about this. She felt that her mother was torn between her daughters and her husband and worried about the outcome of their relationship and their marriage.

Marie was also evaluated individually. Like her sister, Marie was attractive, intelligent, and articulate. She was tearful during most of the interview. Marie described the same type of fondling as Ann (as stated above, the two girls occasionally discussed the abuse with each other). As Marie got older, the father would perform oral sex on her as well. In describing this, Marie became quite tearful and felt guilty and dirty because of this particular abuse. She wondered if it was her fault and if she should be blamed for not stopping her father sooner. She was angry at him, but also sad that he had lost his wife, children, and possibly his job over this disclosure. She was also fearful that he would go to jail and wondered what would become of her mother and the family. She reported an inability to concentrate in school and some sleep disturbance. She stated that it took several hours for her to fall asleep at night, and frequently she would awake in the middle of the night or early in the morning. She reported constant sadness and frequent tearfulness since the disclosure as well.

Marie was extremely angry that her father continued to abuse her (and not Ann) even after he promised to stop. She said this was why she began fighting and being noncompliant with the father in the last several months. She was relieved and glad that she had at last followed through on disclosing the abuse, because this would finally make it stop.

Medical Issues

It may be helpful to digress from the case study at this point in order to discuss general medical issues in the case of incest. (For the purpose of this discussion, the collection of medical evidence for legal proceedings will not be addressed.) The medical approach to incest is basically the same as in any other case of child sexual abuse. The type of sexual activity experienced will determine whether and what type of a medical examination is indicated. For venereal disease to be contracted, the child must have had contact with the perpetrator's bodily fluids.[1] If one is confident that there has been no contact with the perpetrator's body fluids and no history suggestive of traumatic injury (i.e., violent penetration), there is probably no medical indication for a physical exam. This is generally true in the case where the child has experienced digital fondling without other sexual contact. However, even in this case, parents sometimes request a medical exam for reassurance that no permanent injury has been incurred; in this situation, an exam is appropriate.

In the prepubertal female child, if there is a possibility that contact with the perpetrator's bodily fluids has occurred, introitus cultures are generally obtained for chlamydial and gonococcal organisms. Blood samples are obtained for syphilis and HIV titres. (If the abuse occurred less than 3 months prior to the exam, HIV titres should be repeated at a later date, since these frequently do not become positive until 3 to 6 months following exposure.) With either a male or a female child, if there is a history or suspicion of anal penetration, anal gonococcal cultures should also be obtained.

In a prepubertal child, there will rarely be significant internal genital trauma without evidence of severe external trauma. If external injury is severe enough to require suturing, or there is significant intravaginal or intraanal bleeding, an internal exam is generally indicated. In the prepubertal child, this should be done under general anesthesia, to minimize traumatization of the child, as well as to assure an adequate exam. The need for such measures occurs only rarely. When this situation occurs, children are often frightened of being put to sleep, and need careful explanations and reassurances about the procedures to be done.

For postpubertal girls, a serum pregnancy test is required in addition to the tests for sexually transmitted diseases detailed above. If possible, an internal exam should be performed. The main purpose of the internal exam in this situation is to obtain cervical cultures for gonorrhea and vaginal cultures for chlamydia, since these are more reliable than cultures from the introitus. However, the risk of further psychological

---

[1]This may occur without ejaculation; there may be exchange of body fluids with any oral-genital, anal-genital, genital-genital, or oral-anal contact. It might also occur if, for example, the perpetrator ejaculated into his hand, then fondled the child's genitals with that hand.

trauma to the child should be carefully weighed against the benefits of performing an internal exam. If the child seems to experience a significant degree of fear or psychological stress about having an internal exam, the exam can usually be deferred. It should go without saying that any medical procedures should be explained to the child in a supportive way, and that no method requiring forcible restraint of the child is acceptable in this situation. If the child is fearful or resistant, the medical examination will simply victimize that child further. Generally, even very young children can cooperate with the medical procedures involved when they are explained with care and a parent or advocate is available for comfort and support during the exam.

If the child has contracted a sexually transmitted disease, appropriate antibiotic therapy must be instituted. The issue of incest resulting in pregnancy is very complex, and a detailed discussion is beyond the scope of this chapter. The medical and psychological risks of bearing a child conceived from an incestuous relationship are significant. Abortion is frequently the best available option in this situation. However, such decisions are generally conflict-laden, and each situation must be evaluated individually.

With regard to the case history, Marie had experienced oral intercourse with her father on several occasions. Ann gave no history of contact with her father's bodily fluids. However, because the abuse had gone on for so many years and it was possible that some such contact had occurred earlier (without Ann's realizing or remembering it), medical evaluations were performed on both girls at a large metropolitan children's hospital. Cultures and blood tests were obtained from both girls to detect the presence of sexually transmitted diseases. All of these were negative. Both girls continued to have regular asymptomatic menstrual periods, and neither girl had any significant somatic complaints.

Legal Issues

When incest has been disclosed, there is usually a great deal of ambivalence about pressing charges against the perpetrator. Many procedural requirements, particularly in the criminal justice system, may further traumatize the child witness (Landwirth, 1987). One group of researchers found that while testimony in juvenile court may be beneficial for the child (in the case of a juvenile perpetrator), protracted criminal proceedings may have an adverse psychological effect on the child victim (Runyan, Everson, Edelsohn, Hunter, & Coulter, 1988). The risks and benefits of the child's testifying in court should be weighed carefully in each individual situation before the decision to press charges is made. Generally, the prosecuting attorney will respect the child's wishes in this matter, although there have been a few unfortunate cases where the child incest victim has actually been held in contempt of court for refusing to testify against the perpetrator.

In the present case, the father was arrested shortly after the sexual abuse was founded by child protective services. Bail was posted by authorities in his church. Child protective services informed the parents that both girls would be removed from the parental home if the father returned. The mother and father agreed that he should move into an apartment, to "keep the rest of the family together."

The family was very ambivalent about pressing legal charges against the father. (Charges included indecent assault, involuntary deviant sexual intercourse, and corruption of a minor.) The mother fretted that pressing charges would shame the family, because it would be on public record that the father had done these things. She did not pressure the girls not to press charges, but she also did not encourage them to do so, saying that "it has to be their decision." This obviously placed the responsibility (and subsequent guilt) squarely on Ann and Marie. They did agree to press charges, at which point the father said he would plead guilty. He claimed this plea was to "spare the girls having to testify," although it clearly also spared his having the details of his behavior come out in court.

A presentencing interview was conducted by the probation office. This involved each girl's talking with an investigator about her own preferences with regard to sentencing. Theoretically, the purpose of this interview is not only to ascertain how much harm has come to the victim but also to determine what sentence would be most beneficial to the victim (i.e., some children would be further traumatized by the perpetrator's being imprisoned).

At this interview, Ann expressed much ambivalence. She said she would feel terribly guilty if her father were sent to jail; she would feel "like I put him in prison." This seemed to be her strongest feeling. However, she was also clear that if he was not put in jail, he would have "gotten off easy, gotten away with doing that to us with no consequences." She then pointed out that he had "lost his family and his job, and that's probably bad enough." (Church authorities accompanied the father to the trial to provide support. However, following the trial, he was dismissed from his job.)

Marie was much less ambivalent than Ann. She felt strongly that the father should be put in jail, no matter what it meant to the family in terms of embarrassment or loss of income. She expressed this clearly to the probation officer. However, Marie later changed her mind about this option; she indicated that her father had "made improvements" in therapy, that he now understood some of his own underlying conflicts, and that he did not need to be punished anymore. (It is not clear how much of Marie's change of heart was actually due to ongoing family pressure on her.) At the time this chapter is being written, sentencing is still pending.

This is a case in which the legal system worked promptly and effectively in the victims' best interests. This was in part due to the fact that the girls were able, and ultimately willing, to testify against the perpetrator. (This is often not true in incest cases, especially when the victim is younger than these girls were.) Although the presentencing investigation may place too much of a burden of responsibility on the young incest victim, in general, it tends to serve the victim's needs as much as possible.

The initial disclosure in this case highlights a shortcoming of the child protective system. After Marie disclosed the sexual abuse to a counselor, she experienced a great deal of pressure from Ann. This caused Marie to refuse to confirm her claims during the actual child protective services' investigation. Accordingly, the case was unfounded. The pathological enmeshment, guilt, and responsibility evident in this and many other incestuous families makes it more likely that these victimized children will not speak out against the parent-perpetrator. In such cases, unless there is other convincing evidence of abuse, protective services are legally unable to intervene. Unfortunately, there are many situations where this occurs and the incest most likely continues. When such a case is unfounded because of lack of evidence, there is no requirement for the family to enter therapy; indeed, such families probably tend to avoid treatment, in part for fear that allegations will be brought up again by the abused child. These children frequently fall through the "cracks" in the legal system and are unavailable for therapeutic or protective intervention.

Social and Family Issues

This family illustrates many maladaptive patterns of interaction and communication, which allowed the father's abusive behavior to persist for a number of years. These patterns include an unrealistic overdependence or enmeshment in the family, to the degree that any threat to family stability was seen as a threat to each member's very survival. There were inappropriate generational boundaries and coalitions, as evidence by a dysfunctional marital relationship and delegation of parental responsibilities to the children. Communication was characterized by ambivalent, mixed messages, the need to not hear statements that are threatening or dangerous, and placating "at all costs" rather than discussing and working out problems constructively. Not only did these problems contribute to the onset and maintenance of the father's incestuous behavior, but they interfered with the family's ability to cope with events subsequent to the disclosure. These familial problems are illustrated in detail in the following discussion.

Ann initially asked the mother about sexual abuse in 1986, when this was a widely publicized subject. The mother had been a schoolteacher prior to the birth of Michele, and should thus have been more likely than some mothers to be sensitive to this kind of "hint." However, the mother made no attempt to pursue the question with Ann at that time. The mother revealed to us that for several years prior to that episode, the father had wanted to do "kinky" sexual things with her. She refused, and the couple had enjoyed minimal sexual contact for many years. Despite this, she denied any suspicions of a problem when Ann raised the subject. Whether this was indicative of collusion (i.e., the mother knew or suspected the abuse was occurring and did nothing) or of the mother's need to deny any threatening communication is impossible to determine.

After Marie disclosed the abuse the following year, the mother did confront the father, and, to her credit, she forced the issue to be addressed by his therapist. However, she did not try to persuade either girl to speak to child protective services workers, preferring to "work it out as a family." She also did not maintain close supervision of where the father slept at night and whether the abuse had indeed stopped. She never encouraged the girls, even at the family meeting where the father promised to stop the abuse, to report any future abuse to her. Marie was clear that had she felt this kind of support and backing from her mother, she would have been more assertive about reporting or stopping the abuse.

Ann and Marie both feared that if they reported their father's sexual activities, the family would "fall apart." This inappropriate sense of responsibility for holding together a dysfunctional family seems to be a common finding in victims of ongoing incest. It was certainly reinforced by the mother's overt and covert attitudes. Even after the trial, the mother tried to influence the girls with regard to the sentencing, saying things like "I don't know how we'll manage if your father goes to jail. I'd have to get a job and I don't know if I can find one. How will we live?" When confronted with this in therapy, she denied wanting to influence the girls. Ann and Marie both genuinely feared what would happen to their family without the father. They were unable to view that scenario realistically, but rather reacted with global feelings of impending catastrophe if the family changed in that way.

The mother did many things to indicate her ambivalence toward family members. She told the girls she was "behind them all the way," but she also said she "couldn't take sides" by supporting the girls over her husband. Ann picked up on this and adopted many of her mother's empathic attitudes toward the father; subsequently, even Marie displayed signs of doing this. A few specific episodes are illustrative of the ambivalent message the mother gave to the father and the girls. Once when the electricity went off in the father's apartment, he called the family home and the mother brought him candles, staying with him for an hour while the lights were out. Marie was angry about this, but both the mother and Ann pointed out that "he's still our family and we should take care of him." Marie wondered why no one felt compelled to protect and take care of *her* during the years she was being abused, and why she should worry about her father when he clearly did not worry about how he was hurting her. She quickly felt guilty for having these "vicious" thoughts, however—a guilt that the mother subtly reinforced.

Another time, Michele had a college event that both the father and the mother wanted to attend. Ann and Marie at that time felt very betrayed by their father, and said they would not go if he was going to be there. The mother tried to coerce them into going despite the fact that Michele said she did not care whether any of the family attended. The mother was unable to side with Ann and Marie, and instead said that if they did not want to go, she and the father would go together. The parents did go together for 3 days (Michele attended college out of town), and Ann and Marie felt that their mother "chose him over us." The therapist tried to point this out to the mother, but she was unable or unwilling to consider this view. She said that Michele deserved to have both of her parents there, despite Michele's repeated statements that she did not care whether her parents were present or not.

(Michele, in fact, disclosed in family therapy shortly thereafter that the father had also sexually abused her for many years, until she was in her midteens. She had never told anyone about this. She refused to press charges, saying, "It's over; I want to forget it and go on with my life.")

It is clear through all of these events that the mother was unable to take a strong position against the father in order to protect the children. They felt much lack of support and later reported that this contributed to their not taking a stronger stand against their father's behavior. They simply felt that mother accepted what he did, so they should as well. The family's religious background probably contributed to this problem. The guilt of getting a family member in trouble or hurting someone else, and the overly developed sense of responsibility these girls felt, was encouraged by their strong religious training. The fact that their father was a respected minister also probably contributed to their hesitancy to become angry at him or report his abusive behavior.

Even at the present time, the mother continues to give mixed messages to her daughters. She cloaks this in the guise of giving them "control over their lives." When Ann became resistant regarding coming to therapy, the mother said, "That has to be Ann's decision, not mine." The mother has been unwilling to encourage her daughters to do positive things for themselves, yet has been perfectly ready to coerce them when it is to her or the father's benefit. The mother has been totally lacking in insight with regard to this pattern, no matter how it has been pointed out to her. No doubt this style enabled the sexual abuse to go on for as many years as it did. The only way Marie was able to break free of this pressure was by rebelling against both parents. She became angry and confrontative with her father prior to her second disclosure, and has continued to be much more symptomatic than Ann, who has felt less anger and has been less assertive about reporting or pursuing the legal aspects of the abuse. Marie has received overt and covert messages because of her actions, being told she has "destroyed the family" and that she is a "troublemaker." At some points, Marie has become suicidal because of this betrayal by her family; the possibility of her being placed outside the home has been discussed recently. Marie's perception is that she has been punished for "rocking the boat" and reporting the abuse. This certainly seems accurate (particularly with regard to the fact that after the first disclosure, the father continued to abuse only her, not Ann). Unfortunately, if the family cannot change this pattern, Marie may have to leave the home in order to maintain any degree of emotional health.

The father has been in therapy at a facility that specializes in treating sexual offenders. According to his therapist and reports from Ann and Marie, he has focused therapy on his own issues, such as conflicts with his mother when he was a child. He has yet to identify himself as a perpetrator of abuse, saying only that he "loved the children too much." He apparently has had no insight into the fact that he caused long-lasting emotional trauma to his daughters. In fact, he has expressed hurt that they do not want him to return home now that he has been in therapy. (In her typical fashion, the mother has left the responsibility for this decision on the girls' shoulders, saying, "He won't come home until you agree that he can.") Ann has felt guilty for hurting her father and would probably agree to his returning home at this point. Marie also has felt sorry that her father has lost his prestige in the community, and has felt that he has been improving in treatment. (He speaks to the family on the phone frequently and has communicated to them the issues he is addressing in therapy.) However, Marie is still angry and appropriately expects the father to have some understanding of the damage he has done to her and the family. A simple apology is not enough for Marie, she says, because he apologized before but then went right on abusing her.

In summary, the family patterns of overenmeshment, poor communication, needing to maintain the family at all costs, and inappropriate responsibility being placed on the children, along with parental abdication of responsibility, all enabled the incest in this case to continue. These patterns have persisted, causing ongoing problems for the victims. In Ann's case, this has been manifested by her need to "be a perfect daughter," requiring herself to care for her mother rather than allowing herself to need nurturance. The only family member who has significantly broken the pattern is Marie. She has been able to do this only by becoming alternatingly angry and depressed. She has been on the verge of being rejected from the family because of her refusal to comply with the dysfunctional "rules" of the family. Unfortunately, neither parent has shown any significant motivation to acknowledge or change the way the family operates.

Assessment of Psychopathology

Ann and Marie were assessed individually. On the surface, Ann appeared to be coping fairly well. She was maintaining her honor grades in high school and continued to be involved in her usual activities. Her main symptoms were anxiety and panic attacks. These were not specifically related to the abuse but to events subsequent to the disclosure.

They occurred in relation to what would happen now that her father had left the home. She worried that the family would have to move, that her father would have a nervous breakdown, that her friends would find out about the abuse, and that her mother would "fall apart." She had panic attacks related to these concerns several times a week. Ann denied any depressive symptoms and also denied that she ever thought about her father's abusive behavior, except when police, her therapist, or other authorities brought it up. She denied dissociative features or flashback phenomena. Ann was diagnosed as having an adjustment disorder with anxious features, and a panic disorder.

Marie was more symptomatic than Ann. Her grades had fallen from A's to B's and C's. She fought with her friends more frequently. Marie had many depressive symptoms, including a significant sleep disturbance, frequent crying, and suicidal thoughts. At stressful times, she thought about cutting her wrists or overdosing to "end the pain." Marie had poor concentration and frequent fatigue. In addition to these depressive features, Marie had significant behavioral problems. She had become oppositional with her mother, and in angry outbursts, she would throw objects around her bedroom or leave the house for hours at a time without saying where she was going. She was very irritable with her sister Ann, as well as with friends. This profile of anger and aggressive behavior in adolescents who have experienced long-term sexual abuse has been well described in the literature (Runtz & Briere, 1986). Often, when such behaviors occur in the context of frequent intense mood changes and suicidal behavior, the adolescent incest victim may be misdiagnosed as having a borderline personality disorder (Briere, 1989). In evaluating adolescents such as Marie, it is important to understand the etiology of the symptoms rather than focusing on the symptoms themselves. Briere (1989) believes many female adolescents are misdiagnosed as "borderline" when in fact they are manifesting problems directly related to long-term sexual abuse.

In addition to the above symptoms, Marie described frequent intrusive memories of her father abusing her. When she became very sad, she would occasionally experience derealization symptoms. Her diagnosis was major depressive episode and adjustment disorder with mixed disturbance of conduct and emotion. A rule-out diagnosis of acute posttraumatic stress disorder was also made.

Treatment Options

Most programs that specialize in treating incestuous nuclear families have very specific requirements, such as the perpetrator's admitting to his or her inappropriate sexual behavior, the nonabusive parent's providing a safe and supportive home situation, and the perpetrator's not having unsupervised access to the children until various treatment goals have been achieved (Meinig, 1989). Most such programs combine several of the following elements: group therapy for perpetrators, group treatment for spouses of perpetrators, dyadic therapy for mothers and child victims, child victims' groups, individual therapy for victims, and eventual family therapy including the victim, perpetrator, nonabusing parent, and siblings of the victim. Unfortunately, the majority of incestuous families do not meet the entrance requirements for such programs because the perpetrator denies the abuse and/or the mother is unable or unwilling to adequately protect the children from the perpetrator. With these families, therapy is frequently a long and frustrating process. It is not unusual in such circumstances for the child victim to be removed from the home. When the victim remains with family members who are ambivalent or unsupportive, he or she frequently becomes more symptomatic and may require hospitalization, as will be seen in this case study.

Ann was referred for individual and group psychotherapy, as well as family therapy (which was provided through her father's treatment center). After a few months, Ann began missing individual appointments, saying she was "over this," and just wanted to "put it all behind" her. The mother has refused to ask Ann to comply with treatment, saying, "It has to be Ann's decision whether she needs treatment or not; you or I can't decide that for her." It is unclear at this time whether Ann will resume treatment.

Marie began group and individual therapy, and established very positive relationships with the other group members. She was able to provide and accept support very constructively. Soon after the 12-week group ended, Marie became increasingly depressed, culminating in a suicidal gesture (an attempt to stab herself, which the mother stopped). Marie was hospitalized on an adolescent psychiatric unit for 3 weeks. In the hospital, she rapidly improved and stated frequently that she did not want to return home because she felt she received no support there. However, as her discharge approached, she reluctantly agreed to return home at the mother's persistent requests. She continues in individual therapy and family therapy. The possibility of placement outside the home is being seriously considered owing to her recurring depressive symptoms and the difficulty her family is having in making significant changes.

Summary and Conclusions

Incest has the potential for causing significant and long-lasting psychological problems for its victims. Children and adult incest survivors exhibit a wide range of psychological responses to the incest experience (Russell, Schurman, & Trocki, 1988); there is no "typical" symptomatology that characterizes most of these victims. Although it does not appear that the child's relationship to the perpetrator per se determines psychological outcome, there are many aspects of intrafamilial sexual abuse that may make the experience more difficult for the victim. Some of these legal, social, and familial issues have been presented in this chapter and illustrated by the case history. As in other cases of child sexual abuse, each child and family must be carefully evaluated to determine the specific dynamics, psychological symptoms, and family issues that are relevant. Treatment should be tailored to address these specific needs. More systematic empirical research is needed in this area to determine what factors may mediate psychological outcome and how treatment can most effectively aid in optimizing recovery for incest victims, perpetrators, and their families.

References

Briere, J. (1989). *Treating adults molested as children: Beyond survival*. New York: Springer.

Cohen, J. A., & Mannarino, A. P. (1988). Psychological symptoms in sexually abused girls. *Child Abuse and Neglect, 12*, 571–577.

Faller, K. C. (1988). The myth of the "collusive mother." *Journal of Interpersonal Violence, 3*, 190–196.

Friedrich, W. N., Luecke, W. J., Beilke, R. L., & Place, V. (1988). *Psychotherapy outcome of sexually abused boys: An agency study*. Unpublished manuscript, Mayo Clinic.

Landwirth, J. (1987). Children as witnesses in child sexual abuse trials. *Pediatrics, 80*, 585–589.

Mannarino, A. P., & Cohen, J. A. (1986). A clinical-demographic study of sexually abused children. *Child Abuse and Neglect, 10*, 17–28.

Mannarino, A. P., Cohen, J. A., & Gregor, M. (1988). Emotional and behavioral difficulties in sexually abused girls. *Journal of Interpersonal Violence, 4*(4), 437–451.

Meinig, M. B. (1989). *A protocol for reunification of families affected by sexual abuse*. Paper presented at symposium "Beyond theory: Tools for practice in treating sexually abused children," Annenberg Center for Health Sciences at Eisenhower, Rancho Mirage, CA.

Runtz, M. T., & Briere, J. (1986). Adolescent "acting out" and childhood history of sexual abuse. *Journal of Interpersonal Violence, 1*, 326–334.

Runyan, D. K., Everson, M. D., Edelsohn, G. A., Hunter, W. H., & Coulter, M. L. (1988). Impact of legal intervention on sexually abused children. *Journal of Pediatrics, 113*, 647–653.

Russell, D. E. H., Schurman, R. A., & Trocki, K. (1988). The long-term effects of incestuous abuse. A comparison of Afro-American and white American victims. In G. E. Wyatt & G. J. Powell (Eds.), *Lasting effects of child sexual abuse*. Newbury Park, CA: Sage.

Wyatt, G. E., & Mickey, M. R. (1987). Ameliorating the effects of child sexual abuse: An exploratory study of support by parents and others. *Journal of Interpersonal Violence, 2*, 403–414.

12

Ritual Abuse

Cheryl Carey Kent

Description of the Problem

Discussions of ritual abuse in the field of family violence have occurred primarily within the past 5 years. Because of the recent emergence of the area, very little information has appeared as yet in the psychological and psychiatric literature. A few papers have been presented at national and state psychological conferences and the National Symposium on Child Sexual Abuse. Some systematic studies of the effects of child sexual abuse, where children have also made allegations of ritual abuse, are under way (McCord, Waterman, Oliveri, & Kelly, 1990), and two overviews of the symptoms of children alleging ritual abuse have been presented at national conferences (Kelly, 1988; Kent, 1988). However, the area of ritual abuse is still in the pioneering stages.

Despite the recent emergence of the field, the issue of ritual abuse has received nationwide media attention as allegations of the ritual abuse of young children in cities and states across the country (Los Angeles, San Francisco, Chicago, and Minnesota) have flashed across the evening news and newspaper headlines. Survivors of ritual abuse have recently begun to appear on television talk shows (the Oprah Winfrey show and the Geraldo Rivera show, to name two). Since its existence was first publicized in large child abuse cases, reports of possible ritual abuse have increased alarmingly over the past 5 years. Roland Summit, M.D., a community psychiatrist at the UCLA School of

Cheryl Carey Kent • Children's Evaluation Center, Los Angeles, California 90020.

Medicine, reports that he has been contacted about more than 40 cases nationwide in which the possibility of ritual abuse has been raised (Summit, personal communication, 1989). Similarly, self-help groups for sexual abuse survivors report that a significant percentage of their members describe being ritualistically abused as children. The Los Angeles County Commission on Women, upon becoming concerned about its prevalence, organized a task force consisting of law enforcement personnel, psychotherapists, and social service agencies.

However, along with the publicity has come controversy. Arguments have been made that these reports of ritualistic activities have been greatly exaggerated. Anton La Vey, founder of the Church of Satan in San Francisco, has argued that the activities described by alleged victims of ritual cults simply do not occur. However, Charles Manson, convicted murderer, has reportedly stated, "Believe them, everything they say is true."

The whole area of ritual abuse is problematic both because of the bizarre and disturbing nature of the allegations and because of the difficulty in obtaining any corroborative information. These difficulties manifest themselves in medical, legal, social and family, and treatment issues as well. Complications in these areas will be discussed later in the chapter.

Before proceeding further, it is important to describe and define ritual abuse. Pazder (1980) first coined the phrase "ritual abuse" and defined it as the "repeated physical, emotional, mental, and spiritual assaults combined with a systematic use of symbols, ceremonies, and machinations designed and orchestrated to attain malevolent effects." Although one purpose of the abuse may be to gain personal spiritual power or to "please Satan," another purpose may be the systematic breaking down of the victim's sense of self in order to assure his continued cooperation with the goals of the group. Police investigators interviewed by Kahaner (1988) described three distinct types of satanic groups. The first are groups that make themselves publicly known—for example, the Church of Satan and Temple of Set. These groups deny that they engage in any abusive practices, and they are generally viewed as operating within the law. Two other types of groups are viewed as engaging in many illegal practices. The second group, the "self-styled Satanists," are loosely knit groups of individuals who band together and "dabble" in occult practices. They are often adolescents who are exploring occult activities, and who may be influenced by heavy-metal music or by certain games, such as Dungeons and Dragons. One case in Long Island is an example of this. An adolescent was killed by a group of his peers who were reportedly dabbling in occult practices. The third level of Satanic involvement appears to be composed of more organized, hierarchical, and secretive groups of people. These latter groups may have national and international connections with one another. Smith and Pazder (1980) and Terry (1988) have both described these possible connections. These reports have been dismissed as suspect by some members of law enforcement. However, many others find substantial similarity in victims' reports and evidence at crime scenes to merit ritual abuses being considered a serious problem. It will be primarily involvement in the latter two levels of activity that I will be addressing in this chapter, as freedom of religious practices is granted to all recognized religious satanic organizations (i.e., the Church of Satan and Temple of Set).

Satanic groups are reported to celebrate feast days at various times of the year that are close to Christian holidays. However, rather than symbolically revering God through prayer and communion, blood sacrifices of various types are made, and blood and flesh are ingested by the congregation to acknowledge Satan's rule. Similarly, various sacraments, like "baptism" or "initiation rites," are practiced with blood rather than water, and the person's "soul" is viewed as being consecrated to Satan rather than being viewed as being "purified of sin" as in the Christian baptism. Similarly, the "Black Mass" celebrations are the opposite of the Roman Catholic version, in that they involve blood sacrifices (often goats, lambs, dogs, and sometimes humans) to Satan. Animals may be sacrificed by new initiates, and the blood and flesh substituted for the wine and wafers of the Christian communion. Finally, there is a satanic alphabet, and there are satanic symbols (i.e., inverted crosses and inverted pentagrams inside a circle) and various numbers that have satanic significance (666, 13). Other practices reported include the abduction and physical and sexual abuse of infants and young children, and the consumption of feces and urine. Smearing victims with blood and feces also is sometimes reported in association with these rituals. Pornographic movies and "snuff" films may be produced for profit. Drugs may also be sold for profit and used extensively. But perhaps the most disturbing events of all are told by women who describe their role as being "breeders" for the cult. They detail how their role has been to become pregnant and deliver children who, at some point during their infancy or childhood, will be slaughtered in ritualistic sacrifices to Satan. Other survivors describe kidnapping children who are then tortured and starved until they are too weak to protest before they are murdered during ritualistic sacrifices.

Members report being threatened with death if they attempt to leave the cult, identify members to authorities, or tell anyone about what occurred. Many report that they have been led to believe that they cannot escape because their location can be tracked through either supernatural or mechanical means (by some implanted device). Survivors further describe being led to believe that the group will always "know" what they are telling others, and that any disclosures will result in swift punishment or death to them. Similarly, they also report being told that no one will believe them if they do tell about what happened to them, and they will be labeled "crazy." Unfortunately, this latter prediction may be borne out in the experience of the survivor. Smith and Pazder (1980) provide in-depth descriptions of the practices and fear-instilling tactics reported by one alleged victim.

Because of the extreme level of trauma that may be experienced over years and because of the consequent level of psychological damage that may occur, victims of ritual abuse are usually reluctant to talk freely about what they have experienced and are at risk for being discounted as "psychotic" because of their psychopathology and reported experiences. These factors combine to leave the victims particularly vulnerable to further abuse or to be disregarded by systems designed to provide protection or help for them (i.e., the legal system, the psychotherapeutic community, and children's protective services).

Case Description

Because the documentation of ritual abuse in the area of family violence is relatively recent and little information has appeared in the professional literature, I would like to describe three brief case studies. These cases illustrate different problems that the clinician may encounter in understanding and treating cases in which allegations of ritual abuse are made. I have chosen cases to represent a range of ages (preschool age, latency-adolescent, and adult), psychopathologies, and various systems' responses to allegations of ritual abuse. Case 1 is of a preschool-age child whose "bizarre" statements led authorities to dismiss his allegations of sexual abuse by his father. His statements were seen as merely reflecting an "active 3-year-old imagination." Case 2 describes the course of treatment of an adolescent who was placed in a foster home. There was consensus about the validity of her statements, and all systems intervened to protect her. Case 3 describes the treatment of an adult suffering from multiple personality disorder who describes being raised by a family high in the hierarchy of a satanic cult. No legal actions were taken.

Case 1

Matthew was 4½ when he was first referred for evaluation and treatment by another clinical psychologist. Matthew's parents divorced when he was an infant. Matthew's mother immediately requested monitoring of visits with his father because the father's behavior had seemed to her to be bizarre, paranoid, and hostile. When Matthew was 3 years of age, unmonitored visits with his father were ordered by the courts. Matthew's mother noticed increasingly wild behavior after visits. Matthew was uncontrollable and would run away from people. He than began having nightmares and refused to sleep alone. However, he continued to agree to visits with his father. He was rarely excited about visits but reportedly went submissively. He then spontaneously stated to his mother that, "my daddy eats my pee pee." She was alarmed by this statement and asked him what he said. He repeated his statement several times. She then asked if he was lying, and Matthew became upset. She called a social worker whom she and her ex-husband had seen for therapy.

The social worker saw Matthew for a sexual abuse interview and began seeing him in psychotherapy. Over the course of treatment, Matthew made a number of other statements. He described his father's eating "poopee" and making him do so as well. He talked about "monsters" and "guns" and "cutting people's heads off," and finally said that the "monsters killed and ate a baby." The local children's protective services gave the mother information about satanic cults, and she became alarmed that this was what Matthew was describing. The family was then referred for a court-ordered evaluation at a local university with an excellent reputation. The evaluation team was divided in its opinions but finally decided (after 1 day of testing and interviews with the family) that there was little substantive basis for concluding that any type of abuse had occurred. The final consensus was that Matthew's talk of feces and urine was consistent with his age and that his mother had probably been unintentionally "feeding" information about sexual abuse to him, thereby "programming" him to make allegations against his father. Children's protective services then dismissed the case and custody was granted to the father. Matthew's mother has been fighting for what she perceives to be the protection of her son in the civil court since then. When I saw Matthew for treatment approximately 1 year later, he appeared an extremely anxious and guarded child. He spontaneously (and compulsively) demonstrated oral-genital contact in play. In addition, he played out themes of defecating and urinating on people, eating feces, shooting people, and cutting off limbs. He stated that his father had done these things, but he would not elaborate with much detail. He repeatedly stated that "the monsters" would kill him, his mother, and me if he told me more. He also stated that the "magic eye" could see everything that he did. These fears persisted over many months of treatment, although separation anxiety and sleep problems and nightmares gradually diminished. However, each time I questioned him about details, the symptoms were exacerbated.

Case 2

Theresa is a 14-year-old who has been living in a foster home since the age of 11. She described being orphaned and cared for by a family member who had inexplicably left when she was first interviewed by authorities. During the course of a hospitalization for acute abdominal pain, she was found to have both anal and vaginal scarring, symptomatic of chronic sexual abuse. When questioned about this sexual abuse, she described events that sounded as if she were being used as a prostitute. She described being drugged, photographed nude, and molested by multiple people. She also stated that she had never attended school or had free contacts with peers. She also described attempting to run away, but said that "they always found me."

Approximately 6 months after her case was originally reported to protective services, her therapist began questioning her about unusual symptoms her foster parents had reported. These symptoms included an aversion to knives (Theresa refused to touch knives and would leave the room if asked to cut anything), intense nightmares from which she would awaken with bloodcurdling screams, a fear of being outside in front of the house, and an aversion to eating meat.

Over the course of the next 6 months, Theresa began to fill in more details of her experiences. She was at first terrified and kept repeating, "I'm not supposed to tell." However, her therapist had seen other victims of satanic cults and was suspicious that Theresa was hiding far more than she had been willing to report. With gentle prodding and reassurances that she would be believed and would be safe if she talked about what had happened to her, Theresa gradually became comfortable enough to allow her tale to unfold. She described being given by her family to the cult at the age of 5. She talked about being punished with "fire needles" for any infraction of their rules, being told she was now a "child of Satan" who belonged to him and would never be free. She described being passed among cult members for sexual use at night and began to talk about cult ceremonies. Theresa first described animal sacrifices and then human sacrifices. She talked about how participants in the rituals drank the blood and ate the flesh of those they slaughtered. She described with particular horror having to stab babies during ceremonies and also described making "snuff" movies, in which she killed other children after performing sexual acts with them. These disclosures were each followed by a series of dreams, repeated over many nights, in which she relived the experiences. These "dreams" had a similar quality to those reported by adult victims of posttraumatic stress, in that, when someone awakened her, she believed herself to be reexperiencing the trauma. Although her openness about these experiences grew, she remained careful about not revealing any information (i.e., names, locations) that she felt would put her or her foster family in jeopardy. Several times she mentioned that some people she saw on evening television news shows who were being tried on drug, molestation, or murder charges were familiar to her from the group.

Over the course of her treatment she has shown a number of symptoms of posttraumatic stress disorder. These include auditory and visual hallucinations and flashbacks. She has major sleep disturbances (for which she has been medicated), self-inflicted injuries (an E Coli bacteria found in feces has been cultured from frequent infected sites), social adjustment difficulties relating to her entry into new family and school environments, and emotional problems including anxiety and depression. She also has a sense of foreshortened future, described by Terr (1983) as symptomatic of children who faced severe trauma and fear of death. Theresa remains convinced that the group will abduct her at some future time and is doubtful that she will be free to live a "normal" life.

Case 3

The third case, that of Leslie (age 34), involves an individual who was amnesic for experiences of satanic abuse by members of her family until adulthood. Leslie entered treatment for problems with depression, social isolation, and low self-esteem. She was able to function adequately in her job as a medical office manager but found herself disturbed inexplicably by cases involving severe child abuse. She reported that when these cases were seen in the office, she would have what she first described as "spells," after which she would become amnesic for what occurred. Prior to the "spells," Leslie reported the altered perception of seeing her surroundings as being at a great distance. Medical work-ups for the symptoms were all negative. During the course of her therapy, it became clear that these "spells" were dissociative episodes precipitated by contact with issues of child abuse. After the death of her mother (whom she later remembered as a cult leader), Leslie began to recover memories of her own past, which had previously been a blank for her. She began to recall being physically tortured, starved, and imprisoned in a box, as well as being urinated on and defecated on. As she began recalling, other personalities emerged who had memories of events and feelings of which Leslie was unaware. Some personalities remembered giving birth to infants who were sacrificed when they were approximately 1 month and 28 months of age. On the anniversary of one of their deaths, a box containing a dead animal was mailed to her. Leslie felt that this was a warning that she should not divulge the secrets of the group. She also reported that on a number of occasions, her brother, whom she believed to be a high-ranking member of the cult, would track her down, beat her, and threaten her. This occurred despite her attempts to keep her address unknown to him.

Medical Issues

Patients with a history of satanic abuse are at high risk for developing a number of medical problems, including sequelae of physical trauma, psychosomatic disorders, sleep disturbances, substance abuse, self-mutilating behaviors that may be conscious or unconscious, suicide, and sexual dysfunctions. Thorough medical evaluation and competent medical treatment are essential concomitants to psychotherapy. In addition, medication for symptoms of anxiety, depression, hallucinations, or sleep disturbances may be useful.

Many patients describe severe physical trauma resulting from beatings, deprivation, and sexual abuse that may require medical attention. Theresa experienced multiple episodes of abdominal pain and weakness and swelling of her joints and limbs. This condition was diagnosed as reflex neurovascular dystrophy and may have been at least partially caused by injuries sustained during beatings. Psychological factors undoubtedly were also present, since Theresa reported being allowed a respite from sexual activities when she had the same symptoms during her time with the cult.

Children may also be worried that they are physically damaged or still have something inside them. Matthew was convinced that his father had put "poopee" in his rectum and that it was still there. He was reassured when a physician told him that he was "normal" and "clean." Theresa was convinced for almost a year that a "tracking device" was implanted in her. She reported seeing "operations" performed on others and was told that these devices were being "installed." Other children report fears of many other things being inside them, including bombs and insects. These fears may be somewhat allayed by the attention of a physician. Although her entire body had been X-rayed, Theresa was not entirely certain that the physicians might just have failed to detect the implanted device.

Psychosomatic disorders that may be precipitated by stress or have a symbolic value often occur. Matthew developed a rash after describing what his father had done to him. Theresa regularly developed physical symptoms (nausea, severe abdominal pain, night terrors, and fatigue) at the anniversary dates of significant events (dates of major satanic feasts, dates of the killing of her relatives).

Patients abused in satanic cults almost universally report severe problems with sleep disturbances and nightmares, and many describe hallucinatory and flashback episodes. They will often avoid sleep because of the dreams. Soporific or antidepressant medications may assist the patients to sleep, although they do not appear to change the quality of their dreams. Patients often will report hallucinations (i.e., hearing voices—often threatening or commanding them) that are extremely disturbing to them. They may be reluctant to admit to hallucinating experiences for fear of being labeled as "crazy" or because they believe that such voices are spirits (i.e., Satan) talking to them. Moreover, they are fearful of breaking the cult's code of secrecy. Although Theresa "heard" members of the Cult talking to her every night, she did not report this in therapy because "they tell me not to talk to you." She also reported that they told her "not to listen to you or do what you say" and that "I belong to Satan." Similarly, Matthew believed that he was visited by "evil spirits" at night. Having his mother pray with him offered him reassurances that "Jesus is in my heart, protecting me." Many patients report that antipsychotic medications do not help these symptoms and merely make them feel "drugged." Many are reluctant about taking any drugs since they report being drugged by the cult. Medications may also trigger memories of past experiences. Similarly, with the affective symptoms of anxiety and depression, each case must be individually considered to determine if medication would be helpful. A trial period of medication prescribed by an experienced psychiatrist may be helpful.

Caution must be exercised in the use of any medications, however, because survivors of ritualistic groups may tend to overmedicate themselves with prescription drugs; adults may have a tendency to self-medicate with alcohol or other substances in an effort to relieve themselves of the pain (both emotional and physical) that they feel.

Legal Issues

Cases involving suspicion of ritual abuse can involve a number of complicated and difficult legal issues during the course of treatment. Some issues, such as the importance of confidentiality and privilege of information, are typical of all therapy cases but are of particular significance in ritual abuse. Because of the extreme nature of the threats, patients must feel that their disclosures will not be openly discussed. This is often a matter of life and death in their view. The intense fears of "telling what I'm not supposed to" may frequently be opposed to the clinician's credo of being obligated to report suspicion of child abuse to authorities. Further complications often result from the victim's experience and/or beliefs that authority figures, such as policemen, judges, and doctors, were members of the group. In many cases this may be true, but in other cases it is staged to procure the child's silence. Either way, patients need to be reassured by the therapist, who must model confidence, that some crimes that they are disclosing need to be reported so that the authorities have a record of them and can protect both the patients and other potential victims. Reporting can also provide a healthy "empowering" experience for patients.

Unfortunately, such "protection" is often not the outcome of reporting the suspicion of abuse. When I have called police agencies to report alleged murders within their jurisdiction, I have often been put on "hold" on the telephone and then had supervisors talk to me and say that they will "look into the matter," but go on to say that they have not as yet had "missing persons reports" and so would not be likely to pursue the issue. This is unfortunately a common experience for therapists involved in these cases as well as for police investigators. Sandi

Gallant, a San Francisco police detective, has described these problems (see Kahaner, 1988). Cases involving ritual abuse allegations produce multiple dilemmas for therapists. Patients describe crimes that often must be reported (e.g., child sexual abuse), but authorities often disbelieve therapist (and patient) reports. This creates dilemmas when therapists who report these cases are dismissed by police agencies, who may have little or no experience with such types of crimes.

Prosecuting ritualistic abuse cases presents further difficulties for police agencies and the legal system. Participating in a satanic religion is not a crime, since freedom of religion is protected under the First Amendment of the United States Constitution. Some ritualistic activities described by survivors certainly do constitute criminal activities (i.e., animal and human killings, child sexual and physical abuse, kidnapping). However, it is often difficult to prove that they occurred, and corroborative physical proof is often unavailable. Typically, bodies used in rituals are not found. Many survivors explain that this is because remains are cremated in a mortuary, saved for future ceremonies, or buried in remote places. However, the fact that physical evidence (bodies, pornographic pictures) are not found often leads investigators to discount the claims of victims. When bodies *are* found with evidence suggesting satanic ritual involvement, this aspect of the case is often downplayed or ignored in criminal proceedings. For example, although Richard Ramirez, the "Night Stalker," left satanic symbols in his victim's homes and shouted, "Hail, Satan," after a hearing in court, the issue of satanic cult involvement has not been an important aspect of the court case and has not been highly publicized. Unfortunately, such lack of prosecution and/or publicity results in a lack of public awareness of the full implications of the crimes involved or of how frequently satanic cult-related crimes occur.

Similarly, when the victim is a child, the child's claims that he or she was forced to eat feces or drink blood, saw hooded figures dancing or chanting, saw someone shot, stabbed, or hanged on a cross are often dismissed as "childhood fantasies" or as "something they saw on TV or in a movie." These statements tend to impeach the child's testimony and provide fertile ground for the defense attorney's cross-examinations. This may leave vulnerable and unprotected the child who was assaulted by someone within the family, even if there is clear medical evidence that sexual abuse occurred (as in the case of Matthew). Although Matthew's spontaneous statements about sexual abuse initially led professionals and authorities to believe him, his later statements about seeing someone shot, eating feces, and seeing a baby killed led authorities to attribute his statements to "an active 3-year-old imagination" and to his mother's "programming" him.

However, highly publicized cases of ritual abuse in Canada (Marron, 1988) and another Florida case (Hollingsworth, 1986) resulted in a number of sensitive and innovative changes being made in how child victims were allowed to testify in court. These may well provide guidelines for protecting child victims in future cases.

Social and Family Issues

Over the past 20 years, there has been a growing awareness and recognition among the professional communities of psychotherapists, social workers, and police agencies about the various forms of intrafamilial violence, including child physical abuse (first identified by Henry Kempe, M.D., in the 1960s as the battered child syndrome), the battered women's syndrome and rape recognition, supported by the women's movement of the 1970s, and child sexual abuse. Russell's (1983) pioneering research led to the recognition of how widespread a problem it was when her data revealed that 33% of women had experienced some form of sexual abuse before the age of 18 and that 2.5% had experienced incestual relationships. In each of these three areas (child physical abuse, child sexual abuse, rape, and the battered wife syndrome), there has been a tendency for both professionals and our society to initially recoil from an awareness that these problems commonly exist. It has only been after careful professional documentation, laws requiring reporting, and professional education about how to recognize and treat these family disorders that both professionals and the society as a whole have begun to accept and recognize their widespread existence. We cannot see or recognize a problem that we do not know about or acknowledge exists and that we do not know how to identify. It is only after professionals begin to identify and document the existence of a disorder that a more widespread understanding of the problem among both professionals and the society becomes possible. The area of ritual abuse is currently in this initial stage, where it is just beginning to be identified and treated in the professional community. This is not to say that it is a "new" social problem. As with all other forms of abuse, its history extends for centuries. It is not new, but it is newly recognized and accepted among a growing number of professionals. No doubt the more that becomes known and documented about ritual abuse, the more professionals and society will become willing and able to identify it.

However, this may be the most optimistic view, that as our knowledge increases, our skill in recognizing or identifying the cases of ritual abuse will increase and a general societal awareness will follow.

It is important to recognize the operation of a second factor—denial. An almost universal first response to being told about how a patient participated in or witnessed animal slaughters, the murder and rape of infants and/or adults, and the consumption of blood, flesh, urine, and feces is to recoil from the horror of their description and experience, and to say to ourselves, "This can't be true." We may then go on to say, "This patient must be delusional/psychotic/lying/must have read this in a book/saw this in a movie and is testing me to see if I'll believe this preposterous story." Such experience of denial is further strengthened if patients go on to describe spiritual experiences (e.g., seeing Satan or demons appear during ceremonies and hearing Satan talk to them). This is the realm of horror movies and nightmares, not of psychotherapy with *our* patients in *our* own offices. Our initial response is to make a psychiatric referral for some effective psychotropic medications. To accept that our patient may have had these experiences in our town with people we may know is often too threatening to accept initially. It is easy to acknowledge that psychopathic killers like Charles Manson, Richard Ramirez (the "Night Stalker"), or David Berkowitz ("Son of Sam") engage in brutal murders, but to believe that we may be encountering some form of this can keep us denying the reality of what the patient is saying rather than accepting it as true or even possibly true. I have struggled with these issues myself over the past years. I have found myself wanting "proof" that was not forthcoming before I would apply a label of "ritual abuse" to these unusual experiences that both children and adults whom I was seeing in my practice were describing. I found it bizarre when children described mock marriages to "a bad Jesus" or "Satan" and described goats being killed and drinking blood and being urinated on. Although I had seen child and adult victims for many years, I remained confused by what was described. This factor of denial operates in society as a whole as well as in communities, within agencies, among professionals, and within families. When a victim makes claims about having been ritualistically abused, people tend to polarize into those who believe the claims and those who do not. The "believers" (whether in the victim's family, in the community, or among professionals working with the victim) tend to be described in a number of pejorative ways (hysterical, naive, overreacting, unscientific, nonprofessional, troublemakers, "gone off the deep end").

What happened in Matthew's case is a good illustration of this. Matthew's mother was initially viewed as overreacting to "statements a 3-year-old makes" by her own family. Although her family later came to believe that she was correct, the children's protective agency felt she was "brainwashing Matthew" and believed the therapist who reported the abuse to be "naively taken in" by Matthew's accusations. The community became polarized into supporters of Matthew's mother versus supporters of his father.

Butler (1978) has documented this effect well. She states that those who try to tell are commanded to silence, and that those people who dare to believe the victims and to help them tell receive the same treatment. The more heinous the crime, the more pressure to keep the secret. We want to deny what victims of ritual abuse are saying, and we want to deny that those who do believe them are correct. In order to clearly understand and help these victims, it is imperative that we push aside the veil that denial and deception drop and carefully listen to and evaluate what they are describing. We must learn to listen to what we do not want to hear and to understand what we do not want to know.

Assessment of Psychopathology

The identification of the type of abuse experienced is a crucial initial step in assessing the psychopathology of the patient. It is important to recognize certain behavioral indicators that may differentiate victims of "typical" sexual abuse from those who also experienced ritual abuse. Sgroi (1982) has described a number of behavioral indicators of childhood sexual abuse. These include overcompliance or aggressive acting-out, pseudomaturity, hints of sexual activity or persistent play with toys and peers reflecting sexual knowledge beyond that expected, poor peer relationships and lack of participation in social activities, difficulties with concentration, school performance, fears of men, seductive behavior, regressed or withdrawn behavior, and depression and suicidal feelings. These symptoms are often present, if in different forms at times, in adult victims as well as in victims of ritual abuse. In addition, the latter victims often show additional symptoms that are not typical of victims of other types of sexual abuse and that may help to differentiate the type of abuse to which they were exposed. Some of these symptoms have been documented (Gould, 1987, personal communication). In young children these symptoms may include preoccupation or play with urine or feces, passing gas, and mutilation themes in play (i.e., the child acts out severing limbs or head, or removing body parts or parts of the face). The child talks of animals being killed or mutilated, is preoccupied with death or dying, particularly on birthdays, fears that foreign objects are inside his body (i.e., insects, a bomb, a microphone), shows unusual fears of going to jail, ghosts, monsters, "bad people," is preoccupied with the devil, supernatural powers, crucifixions, numbers, phases of the moon, makes unusual references to people in scary costumes (monsters, ghosts, devils, Dracula, clowns), describes sexual activity with other children or multiple adults, asks unusual questions about eating people, feces, drinking blood, and makes unusual drawings (figures with horns, Satanic symbols).

As some of these behavioral indicators of both sexual or ritual abuse are observable in normal as well as abused children, they should not be taken, by themselves, as being diagnostic of ritual abuse. However, when they are observed to occur with great frequency or intensity in a child where there are few other explanations (i.e., family psycho-pathology, intensely religious background), the clinician would be well advised to explore the issues further.

In questioning children (or adults) about ritual abuse it is necessary for the clinician to be aware of both legal and clinical implications. In general, it is crucial that the questioning be done in a nonleading fashion that does not provide detailed information to the patient. Similarly, questioning should be done in a neutral fashion that does not imply that one answer is "right" and another "wrong." Sgroi (1982) and Mac-Farlane and Waterman (1986) both include excellent chapters about ap-propriate interviewing techniques for suspected cases of child sexual abuse. The clinician should be thoroughly familiar with these techniques before attempting any interviews that could have complicated legal and clinical ramifications. Similarly, it is also good clinical practice to seek consultation with another professional experienced with ritual abuse when it is suspected that this issue may be involved in a case.

The clinical assessment of older children and adults is somewhat less complicated, in that they are developmentally more capable of de-scribing their experiences and are less likely to be viewed as highly suggestible in court cases. However, they may be just as fearful of talk-ing as young children. Theresa did not explain much about her life experiences until she had been away from the group for more than 6 months. Similarly, adults may be unable to recall their experiences in cases where significant dissociation is present. Unusual fears or con-cerns of adults often provide clues to the possibility of experiences of ritual abuse. These include excessive aversion to guns, knives, blood, eating red meat, churches, Satan, or dead animals. Unusual concerns may include a conviction that they are bad or evil, have "lost their soul," or have been "given to Satan." These symptoms in older children or adults should also be explored further, since they are possible indicators that the patient has been exposed to ritual abuse.

When a determination is made that a patient has been ritualistically abused, an assessment of the consequent psychopathology is important, since this will determine treatment strategies and options. Sexual vic-timization alone will usually result in a configuration of issues that are produced by the experience. These include the "damaged goods" syn-drome, guilt, fear, depression, low self-esteem, and poor social skills. Additional issues that also should be clinically assessed include re-pressed anger and hostility, impaired ability to trust, role confusion, and problems with self-mastery and control. Sgroi (1982) and MacFarlane and Waterman (1986) both discuss the assessment of these areas of concern in victims of child sexual abuse.

These issues are all relevant for victims of ritual abuse and should be assessed. Often, because of the more extreme and perverse nature of the sexual activities, threats, and the victim's participation in physical mutilation and/or murder, some issues (i.e., fear, guilt) are more intense than for other victims.

Other areas that should be assessed are more unique to victims of ritual abuse. These include (1) confusion about values, (2) a deep mistrust of authority figures and social structures, (3) concerns of a spiritual nature, (4) fears of being abducted or killed by the cult, and (5) concerns about being "different" and forever "unacceptable."

Survivors report that many cults preach that self-indulgence and obedience to "Satan's ways" are good while traditional social values are "false" or "weak." Similarly, survivors may have been told that their pain is good for them and that Satan wants it. The conflict between these cult values and those of society leaves the survivor confused and lacking a basic ethical system that most people have internalized. Similarly, because survivors report that many authority figures (judges, doctors, policemen, pastors) were members of the cult, it is often difficult for victims to trust others in these roles. Spiritual matters are of great concern to victims. They may feel that they are being watched or threatened by evil spiritual forces or demons and often find it hard to believe in a God. Theresa repeatedly asked how anyone could believe in God when so many bad things happen in the world. Many survivors also have experienced such intense threats and experiences of helplessness and victimization that it is difficult for them to develop a sense of security and confidence in their own ability to develop a productive lifestyle. They may remain fearful that the cult will reappear at any moment. They may have little or no confidence that they could refuse to return and still live. Finally, survivors have often been told that they are worthless and will always be unacceptable to others. This threat, along with the knowledge of the acts they have committed, leads to their feeling cut off from others and also to their sense of being "damaged goods."

All of these issues should be accurately assessed in anyone suspected of having been ritualistically abused because addressing and resolving these issues will form the basis for treatment and recovery.

Making an accurate clinical diagnosis is also important and will determine the type of treatment. Many victims of ritual abuse suffer from some form of posttraumatic stress disorder. Dissociation and hallucinations may be present. Among both adults and children, multiple personality disorders may result. These diagnoses and subsequent treatment will be discussed in the next section.

Treatment Options

The type of treatment that will be most effective for any victim of ritual abuse must always be determined on an individual basis, taking into account the patient's age, the degree of involvement in ritual practices and abuse, and the degree and type of psychopathology involved. However, there are some general guidelines that seem to apply to all cases. The length of treatment necessary will increase for patients with more intense or lengthy involvement and with more severe psychopathology. In general, long-term intensive individual psychotherapy is necessary to help most patients recover from their experiences. With young children, play therapy focused on their experiences and feelings is usually effective. With adolescents and adults, individual therapy also focusing on their memories of what happened and feelings about themselves and others is called for. Most victims of ritual abuse will show evidence of posttraumatic stress disorder, and many victims of intense and/or lengthy involvement will show evidence of multiple personality disorder. When the latter diagnosis is made, specialized treatment techniques that involve having the various "personalities" come to know one another, share memories and feelings, value one another's special strengths and needs, and finally "integrate" into a single functioning unit are called for. Klupft (1985) has described the identification and treatment of this disorder. When this diagnosis is made or suspected, such patients are best seen by a psychotherapist with special training and experience. Treatment should not be attempted by therapists without this expertise.

During the course of treatment, a number of issues must be addressed. As in any psychotherapy, the necessary climate of trust, respect, and empathy must be established before the psychotherapeutic process can begin. The first issue that must be addressed is the patients' intense fear of telling their secrets. Unless the fears are addressed and alleviated (at least to some extent), they cannot begin to describe their concerns. Similarly, unless the patients feel that they will be believed and that the therapist will not be shocked or judgmental about what they are describing, they cannot be free to talk. These issues can all be addressed by the therapist's establishing himself/herself as someone who has seen many people who were afraid to talk about what they had experienced but who were eventually helped by becoming able to do this. Sgroi (1982) has described the importance of this therapeutic stance in the treatment of child sexual abuse. When the patient begins to describe the abuse which was experienced, disclosures often follow a hierarchy of least to most gruesome. Physical abuse and neglect are first described, and then sexual abuse. It is usually later in treatment that patients describe rituals with animal killings, then urine and feces. The sacrifice of humans is often described later and may be followed by the patient's acknowledgment of his/her own participation in such killings. Describing feelings that they have seen or heard Satan is often most threatening and usually appears last. As children often describe how they "heard these things from someone else" or "saw it happen to someone else" or "dreamed that these things happened" before they will acknowledge that it happened to them, these minimizing statements should not be accepted at face value but should be explored further. For example, Matthew would play out scenes from his memories, but when asked if he had seen that happen, he at first said, "I'm not sure if I remember that," and only later talked about what "really happened" to him. Similarly, adult victims of ritual abuse may have blocked or repressed most conscious memories of what occurred, and may be puzzled and troubled by symptoms that are triggered by sights, smells, or circumstances. They may not know how the symptoms are connected to past events and must be helped in treatment to uncover the connection for themselves. An adult victim described this in a newsletter published by *Believe the Children* (1988), a self-help organization for parents of children who have made allegations of ritual abuse:

> There are certain things survivors, whether adults or children, endure and experience. The sight of an animal that has been hit on the road can throw me into a panic. Things trigger memories. When something triggers a memory, my behavior becomes erratic. I will start crying for no reason, or become horribly afraid. Often a memory comes out of it, other times nothing.

Some of the common "triggers" that patients describe include blood (including menstrual blood), dead animals, people dressed in dark colors or costumes, times of the year associated with satanic holidays and phases of the moon (rituals often occur during the full moon), and a fear of drug-induced states, spiders, and other bugs.

A number of issues about the patients' feelings about themselves must also be addressed over the course of treatment. These issues include shame, guilt, and feelings of being bad, evil, and unworthy of love. Problems often stemming from these feelings must also be assessed and addressed. These include alcohol/drug abuse and self-mutilating or suicidal thoughts or feelings.

Finally, their experiences of abuse often make it difficult to trust others and to form close relationships. Sexual dysfunctions are often commonly described. These issues must also be addressed in treatment.

Overall, the victim must be helped to regain or establish positive feelings about their own identity and a sense of optimism about being able to go forward in a healing and productive life.

Finally, it is beneficial for the therapist to use as many other resources as possible. Noninvolved parents should be included as a valuable and integral part of the treatment (and will often benefit from their own treatment). With child victims, noninvolved parents can become the most effective treatment resource for the child when they can be included as cotherapists. This may be precluded in cases in which the parent is viewed by the court system as influencing the child to make allegations. Other sources of support can be found in social workers and police who may be involved. Ministers, priests, and religious communities are often invaluable resources in dealing with spiritual issues outside of the realm of psychotherapy. Theresa was greatly reassured after being told by priests and nuns that she was a child of God and not of Satan, and Leslie in times of crisis stayed with a nun in a convent and gained a sense of security and belonging from her.

Summary and Conclusions

In the past 5 years, allegations of ritual abuse from hundreds of children in cases across North America against teachers and other school personnel, parents, and neighbors have left a storm of controversy in their wake. They have also raised the issue of how widespread ritual abuse, or groups using its trappings, may be. There are striking similarities among the cases, in what children describe, in therapists' impressions, and in the eventual outcome in the courts. Although many individuals have been investigated and/or charged, few cases have been tried in court. Typically, a lack of corroborative physical evidence (i.e., photographs, bodies, traces of blood) contributed to the children's allegations being discounted.

In Manhattan Beach, California, seven teachers were originally indicted in March 1984 in conjunction with the McMartin case. Although the judge ruled at the end of a preliminary hearing in 1986 that all seven should be tried, the newly elected Los Angeles district attorney, Ira Reiner, dismissed charges against five of them, stating that evidence against them was "incredibly weak." Although more than 5 years had passed since the original charges were made, the trial on charges against two remaining defendants resulted in an aquittal on most counts. Members of the jury stated that, although they believed some of the children were molested, the prosecution had not proved "beyond a reasonable doubt" that the defendants were guilty. Charges were then refiled for three children on whose counts the first jury could not agree, and a second trial began in April of 1990. The jury for the second trial also failed to deliver a verdict and reach an agreement on any of the counts. In a large-scale investigation of other preschools in the Manhattan Beach area, scores of other adults were alleged by children to have molested and photographed them, killed animals in their presence, threatened them with death, and performed mock ceremonies in homes and churches. Some children also described murders. Five other preschools closed or were closed, but the investigation resulted in the trial of only one defendant. The jury was unable to reach a decision and the case was not retried. However, the Los Angeles chief of police, Sherman Block, made a public statement that there was evidence to believe that hundreds of children had been sexually molested. In Bakersfield, California, 9 arrests were made and 21 children were removed from their homes. One defendant was convicted and two other defendants pleaded guilty, but charges against all others were dropped because of insufficient evidence. In Jordon, Minnesota, police arrested a 26-year-old garbage collector who had four prior sexual abuse convictions, and charged him with molesting two children. The investigation uncovered a number of other children who described being molested by parents, friends, and relatives who appeared to be part of a sex ring. By the summer of 1984, 24 arrests were made. The trial of the first defendants ended in acquittals, and one of the victims in cross-examination stated he had lied during the direct examination. During this investigation children also described ritual abuse, and some said they had seen murders. The original defendant pleaded guilty, but eventually all charges against the remaining defendants were dropped. The FBI and the Minnesota Bureau of Criminal Apprehension investigated the case and concluded that "cross-germination" or passing of information among victims discredited their statements. Another report issued by a special panel appointed by the governor of Minnesota stated that some of the cases could have been successfully prosecuted. They concluded that "those defendants who were guilty went free and those who were innocent were left without the opportunity to clear their names" (Moss, 1987). In Rogers Park, Illinois, a janitor was arrested and charged with molesting children in a Jewish community center. Twenty-five children alleged that he had molested them and ultimately made 246 allegations of abuse, which included a number of other adults at the center. These children also described ritual abuse and then the murder of babies. However, the janitor was acquitted and no other charges were filed.

What is happening in these cases in which ritual abuse allegations are made? Clearly the courts have had difficulty in drawing conclusions. It appears that the children's bizarre allegations of abuse have been difficult for judges and juries to accept "beyond a reasonable doubt," which is the necessary criterion in criminal courts. The lack of any corroborative physical evidence (i.e., photographs, bodies) has for many posed additional questions about the children's credibility. In each of these cases, however, police investigators were criticized for not doing more thorough and immediate searches. In each of the cases, some children have also made statements that were proved to be untrue or that they later recanted.

What should we make of this? Do these cases represent a national mass hysteria where otherwise sensible adults are believing exaggerated statements and fantasies of young children? This is the view of Ralph Underwager, a psychiatrist who testified as an expert witness for the defense in a number of these cases. He is quoted in Marron (1988): "This information comes from the fantasy world of children. It will come out when gullible adults, predisposed to belief in a Satanic conspiracy theory, delve into the children's fantasies producing more and more allegations that they reinforce with their belief. . .. What we are trying to fight is stupidity on such a massive scale." If this is true, then scores of innocent adults have been wrongfully charged. This view, however, does not explain why so many of the alleged victims had physical evidence of sexual abuse.

Another possibility is that these cases are at their core conventional instances of sexual abuse in which exaggerated claims were made by the victims. Repeated criticism of interviews of the children in all of these cases is that they were suggestive, excessively demanding of information, and reinforced the children's disclosures, or that too many interviews were done. Forrest Lattimer, a defense attorney in the McMartin trial, feels that the children are playing a game of "Can You Top This?" "If one kid said they slapped a rabbit, the next kid had the rabbit's ears cut off, and the next kid said the rabbit was cut up altogether. The next kid said, 'that's nothing, they took me to a farm and killed a horse.' Another said, 'well, they took me in a hot air balloon'" (Moss, 1987).

If this explanation is true, it does not explain why the children in all of the cases seem to describe such similar events (animal killings, eating feces or flesh, being stuck with pins or sticks, mock ceremonies in homes or churches, the killing of babies) or why the disclosures in all of the cases seem to follow the same pattern (i.e., first describing sexual abuse, then animal killings, then ritual abuse, then the murder of babies). Therapists who treated children in such cases all have described this pattern to me. Also, the therapists have found the children to be credible, in that these disclosures are accompanied by genuine distress and are often followed by periods of disruptive behavior, nightmares, and increased fears. Moreover, symptoms have often persisted for months and years. Similarly, the children's descriptions also match quite closely the descriptions of events given by adult survivors of ritual abuse.

Are they all exaggerating? If there is truth to their statements, the worst case scenario is, that the ritual abuse of children, or the abuse of children by groups using the trappings of rituals, is far more widespread and lethal than is commonly imagined. Ritual abuse may not be readily identified, and if identified not readily believed, and if believed not readily prosecuted. We may hope that, over the next few years, some of the confusion will clear as we learn more through continued research and treatment.

References

Believe the Children Newsletter. (1988). Manhattan Beach, 7, 1–4.

Butler, S. (1978). *Conspiracy of silence: The trauma of incest.* San Francisco: New Glide Publications.

Hollingsworth, J. (1986). *Unspeakable acts.* New York: Congdon & Weed.

Kahaner, L. (1988). *Cults that kill.* New York: Warner Books.

Kelly, S. (1988). *Ritual abuse.* Paper presented at the National Symposium on Child Victimization, Anaheim, CA.

Kent, C. (1988). *Presenting symptoms and three-year followup data on children alleging abuse during pre-school years in multi-victim, multi-perpetrator circumstances.* Paper presented at the National Symposium on Child Victimization, Anaheim, CA.

Klupft, P. (1985). The treatment of multiple personality disorder. Current concepts. *Directions in Psychiatry, 5,* 1–9.

MacFarlane, K., & Waterman, J. (Eds.). (1986). *Sexual abuse of young children.* New York: Guilford Press.

Marron, K. (1988). *Ritual abuse.* Toronto: McClelland-Bantam.

McCord, J., Waterman, J., Oliveri, M., and Kelly, R. (1990). *Ritualistic and non-ritualistic sexual abuse of preschoolers: A comparison of symptom patterns throughout treatment.* Paper presented at the 1990 National Symposium on Child Victimization, Atlanta, GA.

Moss, D. C. (1987). Are the children lying? *American Bar Association Journal.*

Pazder, L. (1980). *Ritual abuse.* Paper presented at the American Psychiatric Association, New Orleans.

Russell, D. E. H. (1983). The incidence and prevalence of intrafamilial and extrafamilial sexual abuse of female children. *Child Abuse and Neglect, 7,* 133–146.

Sgroi, S. (1982). *Handbook of clinical intervention in child sexual abuse.* Lexington, MA: D. C. Heath.

Smith, M., & Pazder, L. (1980). *Michelle remembers.* New York: Congdon & Lattes.

Terr, L. C. (1983). Chochilla revisited: The effects of psychic trauma four years after a school-bus kidnapping. *American Journal of Psychiatry, 140,* 1543–1550.

Terry, M. (1987). *The ultimate evil.* New York: Doubleday.

13

Maltreatment of Handicapped Children

Robert T. Ammerman, Martin J. Lubetsky, and Karen F. Drudy

Description of the Problem

As professional and public awareness of the problem of child maltreatment expands, increased attention is being directed toward abuse and neglect of handicapped children. Indeed, in the initial stages of controlled empirical research on child maltreatment, several authors speculated that handicapped children are at greater risk for abuse and neglect relative to their nonhandicapped peers (Helfer, 1973; Solomons, 1979). This belief was derived, in large part, from the growing literature reporting a disproportionate number of handicapped individuals in samples of abused and neglected children (e.g., Birrell & Birrell, 1968; Lightcap, Kurland, & Burgess, 1982). Methodological shortcomings in much of this literature, however, have prompted some authors to reject the link between handicap and subsequent maltreatment (Starr, Dietrich, Fischhoff, Ceresnie, & Zweier, 1984). In contrast, others have acknowledged the relative paucity of and methodological limitations in much of the research conducted to date, but argue that there are compelling reasons to suspect that a significant number of handicapped children are at

Robert T. Ammerman • Department of Research and Clinical Psychology, Western Pennsylvania School for Blind Children, Pittsburgh, Pennsylvania 15213.   Martin J. Lubetsky and Karen F. Drudy • John Merck Program, Western Psychiatric Institute and Clinic, University of Pittsburgh School of Medicine, Pittsburgh, Pennsylvania 15213.

heightened risk for maltreatment in general, and physical abuse in particular (Ammerman, Van Hasselt, & Hersen, 1988).

Most theoretical models of child abuse and neglect outline the contribution of certain child characteristics to the etiology of maltreatment
(see Ammerman, 1989). In general, these factors consist of severe behavior problems (e.g., oppositionality, aggression, defiance) or variables
that often elicit negative reactions from caregivers (e.g., prolonged crying). The relationship between handicap and maltreatment is based
upon the similarity between hypothesized "abuse-provoking" behaviors
of some maltreated children (deLissovoy, 1979) and those often exhibited by children with disabling conditions.

Ammerman, Van Hasselt, and Hersen, (1988) describe three processes whereby handicapped children are at heightened risk for maltreatment: (1) disruption in the formation of infant–caregiver attachment, (2) prolonged stress associated with raising some children with
disabilities, and (3) increased vulnerability to maltreatment. Insecure
attachment is a common finding in maltreated children and their caregivers, and is primarily thought to be a consequence of abuse and neglect (Cicchetti, 1988), although some authors have suggested that it can
play a causative role in maltreatment as well (Ainsworth, 1980). A
number of factors may impede the formation of secure attachment in
handicapped children, including frequent mother–infant separations
secondary to illness, and deficits in specific attachment-promoting behaviors (e.g., gaze, responsiveness) in physically and sensory-disabled
children.

Stress is an additional risk factor in families with handicapped children. Many of these children, especially those with multiple handicapping conditions, display difficult-to-manage behavior problems that are
resistant to intervention. These consist of stereotypies, self-injurious
behaviors, aggression, hyperactivity, crying, and screaming. Moreover,
handicapped children often require increased care and supervision that
further adds to caregiver stress. The frustration engendered by these
difficulties may contribute to subsequent abuse.

The final risk factor associated with maltreatment in handicapped
children is vulnerability. Specifically, many handicapped children are
more vulnerable to maltreatment in that cognitive or communicative
deficits prevent them from revealing to others information regarding
possible mistreatment.

Of course, the degree to which the aforementioned factors contribute to risk for maltreatment is dependent upon the type of handicapping
condition, its severity, the functional limitations of the child, and the
course of disorder (stable vs. degenerative). Furthermore, it is acknowledged that other variables (e.g., social isolation, financial hardship, substance abuse) are more influential in the etiology of maltreatment than

the presence of a handicap. Risk for abuse and/or neglect is posited to increase when a handicapped child is introduced into a family that *already* displays those characteristics that can lead to maltreatment (e.g., poor parenting skills, impulse control deficits, unemployment, past experience of abuse).

Unfortunately, little research directly examines the incidence of abuse and neglect in handicapped populations. In one study, Diamond and Jaudes (1983) retrospectively investigated the medical charts of children with cerebral palsy admitted to a hospital clinic. Results indicated that 9% of their sample had been maltreated, and an additional 14% were at "high risk" for maltreatment. In another study, Ammerman, Hersen, Van Hasselt, McGonigle, and Lubetsky (1989) conducted a retrospective review of 150 handicapped and multihandicapped children admitted to a psychiatric hospital. Thirty-nine percent of the sample either had been maltreated or warranted high suspicion of abuse and neglect at some point in their lives. These studies document an alarming percentage of handicapped children that experience maltreatment, although methodological shortcomings (e.g., retrospective design) preclude determining that handicap per se directly adds to risk for abuse and neglect.

Regardless of whether or not handicapped populations are at higher risk for maltreatment, the fact remains that a significant proportion of these children are abused and/or neglected and are in need of intervention (Ammerman, Lubetsky, Hersen, & Van Hasselt, 1988). Clinicians and other professionals involved in helping these families must be sensitive to the unique issues encountered in treating the abused and/or neglected handicapped child. Although there is an overlap in the assessment of and intervention with families who maltreat their handicapped children and those who abuse or neglect their nonhandicapped children, a number of special considerations must be taken into account when working with this population. The complexities associated with such families are illustrated in a case involving a young developmentally disabled child with a past history of abuse and neglect as well as current risk of additional physical mistreatment.

Case Description

Peter L. was a 6-year-old white male who lived at home with his mother (Ms. R., age 24) and younger brother, Nick (age 3). Peter's father (Mr. L.) and mother had lived together for 7 years, and then separated 1 year prior to Peter's hospitalization. Up until 5 months prior to admission, Mr. L. maintained contact with the family, but had since left the state. Ms. R. received public assistance and lived in a subsidized housing project. Peter was referred to the John Merck Program for Multiply Disabled Children at Western Psychiatric Institute and Clinic by a local mental health center for overactivity, impulsivity, and inattentiveness. Because of the severity of these problems, and their resistance to prior treatment (see below), an inpatient evaluation was recommended. This was Peter's first psychiatric hospitalization.

A comprehensive neuropsychiatric assessment revealed a variety of disruptive behavior problems and concomitant physical conditions. Peter was observed to be impulsive, oppositional, inattentive, and hyperactive. These problems were reported to occur both at school and at home. In addition, Ms. R. complained that he was aggressive, especially toward his younger brother. Ms. R. also reported weekly occurrences of nighttime enuresis. Finally, Peter exhibited self-injurious behavior (self-biting), masturbation, bolting from his mother and running away, recklessness, and a lack of awareness of danger. Examples of the latter include an incident in which he swallowed an entire bottle of aspirin, and another where he jumped into a frozen pond because "he wanted to swim."

Upon admission to the John Merck Program, Peter was receiving 10 mg of methylphenidate three times per day to treat his inattention and overactivity. Moderate improvement in attention span was noted both at home and at school, although no changes occurred in Peter's aggressiveness, defiance, and noncompliance. One year prior to admission, Peter was prescribed 100 mg of Pemoline once per day. This was discontinued owing to several negative side effects, including irritability, lethargy, and increased noncompliance and aggression.

Ms. R. was distraught over her difficulties in handling Peter and managing his behavior problems. In particular, she was quite concerned about his aggression, which she described as being unpredictable and severe. Typically, she responded to his aggression with physical restraint. Upon being released, he would often continue to aggress against his younger brother. She also expressed frustration that, because of his language and cognitive limitations, she was unable to "reason" with him. Ms. R. reported frequent use of moderate to severe corporal punishment. These involved slapping Peter in the face, and spanking him on the buttocks and legs with a stick, paddle, fly swatter, or belt. Although Peter's younger brother "did not need" this form of discipline, Peter's misbehavior was "serious enough" that Ms. R. resorted to physical punishment at least once a day. In addition, on one occasion during which Peter was biting other children, she instructed the other children to "bite him back, to teach him what it is like." Ms. R. acknowledged that these methods were rarely effective in managing Peter. In addition, she described two incidents, the last occurring 6 months prior to admission, in which she had "lost control" and spanked Peter until he had black-and-blue marks on his buttocks that lasted for several days.

Ms. R. was raised in an intact family with two sisters. Her father was an alcoholic, and she witnessed his physical battering of her mother that often resulted in facial marks and bruises. Ms. R. was disciplined, primarily by her father, with a belt, paddle, and hair brush. During high school, Ms. R. excessively used drugs (i.e., marijuana, amphetamines) and alcohol. She quit on her own at the age of 17 because she "wanted to have children." At the age of 18, she moved in with Peter's natural father. When she was 20, Peter was born.

Peter was 6 weeks premature and weighed 5 pounds 6 ounces. He had respiratory problems at birth that required oxygen treatment. Ms. R. described Peter as a "jittery" baby who was difficult to comfort, did not like to be held, and had problems sleeping through the night during his first year of life. Shortly after Peter's birth, Mr. L. became physically abusive toward Ms. R. and Peter. He did not accept Peter's medical problems and developmental delays, and would frequently hit Peter to "toughen him up." This abuse lasted from age 1 to 5, often resulting in welts and bruises that lasted for up to 2 days. These incidents were more likely to occur when Mr. L. drank alcohol excessively. Ms. R. also was physically abused by Mr. L. approximately every 4 months, resulting in facial bruising. On one occasion, Ms. R. took Peter and hid in the woods next to their home when Mr. L. returned home drunk. Ms. R. reported that both children witnessed the physical violence directed toward her.

Also around this time, Ms. R. had a variety of odd jobs in order to support the family. While she was working, Mr. L. was responsible for care of the children. She reported that during these times the children were neglected, and she described several accidents to underscore his lack of supervision of the children. For example, at one point, Peter cut his foot on a piece of glass while walking barefoot through some garbage near the home. On another occasion, he put his hand in a blender and was seriously cut.

Ms. R. was evaluated by the Child Assessment and Management Project, a comprehensive assessment and treatment program conducted in collaboration between Western Psychiatric Institute and Clinic and the Western Pennsylvania School for Blind Children. Because of her serious parenting difficulties and high risk for abuse, she was offered treatment in conjunction with the psychiatric interventions that were implemented during Peter's hospitalization.

Medical Issues

Peter presented with a history of multiple medical and psychiatric problems and interventions. He was born 6 weeks premature and his lungs were not fully mature, resulting in respiratory difficulty. This also required care in a special nursery involving oxygen treatment and other medical interventions. This, in turn, led to multiple caregivers' involvement in an environment with constant stimulation by individuals other than his mother. It is unclear what impact this disruption had in the early formation of infant–mother attachment. However, such separations are common in congenitally handicapped and medically fragile children, and may play a role in subsequent maltreatment (see Ammerman, Van Hasselt, & Hersen, 1988).

In addition, it is not uncommon for parents of ill newborns to see their infant as vulnerable or susceptible to future catastrophic events. As Green and Solnit (1964) have described, parents of a newborn or infant who was ill or had an accident have persistent overconcern. This may engender distorted perceptions and confused parental expectations. Peter's parents began parenthood with such fears, misunderstandings, anger, and exhaustion as they were guided through a maze of medical interventions and confusing terminology.

As an infant, Peter was described as being difficult to comfort. Parents are typically reinforced by an infant who cuddles, coos, and feeds well. Peter's parents, on the other hand, were frustrated by his apparent frailty and irritability and their inability to soothe and satisfy him. Chess (1970) has described infants with different personality styles and their impact on parents' coping abilities. Peter would be categorized, at best, as the "slow-to-warm-up" child who presents as negative, has intense reactions to new stimuli, and needs extensive encouragement. At other times, he could be categorized more as the "difficult" child who has unpredictable sleeping and eating habits, rejects new toys or foods, and tantrums in response to frustration.

By the age of 1 year Peter was diagnosed as visually impaired. His parents questioned why he was not responding to toys placed in front of him. At that time, they had to cope with a child that was difficult to satisfy, had received early medical interventions (and survived), but would have an intractable visual impairment. It was about this time that Peter's father became physically abusive toward Peter and his mother, possibly in response to the frustration related to his special needs.

At age 3, Peter was diagnosed with a seizure disorder. It was first noticed when he had staring spells, cessation of activity, and drooling. This led to multiple appointments with neurologists for EEGs, another CT scan of the brain, and introduction of anticonvulsant medications. Although Peter's parents had heard of seizures, they had to learn to observe and document these episodes, give medication three times a day, watch for side effects, and return for neurology appointments. In addition, Peter was "always on the go," fidgety, and "getting into everything." Peter's father did not accept that he needed extended attention and care, but contended that he would "overcome" or "outgrow" it.

By this time, Peter's parents and physicians also questioned why he was not speaking and why developmental milestones of walking and toilet training were delayed. Further evaluations revealed developmental speech and language disorders and mental retardation (which was specified as mild a year later). Having a child who could neither reason well nor clearly communicate wishes or needs when compared with other same-age children may have further impeded Mr. L.'s ability to cope.

In addition, Peter continued to contract respiratory infections resulting in bronchospasm and recurrent asthma. His medical problems not only frightened Peter's parents but also required frequent emergency room visits, clinic appointments, and medications when ill. The fear aroused by a child displaying respiratory distress or having a seizure, and especially being unable to effectively communicate, may have reactivated the early fears of the parents having a "vulnerable child."

By age 5, Peter was seen by a child psychiatrist for overactivity, impulsivity, inattention, distractibility, oppositionality, noncompliance, and temper tantrums. In spite of medication trials of Pemoline and methylphenidate, his difficult-to-manage behaviors persisted. His mother reportedly was fearful of Peter's getting into dangerous situations. This fear was substantiated by his actions, including falling into a pond and taking his mother's pills in one occasion in the past.

As exemplified by Peter, handicapped children commonly have more medical evaluations and interventions than nonhandicapped children. Approximately 67% of handicapped children present with more than one handicap (33% have one handicap, 33% have two handicaps, and 33% have three or more handicaps) (Gottlieb, 1987). The combinations of varied forms of disabilities can result in a severely impaired child with multiple handicaps. In addition, dual diagnosis is another form of multiple disability in which mental retardation and mental illness coexist (Corbett, 1985). This was the case with Peter, who had multiple handicaps *and* severe psychiatric/behavioral problems.

Even if only one handicap exists, there are numerous medical interventions necessary for maintenance of good health and prevention of complications that can occur (Lubetsky, 1990). These medical complications may include contractures for those with cerebral palsy; chronic pain primary from the handicap or secondary to complications that arise, or from surgical procedures in order to alleviate or remediate the problem; newly diagnosed epilepsy, seizures that progress to other types, or those that do not respond to conventional anticonvulsant therapy; and congenital syndromes such as Down's syndrome, which has the enhanced risk of future heart disease, hypothyroidism, cataracts, myopia, and hearing loss (Nelson & Crocker, 1983). In addition, maintenance of good health care for a child with spina bifida, for example, may require such procedures as surgical repair of the spinal malformation and shunting of hydrocephalus if present, urologic care for bladder control, gastroenterologic care for bowel control, or physical therapy for ambulation and strength (Liptak, 1987).

The child's handicap frequently leads to delayed development and requires increased intervention to maximize progress. For example, the visually impaired child may have other coexisting medical conditions that interfere with normal development (i.e., hearing impairment, ambulating problems, mental retardation, seizure disorder). They also may have delays in attachment, gross motor skills, locomotion, language, and social development (Fraiberg, 1977).

Such added medical needs can heighten vulnerability to maltreatment, since they require so much additional time, money, commitment, and energy from parents. In handicapped children, the potential for neglect can arise more frequently by ignoring the need for additional medical care. There are certainly more opportunities to be neglectful when so much care is required (Morgan, 1987). Ignoring of simple child care issues for a normal child may be far less dangerous than for a handicapped child. For example, severe contractures can occur in a child with severe cerebral palsy, and skin breakdown, open sores, and infection must be avoided in the child with spina bifida. Further, environmental dangers must be identified and corrected. Examples of these include open room heaters that can lead to burns, open doors to stairways that can be a hazard for falling, and cigarettes left in ashtrays that can be used for firesetting. For those children who cannot verbally report danger or pain, considerably greater supervision and patience is needed.

Recognition of physical abuse is elusive in children who already have bruises or scars due to clumsiness, ataxia, poor coordination, hyperactivity, or impulsivity, or who lack the awareness of dangers (Ammerman, Van Hasselt, & Hersen, 1988). Such children frequently may be injured as a consequence of their handicaps, or inadequate protection and supervision, rather than direct physical punishment. It may be difficult for parents to know what an adequate level of supervision is for their handicapped child, as compared with a nonhandicapped child, without appropriate professional education and training. Also, the child with language impediments may be unable to communicate when physical or sexual abuse or neglect has occurred.

In summary, the multiply disabled child may have more medical needs and hence responsibilities for the parent. Ignoring of these needs or poor supervision definitely can lead to neglect. The multiply disabled child may also be less capable (owing to lower cognitive ability, lack of communication, hearing or vision impairments) of alerting others to ongoing physical or sexual abuse.

Legal Issues

The role of the legal and criminal justice systems in abuse and neglect of children begins with child protective service agencies. Such organizations exist in most developed countries in one form or the other. They are responsible for the investigation of suspected abuse and neglect, and for providing temporary emergency shelter for children in acute danger. In the case of Peter and Ms. R., the family had been involved with child protective services because of the past abuse and neglect by Peter's father. Although the family was monitored by a caseworker, the father was not removed from the home and additional support services were not provided. Unfortunately limited resources and the excessive caseload carried by child protective service agencies curtail efforts to implement comprehensive interventions with many families (as occurred with Peter and his family). Although Ms. R. was found to be at high risk for engaging in physical abuse, the clinical team working with Peter and his family did not find sufficient reason to file additional reports of incidents of mistreatment.

Existence of a handicap complicates the already difficult process of investigating suspected cases of abuse and neglect and providing needed services. As previously mentioned, cognitive limitations of the child and injuries secondary to the handicapping condition rather than abuse per se impede accurate identification of abuse. Also, for handicapped children who are aggressive, physical restraint procedures may inadvertently lead to bruises or hand marks that are mistakenly attributed to mistreatment. Of course, such restraint procedures must be used sparingly and only when the children are in danger of hurting themselves or others. An additional problem in recognizing abuse and neglect in handicapped children is the frequent presence of multiple caretakers for the child. These include other family members, babysitters, respite caseworkers. special education teachers, and support staff. Therefore, caseworkers must be thorough in their investigation of possible perpetrators and must also be vigilant for false allegations of mistreatment directed toward nonparental care providers.

Child protective service agencies must also contend with finding appropriate services for handicapped children and their families. Depending on the type and extent of impairment, these might include medical and psychiatric services, parent training, and parent support groups. Accessibility to needed organizations varies considerably across localities. For low-incidence conditions, proper facilities may be unavailable in most communities. For children who are removed from the home, foster care and adoption services may be unprepared and untrained to address the special needs of handicapped children.

Additional legal issues with abused and neglected nonhandicapped children are present as well in their handicapped counterparts. Custody questions often arise, and court assumption of parental rights may be required when the child's needs are not being met. In cases of severe mistreatment, criminal proceedings are pursued. The special considerations associated with handicapped children must be taken into account at each step of the legal process.

Family and Social Issues

Peter's family history and home environment revealed vulnerabilities for potential abuse and neglect. Peter's mother grew up in a low-income home with an abusive and alcoholic father who physically mistreated her and her mother. Ms. R. not only experienced this abuse but observed it frequently in the home. Peter's own parents were poor and socially isolated from their own family and friends. Peter's father drank alcohol frequently and was more abusive when intoxicated. Peter's parents fought often over many issues, particularly about his special needs. They separated 1 year prior to his psychiatric hospitalization, and his father had no contact with the family after 7 months. In addition, Peter was left with multiple caretakers, whose skills were questionable, while his parents were periodically working.

Peter reportedly observed his mother being hit by his father on numerous occasions. He was also a target of severe physical punishment by his father. His mother reported "feeling like losing control" and feeling more frustrated and stressed when Peter was disruptive. This led to her use of harsh physical punishment on several occasions.

As in Peter's case, the social, economic, and emotional burden on a family with a handicapped child are great. The stresses may become unmanageable. As Goldfarb, Brotherson, Summers, and Turnbull (1986) have summarized: "Obviously a disability or illness is itself a major life crisis. . . . But disabilities and illnesses also carry with them a number of side effects that cause stress to add up. There may be an unrelenting demand for physical or nursing care or supervision. . . . And in the back of everyone's mind there is an undercurrent of stress . . . [there are] too many bills, [and] not enough time to get everything done" (p. 21).

It is clear that the birth of a handicapped child can affect a marital relationship and the subsequent care of the child. Pueschel, Bernier, and Weidenman (1988) have found that "the birth of a handicapped child is bound to affect a husband and wife's relationship . . . when the baby has special needs, an extra dimension of stress is added. Some marriages, however, have problems unrelated to child's disability that may become more evident during this period of stress" (p. 17).

It is important to address the impact of a child with handicaps on the family system as a whole. The requirements for a family to survive stress points in which breakdown can occur have been described by Goldfarb *et al.* (1986). These family needs include such areas as (1) economic, (2) health and security, (3) physical caretaking, (4) social, (5) recreational, (6) affectional, (7) self-definitional, and (8) educational. For example, not only are there more costs incurred depending upon the type of handicap, but parents may have less time to earn an income as caretaking needs increase. The family may have less recreation time, which usually in most families serves to reduce stress and improve cohesion and cooperativeness among the members. Frequently, parents and siblings are embarrassed or isolated by the appearance of the handicapped child, and this, of course, can result in resentment, anger, and guilt. Family members' sense of self-worth may be lessened by the stresses or perceived stigma that may result from having a handicapped child in the milieu.

In assessing and understanding maltreatment, it is important to explore specific family stressors. Bittner and Newberger (1981) have described these stresses as child-produced, social-situational, and parent-produced. The child-produced stresses can include the following: physical handicaps, congenital disabilities, mental retardation, neurologic damage, language deficits, schizophrenia, hyperactivity, low birthweight, and prematurity (Snyder, Hampton, & Newberger, 1983).[1] Friedrich and Boriskin (1976) reported that abuse is associated with the child who displays behaviors that make him difficult and also with the child whose parents perceive him as different.

The coping styles of families with a handicapped child vary considerably and are mediated by a number of factors. Some of the "parent-produced" vulnerabilities that affect these coping capabilities include having been abused as a child, low self-esteem, depression, substance abuse, other psychiatric illness, ignorance of childrearing, or unrealistic expectations (Bittner & Newberger, 1981). Parents who were abused as children may themselves have failed to learned nonviolent coping methods under stressful situations (Burgess, Anderson, & Schellenbach, 1980).

---

[1]This is not to say that these conditions directly cause abuse and neglect. On the contrary, it is evident that most children who display these features are *not* subsequently maltreated (see Ammerman, Van Hasselt, & Hersen, 1988). Rather, characteristics associated with handicapping or disabling conditions (e.g., difficult-to-manage behavior problems, uncontrollable crying) may increase the likelihood of abuse in families already at risk.

The third set of family stressors, social-situational, include structural factors such as poverty, unemployment, mobility, isolation, and poor housing; problems in the parental relationship; and parent–child relationship difficulties (Bittner & Newberger, 1981). One such parent–child problem may be an impaired attachment resulting from the handicapped child's difficulty to be responsive and reciprocal in this relationship. It is postulated that some parents may be unable to elicit the response that they would like to elicit from their handicapped child and react with more anger, negativity, or violence than with their nonhandicapped child (Ammerman, Van Hasselt, & Hersen, 1988).

In summary, the impact of a handicapped child on the family can create significant stress in many areas. The parents' own family history and experiences, interpersonal relationships, outside supports, and individual self-esteem all further influence the risk for abuse and neglect.

Assessment of Psychopathology

Comprehensive assessments of Ms. R. and Peter were conducted via (a) Ms. R.'s participation in the Child Assessment and Management Project, and (b) the standard assessment procedures utilized by the hospital treatment team. As part of the CAMP, Ms. R. participated in several clinical interviews in addition to completing a variety of questionnaires evaluating psychopathology, parenting stress, social functioning, and child abuse risk. The inpatient evaluation of Peter involved clinical and psychometric assessments conducted by members of the treatment team, including an attending psychiatrist, psychiatric resident, psychodevelopmental specialist, clinical psychologist, physical therapist, and several psychiatric and pediatric nurses.

Parental psychopathology was measured using three instruments examining psychiatric disorders and personality dysfunction: the SCL-90-R (Derogatis, 1983), the MMPI (Hathaway & McKinley, 1940), and the Beck Depression Inventory (Beck, Ward, Mendelson, Mock, & Erbaugh, 1961). The SCL-90-R contains items reflecting specific symptoms of psychiatric disturbance and yields scale scores reflecting subtypes of psychopathology (e.g., depression, paranoia). Ms. R. obtained T scores within the normal range ($T < 70$) for all of the SCL-90-R scales. Her BDI score (19), on the other hand, placed her in the moderate range of depressive symptomatology. The MMPI yielded a 4–6 two-point code, suggesting a long-standing characterological disturbance. Individuals with this profile are often described as egocentric, self-centered, and narcissistic. They have difficulty in interpersonal relationships and are noted for their lack of insight into the nature of their maladjustment.

A clinical interview confirmed Ms. R.'s interpersonal difficulties. She reported having no close friends, and she was estranged from her family. Her employment history was sporadic, and she rarely remained in a job longer than 3 months. She exhibited little insight into the nature of her problems, focusing instead on the characteristics of others (including her children) that she believed were the causes of her difficulties. Although reporting several depressive symptoms, Ms. R. did not meet criteria for Axis I or Axis II psychiatric diagnoses.

Risk factors for child abuse were examined using the Novaco Provocation Inventory (NPI; Novaco, 1975) and the Child Abuse Potential Inventory (CAPI; Milner, 1986). The NPI is a measure of anger responsivity and is often used to assist in the detection of parents who exhibit poor impulse control. Ms. R.'s summative score of 182 was within the normative range on this measure. The CAPI, a measure of child abuse risk, yielded elevated scores on subscales reflecting abuse risk (288), distress (192), problems with child/self (20), and family (38). Additional measures documented further parenting difficulties. The Parenting Stress Index (PSI; Abidin, 1986) revealed high levels of stress, especially involving problems encountered with Peter. Indeed, subscale scores in the 99th percentile were noted in the following areas involving Peter: adaptability, acceptability, demandingness, mood, and hyperactivity. Furthermore, her total stress score (307) was more than 2 standard deviations above the mean for the normative sample.

Supplementary evaluations included the Child Abuse and Neglect Interview Schedule (CANIS; Ammerman, Hersen, & Van Hasselt, 1988), the Social Provisions Scale (Russell & Cutrona, 1984), and the Shipley Institute of Living Scale-Revised (Zachary, 1986). The CANIS is a semi-structured interview designed to identify factors associated with child maltreatment. It contains over 100 questions examining such topics as family stress, neglect, child behavior problems, disciplining practices, past history of family violence, sexual abuse, and parental substance abuse history. Detailed information about Peter's past maltreatment by his father (see Case Description) was adduced with the CANIS. In addition, Ms. R. reported her tendency to use physical punishment techniques (slapping, hitting with an object) to manage Peter, despite their ineffectiveness. As a child, Ms. R. was physically disciplined by her parents with brushes, paddles, and belts. Ms. R.'s mother also was a victim of spouse abuse, which often resulted in facial bruising. There also was vague suspicion that Peter might have been sexually molested at the age of 4. At this time, he began to masturbate at inappropriate times and with high frequency. His father, too, masturbated frequently, often in front of the children. Peter's behavior may have been instigated by modeling of his father. On the other hand, inappropriate genital play is a relatively common behavior in developmentally delayed children. Ms. R. denied any direct evidence that Peter and his father had any direct sexual contact (although Peter's observation of his father's masturbation was certainly highly inappropriate). Finally, Ms. R. described her past abuse of alcohol and other drugs, and denied current usage.

The specific assessment strategies carried out in this case reflect the general considerations that should be taken into account when working with abusive and neglectful families of handicapped children. In particular, it is critical that the assessment be comprehensive and multidimensional. The complexity of child abuse and neglect cannot be overemphasized, and a thorough evaluation of the numerous factors that can contribute to etiology and maintenance of maltreatment is critical to effective treatment planning. A comprehensive assessment serves two purposes. First, it permits the clinician to identify deficits of functioning that can subsequently be targeted in treatment. Second, it provides a screening for severe psychopathology that may need concurrent intervention or treatment prior to addressing the abuse and neglect. As such, it is necessary to use a variety of assessment strategies and multiple sources of information. These include administering questionnaires, conducting clinical interviews, and observing family interactions. Likewise, data should be gathered from professionals involved in the case, as well as significant others and extended family members. On the whole, assessment is parent-focused, given the fact that abuse and neglect is primarily defined by parent behavior. Other family members, however, should not be ignored. On the contrary, their involvement in assessment and treatment may make the difference between success and failure (Ammerman, 1989).

As was mentioned in the introduction, relatively little is known about maltreatment in handicapped and developmentally delayed children. It is likely that there are many similarities between handicapped and nonhandicapped populations that warrant use of similar assessment approaches. There are, however, several special issues associated with handicapped children that require meticulous attention and careful consideration. The medical status of the child is very important. Many children with handicaps exhibit chronic medical conditions that require frequent monitoring. The amount of medical involvement is dependent upon the type of impairment, extent of impairment, and course of the handicapping condition. All of these are critical in the family assessment of maltreatment, particularly as they pertain to neglect. Since these children require frequent medical follow-up, it is imperative that parents attend to their needs. A second consideration in assessing maltreatment in handicapped children is to identify the types and severity of behavior problems. Many children with profound handicaps display severe behavioral disturbances that are both quantitatively and qualitatively different from those of their nonhandicapped peers. For example, such behaviors as head banging, eye poking, and self-scratching are especially stressful for parents and resistant to change. Physical intervention may be required to control such behaviors, thus increasing the overall likelihood of abuse occurring as a result of heightened frustration and physical proximity of the parent and child. An interview, such as the CANIS, is especially useful in gathering information about parenting practices in general, and behavior management techniques used during these kinds of situations in particular. Finally, because these behavior problems are so difficult to manage, it is important to determine whether or not the parent has the appropriate skills to deal with these behaviors.

An additional focus of assessment is the parent–child relationship and parent–child interactions. Some parents exhibit negative reactions to the birth of a handicapped child and fail to resolve these as the child matures. Hostility toward the handicapped child may contribute to the overall likelihood of abuse. In addition, severely handicapped children are often characterized by a paucity of those behaviors that strengthen the parent–child bond. Such children sometimes do not like to be played with or touched. As a result, parents must be especially sensitive to cues and need to use a variety of techniques to engage the child. Parents who lack these skills are at especially high risk for having nonrewarding relationships with their children.

Treatment Options

When treating abusive families, there are several variables that must be taken into account regardless of whether or not the child is handicapped. Often, abusive parents evidence basic skill deficits that differentiate them from their nonabusive counterparts. For example, abusive parents are frequently inconsistent disciplinarians, who attend more often to negative child behaviors and communicate less positively with their offspring. Abusive parents' knowledge about childhood in general and their expectations about specific needs of the child also tend to be distorted. Further, there are other factors that can contribute to the etiology of maltreatment, including substance abuse, poverty, social isolation, past history of abuse, and stressful life events (e.g., marital conflict, single-parent status). All of these elements must be considered when designing a treatment plan.

In addition, families with a handicapped child are often faced with numerous difficult situations. Some handicapped children evidence unique and recalcitrant behavior problems demanding extensive physical contact for appropriate management or intrusive management techniques. Attitudes and expectations about their handicapped children who may develop slowly and atypically may further complicate parenting. For instance, the wish for a "normal" child or embarrassment about their child's behaviors or appearance may arouse guilt or anger. Added to this are the extended care requirements that can increase already heightened levels of family stress. As previously mentioned, a thorough assessment is required to address the multiple issues that may be associated with the cause and maintenance of maltreatment. Data from the assessment are, in turn, used to construct an intervention approach.

Comprehensive Behavioral Treatment (CBT) was used to treat Ms. R. CBT is a skills-based intervention targeting parenting difficulties in maltreating parents of handicapped or multihandicapped children. It consists of 16 sessions followed by 3 biweekly booster sessions, and it comprises five intervention components: (1) problem-solving skills and stress reduction training, (2) child management skills training, (3) parenting skills training, (4) anger control training, and (5) leisure skills training. Data from the assessments are used to determine appropriate targets for treatment. On the basis of Ms. R.'s assessment, the following areas were selected for treatment: (1) anger control training, (2) behavior management training, and (3) problem-solving skills training.

Anger control training involved having Ms. R. keep an Anger Incident Diary. She was instructed to record 10 incidents each day that were anger-provoking. Ms. R. was to describe cognitive, physical, and behavioral cues indicative of arousal. Along with this, she was to report her level of arousal using a 5-point scale. This task enhanced Ms. R.'s awareness of anger arousal and prevented such anger from building up to the point of losing control. Upon identification of self-statements associated with arousal, the next step was to teach Ms. R. to substitute positive for negative self-statements as a means of more effectively mediating anger.

As Ms. R. continued to monitor anger arousal, she became aware of Peter's behaviors that were most often provoking. In behavior management training, Ms. R. was instructed to observe and record the antecedents, behaviors, and consequences during problematic episodes. We identified that Ms. R. would spend close to 3 hours, at any one time, yelling and threatening her children in an attempt to achieve compliance. It was expected that through careful observation Ms. R. would be able to predict the onset of undesirable behaviors. In this manner, she would learn ways in which to interrupt and redirect them at the beginning, rather than allowing them to worsen beyond the point of becoming unmanageable.

There were a variety of coexisting problems, however, that interfered with the conduct of therapy. Particularly, Mr. L. (the father of Ms. R.'s children) returned to the home. Also, Ms. R. chose to confront her father about the past occurrence of sexual abuse. These situations were crises that drew Ms. R.'s attention away from the needs of her children. Indeed, it is this pattern of "jumping" from problem to problem that necessitated inclusion of problem-solving skills training in CBT. Our treatment plan included teaching Ms. R. to reevaluate and clarify personal situations, determine priorities, and organize her life-style so as to prevent future problems. Unfortunately, Ms. R. regretfully missed appointments during many of these "crisis" periods. She chose to withdraw from treatment after confronting her father about being molested as a child, insisting that she "could not concentrate on anything else" at that time.

The process of treatment for Ms. R. is most representative of these interventions with maltreating parents. Because there often are so many difficulties faced by the family, clinicians must divide their time between addressing acute crises and maintaining the focus of treatment. When the crisis is predominant, as with Ms. R., the parent may leave treatment prematurely. Thus, ensuring compliance with treatment protocols can be the primary theme in therapeutic interventions.

There are additional complex issues in the treatment of child abuse and neglect that are further compounded by factors associated with the handicapping condition. Specifically, five areas must be addressed in treatment: (1) behavior management, (2) medical and psychiatric intervention, (3) parental attitudes and expectations, (4) problem-solving skills, and (5) parental psychopathology.

Behavior Management

Parents who engage in abusive behaviors are inconsistent disciplinarians who attend to negative rather than positive child behaviors. Training these parents in the use of positive reinforcement and structured management procedures (e.g., time-out, extinction) can help circumvent abusive episodes and build positive parent–child interactions (see Wolfe, 1987). This is especially true in families of children with severe handicaps. Handicapped children often present with aversive and, at times, unique behavior problems rarely seen among nonhandicapped children. Managing such behaviors as self-injury (eye poking, head banging), extensive crying and/or tantruming, stereotypies (twirling, hand flapping), often coupled with hyperactivity and aggression, may require intrusive physical contact. These methods include basket holding, visual screening, and holding hands down, and are most often used during episodes of heightened arousal. The combination of increased emotionality and intrusive physical management may increase the possibility that more serious physical punishment will occur.

Medical and Psychiatric Interventions

Medical and psychiatric conditions must be addressed before one can attempt parent training. Prolonged and frequent medical attention is an essential part of caring for many handicapped children. Some conditions require continuous medical visits or caretaking procedures that are both costly and stressful. Other medical procedures may be painful, generating stress for both parent and child. Teaching parents to use stress-reduction techniques can be of assistance.

Psychiatric status of the child also requires attention. Pharmacological interventions for attention deficit hyperactivity disorder or organic brain syndromes reduce the likelihood of provocative child behavior, and facilitate parent training with abusive caretakers.

Parental Attitudes and Expectations

Parental attitudes and expectations about having a handicapped child produce a further impact on parenting. The initial disappointment and discouragement upon the birth of a handicapped child can lead to insecure attachment and possibly subsequent child-abusive behavior. Sometimes parents will deny their child's disabilities and believe that he/she will outgrow any limitations. Such expectations are followed by growing frustration. Also, parents may be rejecting or feel embarrassed about their child, leading to withdrawal or open hostility. Indeed, parents must first understand and accept their child's condition before they will be able to improve their behavior.

Problem-Solving Skills

Many families that engage in maltreatment live in a continual state of crisis and chaos. Indeed, it is such a high state of emotion and stress that at times contributes to the occurrence of abuse. Problem-solving skills training is designed to teach parents to better manage the stress associated with daily problems and to organize their life-style in order to minimize the impact of future problems. Stress management may include teaching parents progressive relaxation strategies and/or cognitive strategies, such as the previously described Anger Incident Diary. Also of import is to teach parents how to engage in enjoyable activities and effectively utilize leisure time to reduce stress.

Often parents are unaware that routine and organization can greatly lessen stress and decrease the opportunity for problems to arise. Prevention, for example, may go so far as to tie the refrigerator shut or bar the windows in order to protect a hyperactive child from injury. Other families may find that simply establishing a structured routine prevents conflict, greatly reducing stress.

Frequently, parents create their own stress in their perception of problematic incidents as crises. Indeed, many such instances deserve immediate attention, but not at the expense of parental responsibilities. Assisting a parent in problem analysis, generating solutions, and decision-making skills will help alleviate the sense of urgency and impatience often associated with crisis situations.

Parental Psychopathology

In some cases, abusive acts are associated with parental psychopathology. In these situations, it may be necessary to refer a parent to specialized programs (i.e., substance-abuse treatment) before involvement in parent training. In other cases, concurrent treatment modalities are an option. For example once a schizophrenic parent is stabilized on psychotropic medication, for example, he/she may benefit from parenting skills training.

Summary

A sizable body of evidence has accrued suggesting that children with handicaps are at increased risk for abuse and neglect. Although well-controlled empirical research in this area is sparse, three characteristics are posited to contribute to this heightened risk: (1) disruptions in the formation of caregiver–infant attachment, (2) increased stress (often related to difficult-to-manage behavior problems and extensive care requirements), and (3) increased vulnerability. These factors, along with the other issues faced in treating families involved in the abuse and neglect of their children, must be taken into account with parents of handicapped children.

Because of the complexity of child abuse and neglect in general, and maltreatment of children with handicaps in particular, it is critical that a multidimensional assessment be carried out. This assessment should address many areas of functioning, including the child's medical, psychiatric, and academic status. Likewise, family functioning, parental psychopathology, and parenting skills need to be closely examined. Moreover, it is essential that treatment strategies stem from such an assessment. It is impossible to utilize one treatment approach with such a heterogeneous population. Therefore, we recommend a multicomponent intervention that uses a variety of skills-based strategies designed to remediate several areas of need. Often, supportive counseling and other forms of psychotherapy may be required in conjunction with our overall approach.

Despite the unique issues found in parents who maltreat their handicapped children, there are many similarities between these families and maltreating families of nonhandicapped children. The pathways leading to maltreatment are complex and interactive. In addition, these families are very difficult to treat. Often, they have so many issues with which to deal that it is most difficult for them to focus intensely on one issue in a treatment setting. Furthermore, motivation of parents to seek and continue in treatment varies considerably.

There is a pressing need for continued research in this area. For example, almost nothing is known about the treatment of neglect in handicapped populations. In addition, we know little about the maltreatment of infants with handicaps, even though, in the general population, infants are more likely than other age groups to be abused or neglected. Although most children with handicaps develop atypically, issues of developmental level and functioning are critical in developing and in carrying out the treatment plan. As continued attention is accorded to this previously ignored population, the future holds promise for helping maltreated handicapped children and their families.

Acknowledgments

Preparation of this chapter was facilitated in part by grant No. G008720109 from the National Institute of Disabilities and Rehabilitation Research, U.S. Department of Education, and a grant from the Vira I. Heinz Endowment. However, the opinions reflected herein do not necessarily reflect the position of policy of the U.S. Department of Education or the Vira I. Heinz Endowment, and no official endorsement should be inferred. The authors wish to thank Mary Jo Horgan for assistance in preparation of the manuscript.

References

Abidin, R. R. (1986). *Parenting stress index* (2nd ed.). Charlottesville, VA: Pediatric Psychology Press.
Ainsworth, M. D. (1980). Attachment and child abuse. In G. Gerber, C. Ross, & E. Zigler (Eds.), *Child abuse: An agenda for action* (pp. 35–47). New York: Oxford University Press.
Ammerman, R. T. (1989). Child abuse and neglect. In M. Hersen (Ed.), *Innovations in child behavior therapy* (pp. 353–394). New York: Springer.

Ammerman, R. T., Hersen, M., & Van Hasselt, V. B. (1988). *The Child Abuse and Neglect Interview Schedule (CANIS)*. Unpublished instrument, Western Pennsylvania School for Blind Children, Pittsburgh.

Ammerman, R. T., Lubetsky, M. J., Hersen, M., & Van Hasselt, V. B. (1988). Maltreatment of children and adolescents with multiple handicaps: Five case studies. *Journal of the Multihandicapped Person, 1*, 129–139.

Ammerman, R. T., Van Hasselt, V. B., & Hersen, M. (1988). Maltreatment of handicapped children: A critical review. *Journal of Family Violence, 3*, 53–72.

Ammerman, R. T., Hersen, M., Van Hasselt, V. B., McGonigle, J. J., & Lubetsky, M. (1989). Abuse and neglect in psychiatrically hospitalized multihandicapped children. *Child Abuse and Neglect, 13*, 335–343.

Beck, A. T., Ward, C. H., Mendelson, M., Mock, J., & Erbaugh, J. (1961). An inventory for measuring depression. *Archives of General Psychiatry, 4*, 561–571.

Birrell, R., & Birrell, J. (1968). The maltreatment syndrome in children: A hospital survey. *Medical Journal of Australia, 2*, 1023–1029.

Bittner, S., & Newberger, E. H. (1981). Pediatric understanding of child abuse and neglect. *Pediatric Review, 2*, 197.

Burgess, R. L., Anderson, E. A., & Schellenbach, C. O. (1980). A social interactional approach to the study of abusive families. In J. P. Vincent (Ed.), *Advances in family interaction, assessment and theory*. Greenwich, CT: JAI Press.

Chess, S. (1970). Temperament and children at risk. In E. J. Anthony & C. Koupernik (Eds.), *The child in his family* (pp. 121–130). New York: Wiley.

Cicchetti, D. (1987). Developmental psychopathology in infancy. Illustration from the study of maltreated youngsters. *Journal of Consulting and Clinical Psychology, 55*, 837–845.

Corbett, J. A. (1985). Mental retardation: Psychiatric aspects. In M. Rutter & L. Hersov (Eds.), *Child and adolescent psychiatry modern approaches* (pp. 661–678). Boston: Blackwell/Year Book Medical Publisher.

deLissovoy, V. (1979). Toward the definition of "abuse provoking child." *Child Abuse and Neglect, 3*, 341–350.

Derogatis, L. R. (1983). *SCL-90-R Administration, Scoring, and Procedure Manual*. Baltimore: Clinical Psychometric Research.

Diamond, L. J., & Jaudes, P. K. (1983). Child abuse in a cerebral-palsied population. *Developmental Medicine and Child Neurology, 25*, 169–174.

Fraiberg, S. (1977). *Insights from the blind: Comparative studies of blind and sighted infants*. New York: Basic Books.

Friedrich, W. N., & Boriskin, J. A. (1976). The role of the child in abuse: A review of the literature. *American Journal of Orthopsychiatry, 46*, 580–590.

Goldfarb, L. A., Brotherson, M. J., Summers, J. A., & Turnbull, A. P. (1986). *Meeting the challenge of disability or chronic illness—A family guide*. Baltimore: Paul H. Brookes.

Gottlieb, M. E. (1987). Major variations in intelligence. In M. I. Gottlieb & J. E. Williams (Eds.), *Textbook of developmental pediatrics* (pp. 127–150). New York: Plenum.

Green, M., & Solnit, A. J. (1964). Reactions to the threatened loss of a child: A vulnerable child syndrome. *Pediatrics, 34*, 58–66.

Hathaway, S. R., & McKinley, J. C. (1940). A multiphasic personality schedule (Minnesota): Construction of the schedule. *Journal of Psychology, 10*, 249–254.

Helfer, R. (1973). The etiology of child abuse. *Pediatrics, 51*, 777–779.

Lightcap, J. L., Kurland, J. A., & Burgess, R. L. (1982). Child abuse: A test of some predictions from evolutionary theory. *Ethology and Sociobiology, 3*, 61–67.

Liptak, G. S. (1987). Spina bifida. In R. A. Hoekelman, S. Blatman, S. B. Friedman, N. M. Nelson, & H. M. Seidel (Eds.), *Primary pediatric care* (pp. 1487–1492). St. Louis: C. V. Mosby.

Lubetsky, M. J. (1990). Diagnostic and medical considerations. In M. Hersen & V. Van Hasselt (Eds.), *Psychological aspects of developmental and physical disabilities: A casebook* (pp. 25–54). Newbury Park, CA: Sage.

Milner, J. S. (1986). *The Child Abuse Potential Inventory* (2nd ed.). Webster, NC: Psytec.

Morgan, S. R. (1987). *Abuse and neglect of handicapped children*. Boston: Little, Brown.

Nelson, R. P., & Crocker, A. C. (1983). The child with multiple handicaps. In M. D. Levine, W. B. Carey, A. C. Crocker, & R. T. Gross (Eds.), *Developmental-behavioral pediatrics* (pp. 828–839). Philadelphia: W. B. Saunders.

Novaco, R. W. (1975). *Anger control: The development and evaluation of an experimental treatment*. Lexington, MA: D. C. Heath.

Pueschel, S. M., Bernier, J. D., & Weidenman, L. E. (1988). *The special child: A source book for parents of children with developmental disabilities*. Baltimore: Paul H. Brookes.

Russell, D., & Cutrona, C. E. (1984). *The Social Provisions Scale*. Unpublished manuscript, University of Iowa, College of Medicine, Iowa City.

Snyder, J. C., Hampton, R., & Newberger, E. H. (1983). Family dysfunction: Violence, neglect, and sexual abuse. In M. D. Levine, W. B. Carey, A. C. Crocker, & R. T. Gross (Eds.), *Developmental-behavioral pediatrics* (pp. 256–275). Philadelphia: W. B. Saunders.

Solomons, G. (1979). Child abuse and developmental disabilities. *Developmental Medicine and Child Neurology, 21*, 101–108.

Starr, R. H., Dietrich, K. N., Fischhoff, J., Ceresnie, S., & Zweier, D. (1984). The contribution of handicapping conditions to child abuse. *Topics in Early Childhood Special Education, 4*, 55–69.

Wolfe, D. A. (1987). *Child abuse: Implications for child development and psychopathology*. Newbury Park, CA: Sage.

Zackary, R. A. (1986). *Shipley Institute of Living Scale: Revised Manual*. Los Angeles: Western Psychological Services.

14

The Child Witness of Family Violence

Mindy S. Rosenberg and Ronita S. Giberson

Description of the Problem

Until recently, the treatment of children who witness their parents' violence has not received separate attention from the mental health community. Far more has been written about children's direct experience of abuse and neglect and the variety of intervention strategies to help maltreated children and their families. While child witnesses may experience psychological issues similar to those of child victims (e.g., parental extremes of emotions and behavior, posttraumatic stress disorder), there are important differences that need explication. In this chapter, we use the case of Maria and her family to highlight the significant psychological issues that emerge when children witness their parents' violence. We begin by describing Maria's family and the circumstances that brought her family to our attention. Next, we expand on the medical, legal, social, and family issues, and assessment of psychopathology that were revealed during evaluation. We conclude with a discussion of treatment options and summary comments.

Case Description

Presenting Problem

The P. family came to the attention of a child and family clinic at the suggestion of an elementary school teacher who was concerned about

Mindy S. Rosenberg • Private Practice, 1505 Bridgeway, Suite 123, Sausalito, California 94965.   **Ronita S. Giberson** • Graham B. Dimmick Child Guidance Service, Comprehensive Care Center, Lexington, Kentucky 40507.

Maria P., the 7-year-old daughter. The P. family includes the mother, Anita (46 years old), the father, Richard (48 years old), and three daughters, Maria (7 years old), Anna (5 years old), and Rosa (3 years old). Mr. and Mrs. P. had been separated for 6 months, and Mr. P. lived in a neighboring state. Maria's schoolteacher contacted Mrs. P. because of concerns about Maria's aggressive behavior toward other children (e.g., hitting, pushing), her lack of school friends, and her difficulty concentrating on academic material. When Mrs. P. contacted the clinic, she had numerous concerns about Maria and her other children, all of whom had witnessed repeated incidents of physical violence by their father against their mother. Mrs. P. was especially worried about her oldest daughter, Maria, who had witnessed the majority of marital violence. Maria cried frequently at home, had aggressive outbursts toward her sisters, and seemed confused about her feelings toward her father. Though the younger daughters were currently not displaying any behavioral or emotional signs of distress, Mrs. P. reported that in the past, both had had difficulty sleeping (e.g., waking up screaming and crying from nightmares, after which they were unable to be comforted).

In addition, Mrs. P. had concerns about her parenting skills. She reported that at times she lost her temper with her children, screaming at them for relatively minor infractions and sometimes spanking them. Mrs. P. was both physically and sexually abused as a child, and although her relationship with her children was not in a crisis state, she was afraid of perpetuating her history of physical abuse with her own children. She also felt that being sexually abused as a child contributed to her own discomfort over bathing, masturbation, normal sexual exploration, and other sexual issues with her daughters. She requested guidance in the areas of discipline, ways to encourage her children's development of appropriate social skills, and how to help them cope with her separation and planned divorce from Mr. P.

Family History

Mrs. P. met and married her husband in Arizona; she is Hispanic and he is Anglo. Whereas the marriage was her first, Mr. P. had been married once before and had five children, with whom he had intermittent contact. His first wife divorced him after years of extreme battering. Although Mrs. P. was aware of her husband's past, she felt he always treated her well and she had his promise that he had changed. She found him to be a warm, charismatic man who shared interests similar to hers.

Once they were married, conflict between Mr. and Mrs. P. increased dramatically as a result of Mr. P.'s infidelities and verbal abuse, and worsened with the birth of their first child, Maria. The first violent incident occurred 3 months after Maria was born and involved Mr. P.'s pushing, slapping, and hitting his wife. The second incident occurred 4 months later in which Mr. P. repeatedly punched his wife's face with his fists. Following this, Mrs. P. was severely battered every few months, with considerable family tension between incidents. Each battering incident left

Mrs. P. with bruises on her face or torso, and necessitated calling in sick to the hospital where she worked as a nurse. Their second and third children were born at intervals of 2 years, and although each child was planned and ostensibly desired by both parents, Mr. P.'s beatings were especially severe shortly after each child's birth.

Maria witnessed the most extensive violence between her mother and father, but there were times when Mr. P. would force all his daughters to watch while he beat their mother. After 10 years of marriage, Mrs. P. insisted that both she and her husband attend marital counseling, which Mr. P. agreed to in order to prevent his wife from leaving. One condition of the counseling was that Mrs. P. would leave if her husband physically assaulted her. Mr. P. violated this agreement within weeks. The counselor discontinued treatment and encouraged Mrs. P. to leave, which she chose not to do at that time. The battering continued until, one evening, Mr. P. beat his wife to the point of her almost losing consciousness. For the first time, he threatened to hurt their children if Mrs. P. did not comply with his every demand. She left with her daughters the next day and went to live with her brother and his family, who lived in a neighboring city. The marital separation created tremendous fear and anxiety for Mrs. P. and her children: They were afraid that Mr. P. would follow them and harm them further. Mrs. P. decided fairly quickly to make the separation permanent and sought counseling for herself. She obtained a job as a nurse in a local hospital, arranged for day care for Rosa, and enrolled Anna and Maria in school. Shortly after Maria entered the new school, her aggressive behavior began to escalate, which prompted the teacher's suggested referral to the clinic.

The P. family was evaluated over a series of sessions. The evaluation included several interview sessions with Mrs. P. to gather information about family history and current family functioning. Mrs. P. completed a developmental history and an Achenbach Child Behavior Checklist for each of her three daughters. Once consent was obtained, phone interviews were conducted with Maria and Anna's schoolteachers, Rosa's babysitter, Mrs. P.'s individual therapist, and her brother. School visits were made to observe Maria and Anna in their classrooms and to meet their teachers. All three children were seen individually and jointly in play sessions to observe their interactions. Family sessions were also conducted to observe the quality of interaction between Mrs. P. and her daughters and among the girls themselves in the presence of their mother.

Medical Issues

Although medical issues were not a primary focus of concern with the P. family, there are instances where the medical profession will come in contact with this population of children and families. For example, it is relatively common for battered women to use the emergency room or other clinic facilities for treatment of injuries sustained during a battering incident (Bergman, 1976). However, battered women do not necessarily report the true cause of their injuries to health care providers (Hilberman, 1979), and, until recently, providers were not trained to ask specific questions about marital violence (Stark, Flitcraft, & Frazier, 1979). Battered women often present with vague physical complaints, minimize the extent of their injuries, and hope that health care providers will ask the right questions or confront the causal logic of the injury. Moreover, it is rare for children of battered women to be brought to the attention of medical staff unless they, themselves, have injuries sustained as a direct or indirect result of the battering. Klingbeil and Boyd (1984) report that battered women typically express relief when health care providers acknowledge directly the presence of marital violence and ask questions straightforwardly to obtain the necessary information.

Children may come to the attention of health care providers in at least two instances. The first instance concerns the overlap between children who witness their parents' violence and those who experience some form of child maltreatment, including physical abuse or neglect, or sexual abuse. A substantial percentage of maritally violent families are at risk for child abuse, particularly during times when children attempt to protect the victimized parent (Barnett, Pitman, Ragan, & Salus, 1980). In these circumstances, children may try to shield their mother from the blows of the batterer or may get in the path of flying objects and inadvertently are injured themselves. Children may also become the direct targets of either parent's anger and frustration. One of the most frequent reasons given by women for leaving a battering partner is that he threatened to abuse the children or already injured them physically (Giles-Sims, 1983). Thus, one of the first medical issues necessitating attention is to determine whether these children have sustained physical injuries, and to treat accordingly. In situations where child maltreatment is suspected or evident, health care providers are mandated to report to the proper authorities in keeping with the established hospital or clinic procedures for child abuse reporting.

In the second instance, children may evidence the psychological sequelae of witnessing their parents' violence, although they themselves have not been physically abused. In this situation, health care providers, particularly pediatricians and nurses, may have a unique opportunity to identify the distressed child witness, given their ongoing contact with the child and his or her family. Parents may first contact pediatricians to discuss noticeable changes in their child's behavior (e.g., increased aggression or withdrawal, nightmares, psychosomatic complaints) or academic problems (e.g., decreased ability to concentrate, refusal to complete homework assignments, school refusal), and it is imperative that pediatricians and nurses be aware of the possibility of marital violence as a potential causative factor.

Legal Issues

Several legal issues may emerge when working with families where children witness marital violence. First, as noted above, child maltreatment may occur in families where there is ongoing marital violence. In those situations, the therapist is mandated to report to child protective services and may then help the family cope with any additional legal intervention to follow. In the case of the P. family, Mrs. P.'s decision to leave her husband was precipitated by an especially severe beating coupled with Mr. P.'s threat to harm their daughters if she did not comply with his future demands. There was no evidence of child maltreatment prior to or after the P.s' separation, so that involvement of child protective services in that capacity was unwarranted.

If the couple decides to separate temporarily or to divorce, as in the case of the P.s, the second, relatively common legal issue that arises concerns child custody rights and visitation arrangements. Making a fair custody determination in divorce cases presents enough of a challenge when marital violence is not a factor (see Weithorn, 1987), but in the context of battering relationships, contested custody determinations are fraught with a myriad of problems (e.g., evaluating how violence in the marital relationship affects each partner's ability to parent). As Walker and Edwall (1987) argue, the legal system can become yet another combat arena for battering men who wish to continue a relationship with their wives. In the case of the P. family, it was clear that Mr. P. did not want sole custody of his daughters and Mrs. P. did, so that contested custody was not a central focus of the divorce.

Problems with visitation arrangements is a third legal issue that might arise when battered women seek separation or divorce. It is not uncommon for the batterer to continue to harass his (ex-)wife by making abusive phone calls, pumping the children for information, refusing to pick up or return the children at the designated time and place, and demanding frequent court appearances to alter visitation arrangements (Walker & Edwall, 1987). Child visitation became the primary battleground for the P. family once Mr. P. realized that Mrs. P. planned to obtain a divorce, and treatment eventually focused on the psychological issues that arose from that battle.

During the first month of the marital separation, Mr. P. focused his attention on trying to get Mrs. P. to give their marriage another chance.

When it became apparent that Mrs. P. was not going to change her mind, Mr. P. began to "work on the girls" to influence their mother's decision. During his weekly visits and telephone calls over the next 2 months with his daughters, he began a campaign to win back his family, first by treating them as well as he could, and then through guilt. He chose Maria as the oldest and most psychologically vulnerable to tell her how he couldn't eat or sleep or work because he missed his family so much, and that he feared he would die unless they lived together again. Maria felt that her father really would die if the family was not reunited, and that it was up to her to save her father's life by trying to change her mother's mind. Once Mrs. P. became fully aware of her husband's manipulative behavior, she said there would be no further contact with her or the girls unless he "straightened up," and told him once again that she was planning to file for divorce. Mr. P. then moved to a neighboring state and was not in contact with his family until shortly after they entered treatment.

Social and Family Issues

Social Issues

It is not uncommon for battered women to become increasingly isolated from their social support systems when they are involved in a violent relationship and the violence escalates over time (Browne, 1987). As ties to friends, family members, and community resources become more tenuous, there is less opportunity for battered women to receive the kind of feedback that could help them reevaluate their intimate relationship and take steps to stop the violence. Without the intervention of outside information and support, battered women often come to have a distorted sense of what is normal, acceptable behavior between spouses. As the violence escalates over time, battered women may become desensitized to all but extreme battering incidents.

This isolation had certainly occurred during Mrs. P.'s marriage. For example, Mrs. P. had few friends of her own while married to Mr. P. Most social contacts were through her husband's family, who either supported Mr. P.'s negative evaluation of his wife or seemed oblivious to the escalating tension and violence in their marriage. In addition, Mrs. P. maintained limited contact with her family of origin to decrease the opportunity for arguments with Mr. P. when they visited family members and to minimize the potential for family members to confront her about her unhappy, volatile marriage. Mrs. P. had always felt socially awkward, and under the best of circumstances she had difficulty making friends and reaching out to co-workers. As the violence in her marriage escalated, she became increasingly isolated from others who could provide emotional support and feedback about the dysfunctional nature of her marital relationship. When Mrs. P. attempted to talk with her husband about the problems in their relationship, he treated her as though she were "crazy" and fabricating information to provoke an argument. Two years into the marriage, Mrs. P. sought help from a clergyman, who counseled her to try and be a better, more obedient wife. She came to doubt her own anguished feelings about the marriage and began to believe her husband's interpretation of their relationship problems (i.e., that any difficulties were caused by Mrs. P.'s inadequacies). It was not until Mrs. P. read a magazine article on battered wives that she realized her situation was not unique and that she must seek help.

Family Issues

In light of findings from the family evaluation and individual interviews with Mrs. P. and the children, several family-level issues emerged for consideration in treatment. First, it became apparent that Mrs. P. and the children were continuing to live as if they were bracing for Mr. P.'s verbal and physical assaults at any moment. Maintaining the home atmosphere at crisis level prevented Mrs. P. and her children from feeling emotionally safe enough to lower their defenses, confront their traumatic memories, and begin to build a new family life. Second, Maria also experienced the effects of marital violence through problems in her relationship with each parent.

Crisis Atmosphere in the Home

Mrs. P.'s pattern of battering experiences and the resulting psychological sequelae exemplifies the cycle theory of violence proposed by Walker (1979, 1984). According to this theory, there are three distinct phases associated with recurring battering incidents: tension building, the acute battering incident, and loving contrition. Over the course of a violent relationship, the tension-building phase tends to predominate while the contrition phase tends to decline. Tension can escalate as a result of the batterer's gradual increase in provocative behavior, which might include trying to start arguments, name calling, temper outbursts, or lesser forms of physical abuse (i.e., pushing). The woman may try to placate her partner, and behave in such a way as to minimize the possibility of future violence (e.g., trying not to respond to his hostility, cooking his favorite foods, keeping the house clean). Children are also pressured to be on their best behavior, and may be told to keep their rooms clean, get good grades in school, and not argue with each other so that their father won't get in a bad mood. It is not uncommon for some children to feel responsible for their mother's assaults when their behavior has somehow been linked with provoking their father's violence.

When the P. family began the evaluation phase, Mrs. P. spoke of needing to be "on guard" in the family to protect herself and her children from the possibility of her husband's violence. She described the atmosphere in the home as perpetually in a crisis state, in which she and her children needed to be prepared to leave at a moment's notice. There were times when the tension between her and her husband became so unbearable that she would not turn her back on him for fear of an unpredictable attack. Maria, in particular, tended to cling to her mother and was fearful of what her father would do if she wasn't around to monitor both parents' behavior. Occasionally at bedtime, Mrs. P. would find Maria asleep in her clothes. Maria explained that she may need to alert a neighbor to help her mother in the middle of the night and she did not want to be seen in her pajamas. What was most noteworthy about Mrs. P. and her daughter's vigilant behaviors is how ingrained they were, and even 6 months to a year after Mr. and Mrs. P. separated, there were many instances where both mother and daughter acted as if they were still living in the crisis atmosphere of the past.

Troubled Parent–Child Relationships

A family systems' perspective would predict that violence and discord in the marital subsystem affects both partners' ability to function in their roles as parents (Minuchin, 1974). There are multiple ways in which a parent–child relationship may be affected by a dysfunctional marriage. For example, it is not uncommon to see parents become emotionally unavailable to their children as a result of their preoccupation with battering, or who rely inappropriately on their children for guidance, support, and affection. In other situations, parents may have difficulty disciplining their children, and may alternately ignore and punish severely their children's misbehaviors. At times, children may be used as outlets for parents' frustrations or as scapegoats for the problems in the marriage. Parents may have particularly negative perceptions of their child that interfere with the parent–child relationship, such as attributing negative qualities to the child that are similar to those of the spouse. Alternatively, parents may focus their efforts on developing positive relationships with their children in an attempt to buffer them from the stressors associated with a violent marriage. Clearly, these are not the only patterns that characterize parent–child relationships, nor are these patterns necessarily mutually exclusive.

Focusing first on the relationship between Mrs. P. and Maria, the following problems were observed: (1) maternal emotional unavailability and reliance on Maria for emotional support, (2) disciplinary problems, (3) negative perceptions of Maria. The most prominent issue in Maria's relationship with her father was trying to understand his behavioral extremes (e.g., loving and gentle on the one hand, cruel and cold on the other) and her conflicting emotional response to him as a result. These are discussed below.

Emotional Unavailability and Reliance on Child for Support

Mrs. P.'s relationship with Maria was characterized by alternating periods of emotional unavailability and intense overinvolvement. Not surprisingly, Maria was confused by her mother's mixed messages. At times, Mrs. P. was preoccupied and did not respond to Maria's distress and need for interaction, while at other times, Mrs. P. would seek out Maria as a confidante and source of emotional support.

Before Mrs. P. entered into treatment, she found it difficult to be sensitive to Maria's emotional needs because her own desire for attention and support predominated their interactions. For example, on one occasion, Mrs. P. said, "I need a hug," to Maria, and when Maria did not respond immediately because she was in the midst of doing something, Mrs. P. became upset and ordered Maria to give her a hug. At other times, Maria clearly desired affection and nurturing from her mother but was rebuffed because Mrs. P. was feeling drained or did not like the manner in which Maria sought the affection.

During her parents' violent marriage, Maria often played the role of nurturer and protector for her mother. Mrs. P. complemented this role by seeking emotional support and strength from Maria, even though she was a young child. For example, after Mr. P. had beaten her, Mrs. P. would often go to her daughters' room to comfort them since they were typically frightened and crying. However, this would often be the time that Maria would soothe her mother. Mrs. P. relates that after the final beating when she almost lost consciousness, Maria came to her, attended to her bruises and cuts, and asked, "What did Daddy do to you this time?" It was at this point that Mrs. P. realized that Maria had taken on a parental role in their relationship and vowed to stop relying on her daughter for support.

After leaving her husband, Mrs. P. actively tried to alter her own and Maria's roles in the family. She stopped turning to Maria for reassurance and discouraged Maria from continuing in the role of protector/nurturer toward her. Maria found it particularly difficult to relinquish her old role, because it was the only way she knew how to be emotionally close to her mother. In an attempt to make sure that Maria understood that "things were going to be different now," Mrs. P. worked to distance herself emotionally from Maria. In response, Maria could do nothing but cling to her mother, fearing that she would lose her mother's love completely. Altering this cyclical interaction pattern of clinging-distancing-clinging became a critical treatment goal.

Disciplinary Behavior

Mrs. P.'s difficulty with child discipline extended to all three daughters. She did not have a repertoire of strategies from which to draw when her children misbehaved, and she often felt "at a loss" as to how to respond. She would alternate between overreaction to her child's slightest infraction (e.g., not clearing the table immediately after dinner) and failing to respond to more severe misbehavior (e.g., Maria hitting her sister in the head with a doll). Because Mrs. P. was unable to set firm, consistent limits with her children, they did not have a clear understanding of what was expected from them. Moreover, as Mrs. P. allowed Maria to continue her aggressive behavior toward her sisters and peers without any form of intervention, her behavior escalated and Mrs. P. became even more frightened, angry, and uncertain of what to do next.

Mrs. P. recognized that she felt "out of control" with her daughters on multiple occasions, although these feelings did not lead to any abusive incidents. She described how difficult it was for her to control her anger once she allowed herself to feel any anger at all, and stated that "any anger led to big anger." Mrs. P.'s ability to discipline her children effectively was further complicated by her guilt over exposing her children to a violent marriage. She reported feeling a sense of explosive range that sometimes came over her in response to fairly minor misbehavior on the part of her daughters. She would yell and scream at her daughters or leave the room rather than physically harm them. The children would cry in response to her anger, which increased her guilty feelings and further compromised her ability to manage their behavior appropriately. She thought of herself as a "terrible" parent and often wondered, "How can anyone as mixed up as me be a good role model?"

Perceptions of Children

Mrs. P. held noticeably different perceptions of Maria as compared with her perceptions of Anna and Rosa. In general, Mrs. P. tended to perceive Maria in an unrealistically negative light while her perceptions of Anna and Rosa tended to be overly positive. The effects of these divergent perceptions contributed to several problems in Mrs. P.'s relationship with Maria. Mrs. P. tended to hold inappropriate expectations for Maria's behavior, she misinterpreted positive information about her daughter, and she identified her as the "problem child" who needed harsher punishment than the other girls. Not surprisingly, there was intense sibling rivalry between Maria and her sisters as a result of their mother's differential treatment.

Because Mrs. P. had divergent perceptions of her three children, her interactional style with each child also was quite different. These varied interactional styles, in turn, affected her children's behavior, which further reinforced Mrs. P.'s perceptions of her children. For example, Mrs. P. had extremely high expectations of Maria but, at the same time, perceived her to be minimally competent in daily activities (e.g., household tasks, self-help skills). Maria was acutely aware of these expectations, felt pressured to succeed at everything she did, and dreaded the possibility of performing below standard. Consequently, Maria often appeared dependent on others to show her what to do and needed enormous guidance and reassurance before approaching new situations. These behaviors only served to reinforce Mrs. P.'s perceptions of Maria as a child who was barely able to get along in the world without a great deal of prodding and attention. Indeed, Maria was rarely praised for her efforts. A second example of this phenomenon could be found in the way Mrs. P. played with her daughters. She was far more playful and spontaneous with her two younger daughters than she was with Maria, and, in turn, Anna and Rosa were playful with her while Maria was solemn and self-conscious with her mother. Again, these differences in interactions only served to reinforce Mrs. P.'s perceptions that her younger daughters were "alive and well" while Maria was a problem child.

Mrs. P. perceived Maria not only as helpless but also as "weird." She had very little psychological understanding of her daughter and tended to project many of her negative feelings about herself onto her child. In fact, Mrs. P. had difficulty perceiving any of Maria's positive qualities and would misinterpret positive feedback about Maria from teachers or other adults that knew her. For instance, when a teacher wrote that Maria did a "good job" on an assignment, Mrs. P. interpreted the feedback to mean that Maria could have done an excellent job if she tried harder, and that "good" was meant to let Maria know that she wasn't working up to her capabilities. In contrast to perceiving Maria from an unrealistically negative perspective, Mrs. P. saw Anna and Rosa as the resilient, "healthy" children and tended to portray them in an overly positive light. Mrs. P. did not recognize that Anna's behavior could become too aggressive at times, or that she liked to get Maria in trouble with their mother. Rosa was depicted to be an "angel," a child that could do no wrong. In terms of discipline, Mrs. P. also tended to treat Maria differently from her other daughters, with Maria typically receiving the harsher punishment.

Mrs. P.'s differential treatment of her daughters led to intense sibling rivalry between Maria and Anna, in particular. The rivalry took the form of resentment, aggression, and competition for their mother's approval and attention. Although Maria and Anna each provoked the other, Anna's behavior tended to be more subtle while Maria's behavior typically involved physical aggression. Maria was blamed more often for "starting" the fight and was told that she "should know better" since she was older than her sister. Mrs. P.'s response served to intensify the conflict between the sisters, and it appeared that the three of them were locked in an escalating battle without end.

Behavioral Extremes

Mr. P.'s behavior with his children swung wildly between nurturance and hostility. His relationship with his daughters could be summarized by the following nursery rhyme phrase: "When he was good, he was very, very good, and when he was bad, he was horrid." At times, Mr. P. would come to comfort the girls after a battering incident when they were crying in their room. He was very athletic and spent long hours with each daughter playing and teaching them the rules of various sports. However, these pleasant interactions usually ended abruptly when Mr. P. became enraged over a seemingly minor incident (e.g., Maria didn't throw a ball according to her father's directions). During these blowups, Mr. P. was often verbally abusive toward his children, and these verbal displays could continue for several days at a time. Then, quite suddenly, Mr. P. would apologize to his daughters, take them out for a McDonald's dinner, and buy them presents. In many ways, Mr. P.'s cycle of nurturance and hostility with his children mirrored his emotional relationship with Mrs. P., with one major difference: Mr. P. was never physically abusive with his daughters. As previously mentioned, however, toward the end of their violent marriage, Mr. P. threatened to hurt the children unless Mrs. P. "behaved" in a particular way. Mrs. P.'s realization of her children's danger led to her final decision to leave her husband.

Child Issues

Although there are multiple issues that could serve as the treatment focus for child witnesses to marital violence (cf. Rosenberg & Rossman, 1990), three core areas of concern emerged for Maria during the evaluation and testing sessions. These problem areas consisted of (1) difficulty coping with the traumatic memories of her father's violence and its emotional consequences, (2) alternating between feeling a profound sense of powerlessness and feeling overly powerful to control people and events, and (3) emotional sensitivity and difficulty with emotional expression. Maria's problems with each of these areas affected her behavior at home, in school, and with her peers.

Coping with Traumatic Memories

Maria was more strongly affected by her father's violence toward her mother than were the other children in the family. She witnessed more abusive incidents than her sisters, and because she was the oldest, she was better able to understand the seriousness of the violence and its implications for her mother's safety. When Maria came to the attention of the clinic, she evidenced many symptoms associated with post-traumatic stress disorder. For example, Maria experienced intrusive, repetitive memories of the violence that interfered with her daily functioning. Maria would often talk about the abuse to others, such as her schoolteacher. Although she was a good student, the intrusive memories interfered with her concentration and overall school performance. Maria would frequently daydream in class, and the teacher felt that she was in "another world" for a significant proportion of the school day. In therapy sessions, Maria described nightmares in which women and little girls were beaten and carried away by monsters; she awoke from these nightmares screaming and shaking with fear. She repeatedly narrated several of the more severe incidents of abuse, but her affect was noticeably flat and she appeared numb. On other occasions, Maria had difficulty recalling violent incidents or refused to talk further about her experiences.

During the evaluation sessions, Maria's play revealed that she saw the world as a dangerous place, full of unpredictable events. She introduced over and over again in her play sudden tragedies and accidents, as, for example, when a family drove their car off an unexpected cliff. There were recurrent themes of needing to be careful in order to avoid these tragedies, although even those play characters who were extremely careful experienced a variety of destructive outcomes. Through play therapy, Maria could begin to work through her experience of unpredictable violence. However, in contrast to real life she would now be able to create and control the dangers around her.

Power and Powerlessness

In the evaluation sessions, Maria often expressed her own sense of powerlessness through play to control other people or events. At the same time, Maria felt a strong responsibility to "make things better" for family members and friends. It was important for Maria to have a great deal of control over what happened to others. Many times she was able to "save" people in miraculous ways, which made her feel strong and happy. However, another frequent theme in these sessions involved several traumatic events occurring one after the other. On one occasion Maria exclaimed, "I can't rescue all these people all by myself, I'm only a little kid!" She began to get angry at the people, stating that it was they who made her feel so bad about herself (i.e., incompetent). After throwing the doll figures around the playroom, she began to cry and talk about how sad and lonely she felt. The juxtaposition of her feelings of responsibility and power to influence people and circumstances with her overwhelming sense of powerlessness contributed to a decreased sense of self-efficacy and self-worth, aggressive behavior, and depressive symptoms.

Another way in which Maria grappled with her feelings of powerlessness was by clinging to external structure. Her way of finding safety in an unpredictable world was to carefully follow all rules, and she often became upset over seemingly minor deviations from any rules. Maria's schoolteacher described this behavior as "perfectionistic," but Mrs. P., who was frequently frustrated by Maria's rigidity, perceived this behavior as additional evidence of Maria's "strangeness." An example of Maria's need to follow rules precisely was an occasion when she cried inconsolably because she was unable to complete a homework assignment on the "proper" paper. A goal in therapy was to help Maria gain some flexibility and feel more comfortable with herself without this excessive dependence on structure.

Emotional Sensitivity and Expression

Maria and her sisters were acutely aware of their mother's emotions, and, in fact, Mrs. P.'s brother compared them to puppets. He reported that both children seemed not to have their own emotions when they were around their mother. Instead, they simply watched and then mimicked their mother's mood when she came to pick them up. For Maria, this fine-tuned sensitivity to her mother's and others' emotions interfered with her ability to identify, understand, and communicate what she was feeling, even in the most innocuous situations.

Initially, Maria's tendency was to "gloss over" and deny her feelings of anger, sadness, and fear. She would report that "everything was fine," despite clear evidence to the contrary (e.g., tears in her eyes, a negative behavioral report from her teacher). This style was so pronounced that at times Maria contradicted herself in one breath in an effort to avoid expression of her distress. For example, she would state, "School's pretty bad, but I like it," or "It makes me sad but I feel better." This tendency was compounded by Mrs. P.'s discomfort with her own feelings of sadness, anger, and fear, or those feelings expressed by her children. She rarely allowed Maria to fully articulate her negative feelings and focused almost exclusively on the positive side of everything that Maria raised (e.g., "But how can you feel that way, things are getting better") or moving quickly to problem solving (e.g., "You should try again").

Maria had difficulty expressing her emotional needs directly and modulating her own distress. She often reacted to distress by becoming angry and aggressive or intensely sad. Maria often sought nurturance from her mother in indirect or inappropriate ways. For example, she would squeeze between her mother and one of her sisters on the couch, clinging to her mother. She had difficulty trying to soothe herself, and relied primarily on emotive strategies, such as crying, biting her nails, screaming, or aggressive behavior. In general, Maria had few effective coping strategies when she felt emotionally needy and overwhelmed.

Not unexpectedly, Maria had particular difficulty expressing anger in appropriate ways, and she tended to alternate between aggressive and passive behavior when she felt angry. The aggression in her daily experiences was mirrored in Maria's early fantasy play. When Maria came to the attention of the clinic, she hit and pushed both sisters on a regular basis. Prior to the teacher's recommendation for therapy, Mrs. P. walked into Maria's bedroom one evening and found her trying to strangle Anna. While Maria's aggression toward her younger sisters was often an expression of anger (whether it was justified anger toward them or displaced anger toward her mother), Maria sometimes hit her peers at school without provocation and, apparently, without anger. She explained that she "hit them so they won't think I'm afraid of them." A focus of therapy was to help Maria express her anger more appropriately and directly, and to respond to peers assertively.

Adult emotions and moods were experienced as unpredictable and confusing to Maria, and she struggled to understand why adults (and she herself) often displayed sudden changes of mood. She initially explained her play characters' behavior in magical terms, such as "he was put under a spell by an evil wizard" or "he drank a magic potion and became a different person" or "a poltergeist entered his body." The confusion in her play clearly mirrored her feelings about her father and his rapid swings between warmth and aggression. Clearly, an important therapeutic goal would be to help Maria explore these different aspects of her father and begin to integrate her discrepant memories of him.

Assessment of Psychopathology

After the initial evaluation procedures were completed, it became clear that Ann and Rosa were functioning well psychologically but Maria was in emotional turmoil. The therapist recommended psychological testing to further assess Maria's cognitive and socioemotional functioning. She was administered the following assessment instruments: the Wechsler Intelligence Scale for Children-Revised (WISC-R), the Pictorial Scale of Perceived Competence and Social Acceptance for Young Children, Conger Children's Sentence Completion Test, and the Rorschach.

Evaluation Findings

Maria's developmental history was unremarkable. She met all developmental milestones at the appropriate ages and was generally a healthy infant and toddler. She was toilet-trained at approximately 2 years, 2 months, and maintained bladder and bowel control without regression. As far back as she could remember, Mrs. P. felt that Maria was particularly sensitive to their marital arguments. She would cry as soon as anyone raised his voice, and it was often difficult to console her once she became upset. Mrs. P. also described Maria as a "slow-to-warm-up" child, who tended to approach novel situations with trepidation until she spent enough time to feel comfortable and to know what to expect. On the Child Behavior Checklist, Mrs. P. reported elevations in Maria's behavior on the Depression, Somatic Complaints, and Aggression subscales. Maria's teacher generally supported Mrs. P.'s perceptions, although the teacher had a more balanced perspective of Maria's strengths and limitations.

On the WISC-R, Maria obtained a Full Scale IQ of 117, which placed her in the high average range of intelligence. A significant difference of 20 points emerged between her Verbal IQ of 106 and her Performance IQ of 126. Whereas there were many possible explanations for this difference, two appeared especially plausible. First, Maria's "slow-to-warm-up" style was painfully evident during the initial play and testing sessions and appeared to compromise her ability to demonstrate the extent of her knowledge. She was noticeably shy, and she hesitated to guess or elaborate on her answers to verbal subtests. She found the nonverbal performance subtests much easier, perhaps, in part, because she did not have to interact verbally with the examiner. Because of Maria's hesitant style, the examiner felt that her Verbal IQ underestimated her true ability. A second, related explanation is the fact that Maria is bilingual, having learned both English and Spanish simultaneously as a young child. It is not uncommon for bilingual children to score significantly higher on nonverbal than on verbal measures of intelligence (see Kaufman, 1979). A third, and least likely, explanation for Maria's significant Verbal–Performance discrepancy was that she had a learning disability. However, Maria consistently achieved good grades in school, and there was no indication that she was having particular difficulty in any of her subjects. According to her teacher, Maria's academic problems at school stemmed from her frequent daydreaming in class. Once the teacher redirected her attention to work, Maria was easily able to complete her assignments. Follow-up educational testing by the school to assess for learning disability confirmed its absence.

Maria's performance was quite even within the Verbal and Performance domains. All Verbal subscores clustered around the average to slightly above average range, while her Performance subscores were significantly higher. Maria's profile did not evidence any relative strengths or weaknesses.

Maria's scores on the Pictorial Scale of Perceived Competence and Social Acceptance were compared with norms for children her age. Her mean score for perceptions of physical competence was highest, followed by her mean cognitive competence score; both were similar to scores obtained by same-age peers in the normative sample. Maria's perceptions of maternal and peer acceptance were much lower than those reported by same-age peers, and appeared to be an accurate reflection of the relationship with her mother and friends when she entered therapy. Interestingly, Maria's answers on the Sentence Completion Test that related to friendships contradicted the responses she gave on perceptions of peer acceptance. For example, in completing the sentence stem "The thing I do best is . . . ," Maria answered "make friends," which was clearly in contrast to her experience at school and in the neighborhood. Additional Sentence Completion items suggested that Maria's potential for self-awareness was quite good for her age (e.g., "The worst thing about me is . . . I get angry at my sister"). She was clearly struggling to make sense of the often discrepant perceptions she had of her father and her parents' relationship (e.g., "When I see my mother and father together . . . I feel good." "I like my father but . . . he was kind of mean." "What I want to happen the most is . . . love in my family").

Maria's responses on the Rorschach lent additional support to the idea that she was depressed, placed too low a value on herself, and was consumed with extreme anger that, at times, masked her sad and lonely feelings. Her protocol reflected her cautious manner and suggested that she invested a great deal of effort into processing information and was prone to approach stimuli with caution and thoroughness. She tended to rely on her inner world of thoughts and feelings for gratification, but she clearly did not have the psychological resources to cope with her overwhelming pain and turmoil. Her repertoire of coping strategies was limited and somewhat rigid. Her affect was not well modulated, and, under stress, she had little or no sense of being able to control her explosive feelings.

Maria's record contained several special scorings of morbid and aggressive where she attributed depressed or angry affect to her percepts. For example, she perceived "a sad cat" and "a lonely bat" on Card IV; "a hungry cat," "a mean wolf," and "someone who's mad" on Card IX; and "a mad dragon" on Card X. She tended to perceive her social environment as marked by aggressiveness and would be likely to express aggression directly. The form quality for each of these percepts was compromised. There were relatively few human responses (one-tenth of the record) in contrast to animal responses, suggesting that even for her age, there was some detachment from people in her environment. In general, the form quality of Maria's responses suggested that she was not perceiving reality in the same way as other children her age, and form quality deteriorated in the presence of uncontained affect. Her responses indicated the presence of complicated internal conflicts and possibly excessive rumination.

In summary, Maria was functioning in the high average range of intelligence, although the combination of her hesitant response style and bilingual background may have underestimated of her true verbal abilities. She was clearly experiencing emotional turmoil in the form of depression, anxiety, and anger that exceeded her available psychological resources and interfered in multiple domains of her life (e.g., academic, social, and familial spheres). The family evaluation revealed several areas of concern, including the family's isolation from potential support systems, a pervasive crisis atmosphere in the home, Maria's troubled relationship with her mother and father, Mrs. P.'s problems with discipline, and the family's difficulty with emotional expression.

Treatment Recommendations

Given the evaluation findings and psychological testing, the therapist recommended two levels of intervention with the P. family. First, child play therapy sessions with Maria were indicated to address the emotional turmoil that resulted in her anxiety, sadness, and aggressive behavior. These sessions would focus on an exploration of Maria's inner experience, with the ultimate goal of helping her understand and integrate her traumatic memories and effects of living with her father's abusiveness toward her mother and the emotional chaos it caused her and her family. Additional goals were to help Maria express her emotional needs more directly and appropriately, find effective ways to communicate anger, build social skills to encourage more positive peer relationships, and, in general, help to boost her self-esteem.

Second, parenting sessions were recommended to extend and strengthen Mrs. P.'s parenting skills, and to develop more appropriate perceptions and expectations of her children. Intermittent family and mother–daughter sessions were also indicated to focus on communication, decreasing sibling rivalry, and improving Mrs. P.'s relationship with Maria.

Treatment Options

Over a 1-year period, Maria made excellent progress toward the treatment goals identified by her therapist. By the end of therapy, Maria's play had grown significantly less aggressive and she had had no aggressive outbursts at home or school for quite some time. Her fantasy play, which was concerned with injury in various settings, also became more realistic: She was able to cope with problems facing her fantasy characters without resorting to magic or unrealistic rescue solutions. Maria was no longer preoccupied with death and violence, either in her play or in her outside world. She seemed to have gained some distance from her traumatic memories of violence and was able to talk about her experiences in a more integrated way.

For example, at the beginning of therapy, Maria never let the dangers in her play world harm her characters. The endings to her fantasy stories usually involved some magical form of intervention that reversed the potentially violent outcome and provided a more acceptable conclusion. Pynoos and Eth (1986) refer to this type of coping as "denial in fantasy," which is a strategy used by some children to modulate their anxiety after experiencing a traumatic event. In Maria's play, children were run over by cars but were miraculously spared; characters were captured by villains but saved at the last moment; meals appeared magically just before characters starved. Maria was remarkably resistant to attempts to consider what would happen if her play situations played out naturally (i.e., if the play had a negative ending). Only much later in therapy was she able to tolerate and talk about the distress created by these traumas and the violent events that she witnessed. Once this occurred, her play became less magical and more realistic. Over time, Maria also introduced fewer dangers and tragedies into her play.

Maria also felt increasingly comfortable and secure with her place in the family and reported that her relationship with her mother was much improved. She was able to express her feelings and experiences more appropriately to her mother, who was in turn better able to meet Maria's emotional needs. For example, during family sessions, Maria was able to tell her mother how she felt hurt and angry when she was made to be the bad one in the family and her sisters were the "good guys." Mrs. P. was able to listen to Maria and validated her feelings without becoming defensive. Maria's sense of competence and self-esteem grew immensely over the course of therapy, and she was able to understand and feel proud about the gains that she had made.

Maria was observed in her classroom several weeks before terminating therapy. Her teacher reported that Maria was an excellent student, and although she continued to have "perfectionistic tendencies," they did not interfere significantly with her work. On the day that she was observed, Maria earned an early recess as a reward for completing all her assigned work correctly. As Maria cleared her desk and prepared to go outside, two female classmates yelled, "Come on, Maria, let's go play jump rope," and Maria hurried out with them. Although the teacher found her shy at times, Maria was able to make friends in her class and was reported to be happier and far less preoccupied with family matters than she had been 1 year ago. Thus, the teacher's perspective clearly supported the therapist's (and Maria's) view of the hard work that was accomplished during individual therapy.

Throughout treatment, the girls' contact with their father continued to be stressful, particularly for Maria. Mrs. P. struggled to distance herself emotionally from her husband, but continued to express sadness over his inability to "pull himself together," and confusion over the role he should play in their daughters' lives. Mr. P.'s phone calls to Maria were often tense, as he tried to extract information from her about Mrs. P.'s current life. After talking with her father, Maria frequently fought with her mother and sisters. Occasional visitation was arranged, but after the first visit, Mr. P. did not comply with the agreements (e.g., he took the girls away from the site that had been prearranged for visitation and was several hours late in returning the children), and there was some concern about the possibility of kidnapping. Mrs. P. found it extremely difficult to set firm limits with her husband and struggled to decide how to proceed with Mr. P.'s blatant disregard for the visitation arrangements. She contacted the court, and visitation was suspended temporarily until arrangements for supervised visitation were made. Mr. P. decided to enter individual therapy at that time and agreed to supervised visitation until he demonstrated his willingness to establish a more constructive relationship with his children rather than using them as revenge against Mrs. P. Maria's anxiety and symptomatic behaviors slowly decreased after Mr. P. entered therapy and made a commitment to understanding and changing his violent interpersonal relationships. However, supervised visitation continued until after the P. family terminated treatment and the P.'s divorce was finalized.

Mrs. P. also made significant progress during the parenting sessions, the dyadic work with Maria, and the family meetings. A major focus of Mrs. P.'s work was to help her see the connection between her past experiences and her present interactions. Mrs. P. wanted intensely to have what she called "clean and clear" interactions with others. For her, this meant responding to others with feelings that were not entangled with previous experiences in her history. "Clean and clear" responses were those that occurred immediately and that were honest rather than distorted by guilt, self-doubt, or fear of rejection.

A second focus of the therapeutic work with Mrs. P. was to help her with the process of integrating opposite characteristics such as good and bad. This splitting seemed to serve a defensive function for her in that Mrs. P. would often begin to feel overwhelmed if she tried to integrate the two extremes. If Mrs. P. was feeling good, then she did not want to contemplate anything unhappy or "bad." Doing so meant running the risk of losing her good feeling. Over the course of therapy, Mrs. P. grew in her ability to integrate opposites. For example, she began to have increasingly realistic perceptions of the positive and negative attributes of all her daughters, rather than seeing Maria as "sick," and Anna and the baby as "healthy." Mrs. P. also became able to view herself and her experiences more accurately, beginning first with her professional self-image and developing a realistic assessment of her strengths and weaknesses. Further along in therapy, she was less likely to perceive herself and her life either with a "Pollyanna-like" quality or with unrelenting pessimism, as she had when therapy began. Rather than dissolving into misery and helplessness, Mrs. P. was able to say as she faced a new problem, "Maybe I'll be able to make a balance with this as I have with other things." Whereas, in the past, previously small concerns ballooned easily into larger concerns, Mrs. P. grew increasingly able to modulate her emotional responses and maintain a balanced perspective.

At the end of therapy, Mrs. P. was able to change her way of relating in many aspects of her life. In the area of discipline, she experienced a great sense of relief when she was able to give logical consequences for the girls' misbehavior, unmarred by her own issues. She worked hard to control her anger and be firm, rather than harsh, in her disciplinary interactions with her daughters. She also began to model more appropriate ways of communicating emotions to the girls and, over time, felt less threatened and angered by Maria's emotional needs from her. As discipline became less problematic, Mrs. P.'s relationship with Maria slowly began to improve. Most important, Mrs. P. no longer relied on Maria for emotional support and was able to accommodate to Maria's need for connection and affection. Gaining distance from Maria enabled Mrs. P. to begin perceiving her more accurately and positively. Mrs. P.'s empathy for and understanding of her daughter grew, and she was less likely to see Maria as "weird." She began to participate in community events, made several new friends, and, toward the end of therapy, began to date men. As Mrs. P. progressed in each of these areas, her sense of competence as a woman and mother also grew, and she began to take real pride in herself and in *all* of her children.

Summary and Conclusions

In many ways, Maria's story clearly illustrates the finding that witnessing marital violence can be a profoundly disorganizing experience for children, with significant effects on their cognitive, emotional, and behavioral functioning. Child witnesses experience these effects directly (i.e., actually witnessing violence perpetrated against a loved one) and indirectly (i.e., parent–child relationships become distorted and compromised as a result of marital violence). Consequently, it is important for therapists to maintain a systems framework during evaluation and treatment of child witnesses and their families.

Child witnesses to marital violence live in a world of extremes and come to understand, and respond to their environment, in terms of dichotomies. Children may experience their parents as emotionally unavailable or overavailable, controlled or explosive, ignoring or overreacting. They may alternately try to deny or ruminate on memories of violence, feel powerful or profoundly powerless, minimize negative emotions or explode with anger and sadness. Child witnesses develop ways of coping that may be quite adaptive in the context of living in a violent family. However, over time, these coping strategies begin to interfere with the child's emotional health and become maladaptive in interactions outside the family. The content of therapy is not limited to helping children confront and integrate their traumatic memories; it also enables the therapist to focus on children's distorted cognitions, emotional reactions, and behavioral responses with the goals of increasing flexibility, modulation, and balance. Therapists must not underestimate the deleterious effects of witnessing violence on children's psychological well-being and must profit by the opportunity to guide child witnesses and their families toward healthier intra- and interpersonal relationships.

References

Barnett, E. R., Pitman, C. B., Ragan, C. K., & Salus, M. K. (1980). *Family violence: Intervention strategies.* Publication No. (OHDS) 80-30258. Washington, DC: U.S. Department of H.H.S.

Bergman, A. (1976). Emergency room: A role for social workers. *Health and Social Work, 1,* 1.

Browne, A. (1987). *When battered women kill.* New York: Free Press.

Giles-Sims, J. (1983). *Wife battering: A systems theory approach.* New York: Guilford Press.

Hilberman, E. (1979). The battered woman. *Emergency Medicine, 2,* 24.

Kaufman, A. S. (1979). *Intelligent testing with the WISC-R.* New York: Wiley.

Klingbeil, K. S., & Boyd, V. D. (1984). Emergency room intervention: Detection, assessment and treatment. In A. R. Roberts (Ed.), *Battered women and their families: Intervention strategies and treatment programs* (pp. 7–32). New York: Springer.

Minuchin, S. (1974). *Families and family therapy.* Cambridge, MA: Harvard University Press.

Pynoos, R. S., & Eth, S. (1986). Witness to violence: The child interview. *Journal of the American Academy of Child Psychiatry, 25,* 306–319.

Rosenberg, M. S., & Rossman, B. B. R. (1990). The child witness to marital violence. In R. T. Ammerman & M. Hersen (Eds.), *Treatment of family violence: A sourcebook* (pp. 183–210). New York: Wiley.

Stark, E., Flitcraft, A., & Frazier, W. (1979). Medicine and patriarchal violence: The social construction of a "private" event. *International Journal of Health Services, 9,* 461–489.

Walker, L. E. A. (1979). *The battered woman.* New York: Harper & Row.

Walker, L. E. A. (1984). *The battered woman syndrome.* New York: Springer.

Walker, L. E. A., & Edwall, G. E. (1987). Domestic violence and determination of visitation and custody in divorce. In D. J. Sonkin (Ed.), *Domestic violence on trial: Psychological and legal dimensions of family violence* (pp. 127–152). New York: Springer.

Weithorn, L. A. (Ed.). (1987). *Psychology and child custody determinations: Knowledge, roles and expertise.* Lincoln: University of Nebraska Press.

15

Psychological and Emotional Abuse of Children

Marla R. Brassard, Stuart N. Hart, and David B. Hardy

Description of the Problem

Psychological maltreatment is increasingly recognized as a core issue in all forms of child maltreatment and as the unifying concept that connects the cognitive, affective, and interpersonal problems that are related to physical abuse, sexual abuse, and all forms of neglect (Brassard & Gelardo, 1987; Brassard, Germain, & Hart, 1987). It is the repeated pattern of behavior that expresses to children that they are worthless, unwanted, unloved, or only of value in meeting another's needs that causes the lasting damage to their selves and their psyches.

The psychological concomitants, more than the severity of the acts themselves, constitute the real traumas and are responsible for the damaging consequences of sexual (Brassard & McNeill, 1987) and physical abuse (Crittenden, 1989; Hart & Brassard, 1989). In cases of neglect it is not simply the parents' failure to provide adequate care but the pervasive psychological unavailability and the lost opportunities for healthy interpersonal involvement that place a child at risk for severe developmental disorders (Farber & Egeland, 1987).

Marla R. Brassard and David B. Hardy • Office for the Study of the Psychological Rights of the Child, University of Massachusetts–Amherst, Amherst, Massachusetts 01030. **Stuart N. Hart** • School of Education, Indiana University–Purdue University at Indianapolis, Indianapolis, Indiana 46202.

While psychological maltreatment is gaining increasing attention, most existing definitions have been judged to be ambiguous and to provide insufficient direction for responsible application. Legislators, judges, child protective service workers, clinicians, and researchers all attempt definitions from different perspectives with different intents. A number of facts confound the issue: Psychological maltreatment is manifested in both acts of commission and acts of omission, there is an absence of physical evidence, it both occurs with other forms of maltreatment and exists alone, it can be defined only within an interpersonal context, and definition is dependent on the developmental stage of the victim. With the lack of an adequately operationalized definition, it becomes problematic to identify psychological maltreatment and to provide appropriate protective services to those families that are in need.

Accurate estimates of the incidence of psychological maltreatment are extremely difficult, if not impossible, to obtain. Psychological maltreatment was recognized as the primary form of abuse in approximately 11% of the 2 million cases of child maltreatment reported in years 1986 and 1987 (American Humane Society, 1988, 1989). It is generally accepted that only a small percentage of cases of maltreatment are reported, and we believe this to be particularly true for psychological maltreatment. Unless they co-occur with other forms of severe abuse, cases of psychological maltreatment are likely to go unreported. If reported, they are less likely to be screened into CPS, less likely to go to court, and less likely to receive serious interventions.

In an attempt to establish an adequately operationalized definition of psychological maltreatment, we used a combination of categories of psychological abuse and neglect conceptualized by ourselves and other researchers (Baily & Baily, 1986; Brassard *et al.*, 1987; Garbarino, Guttman, & Seeley, 1986; United States Department of Health and Human Services, 1988). We have subsequently empirically identified and articulated five distinct subtypes of psychological maltreatment.

Spurning is a type of verbal battering that is a combination of rejection and hostile degradation. The parent may actively refuse to help a child or even to acknowledge the child's request for help. Spurning also includes calling a child debasing names, labeling the child as inferior, and publicly humiliating the child.

Terrorizing is threatening to physically hurt, kill, or abandon the child if he/she does not behave. It also includes exposing a child to violence or threats directed toward loved ones and leaving a young child unattended.

Isolating entails the active isolation of a child by an adult. The child may be locked in a closet or room for an extended length of time, or the adult may limit or refuse to allow any interaction with peers or adults outside the family.

Exploiting/Corrupting involves modeling antisocial acts and unrealistic roles or encouraging and condoning deviant standards or beliefs. This includes teaching the child criminal behavior, keeping a child at home in the role of a servant or surrogate parent in lieu of school attendance, or encouraging a child to participate in the production of pornography.

Denying emotional responsiveness includes ignoring a child's attempts to interact and reacting to a child in a mechanistic way that is devoid of affectionate touch, kiss, and talk. Parents who behave this way communicate through acts of omission that they are not interested in the child and are emotionally unavailable.

Consequences of Psychological Maltreatment

Current research strongly associates psychological maltreatment with a wide range of emotional and behavioral problems for children (Hart, Germain, & Brassard, 1987). Empirical cause and effect evidence, although sparse, exists for a small sample of children whose parents were verbally abusive/hostile and/or provided psychologically unavailable caretaking. These children, subjects in a prospective longitudinal research project, have shown serious social, emotional, and learning problems beyond other general effects of their environments (Egeland, Sroufe, & Erickson, 1983; Erickson & Egeland, 1987). On a national level, the American Humane Association (Wald, 1961) and the National Center for Child Abuse and Neglect (Broadhurst, 1984) have presented the following list of possible negative consequences of psychological maltreatment: behavior extremes, habit disorders, conduct disorders, neurotic traits, psychoneurotic reactions, overly adaptive behaviors, lags in development, and attempted suicide (see Hart *et al.*, 1987, for further clarification).

Case Description

Introduction to the Case
The case described here is an actual family that participated in our research project on psychological maltreatment (Hart & Brassard, 1989); however, all names and identifying characteristics have been changed to ensure confidentiality. The D'Niale family is a multiproblem family that has clearly experienced for several generations the problems related to poverty, unemployment, substance abuse, criminal activity, domestic violence, and the physical abuse and neglect of children.

The D'Niale family was chosen as a case study because the family as a whole functioned as a powerful but destructive force that undermined the healthy development of identity, self-esteem, and autonomy in all of its members. The D'Niale family, with its constant crises and pathogenic functioning, failed to provide even the bare minimum of psychological support, cognitive stimulation, and encouragement that is necessary for normal child development.

The second criterion that led to selection of this family as a case study is that during our assessment we witnessed incidents of all five subtypes of psychological maltreatment. We will describe the examples we identified and attempt to articulate the connections between the specific parental behaviors and the developmental outcomes exhibited in the children's behavior.

In July of 1987 the State Department of Social Services (DSS) received a report from a preschool teacher concerning the possible abuse of a 4-year-old named Joey D'Niale, who had arrived at school with multiple bruises. During the investigation, Joey's mother, Blanche D'Niale, blamed her mother, Beatrice Gelid, who in turn blamed Blanche, and both finally resorted to blaming Joey's 20-month-old brother, Sonny Jr. Charges of physical abuse were substantiated, although a perpetrator was not identified.

Blanche D'Niale and her family were not new to DSS; they had been in and out of the system since shortly after the birth of Blanche's first child in 1980. Joey had personally received services from eight social service agencies in addition to the protective services received from the department. The D'Niale family file at DSS was also cross-indexed with the files of several members of Blanche's extended family, indicating that interfamily as well as intrafamily patterns of maltreatment existed.

Assessment

Our family research assessment, described more extensively later in this chapter, lasts about 4 hours. It involves the collection of information on physical condition of the home, mother's psychological functioning, her satisfaction with her relationships, current life stressors, and information on her family of origin. The mother is also videotaped interacting in a structured task with one of her children.

While Blanche was more than cooperative throughout the assessment, which not only taxes one's endurance but demands significant self-disclosure, there were constant interruptions created by her 20-month-old son, Sonny Jr. Oscillating between ignoring him entirely, threatening to break his fingers, promising to buy him presents, and demanding that he not act like a baby, her responses only seemed to escalate his oppositional and aversive behavior. Sonny Jr. became extremely active, continually climbing on and poking the two members of our assessment team, crumpling up completed questionnaires, and then spilling milk all over the table.

Blanche's mother arrived and immediately monopolized the assessment. She insisted on answering questions on marital satisfaction and parenting practices that were clearly directed toward Blanche, often contradicting or discounting Blanche's responses. Her insensitive and intrusive behavior toward Blanche was markedly similar to Blanche's behavior toward her own children.

In our assessments, we always start with an attempt to identify who the significant players in the family and home are and how they are related. This proved to be no easy task in the D'Niale family. The family has moved seven times in the last 2 years, with the composition of the household changing constantly, as extended family members move in and out. The structure of Blanche's family matched what her caseworker described as an "extremely enmeshed matriarchy." The stable relationships in the family seem to exist among Blanche; her sister, Barbie Gelid; her mother, Beatrice Gelid; and her recently deceased maternal grandmother. Blanche is currently married to Sonny Jr.'s father, but all three of her children have different fathers; all of her relationships with men seem unstable and full of conflict: a configuration that closely resembles her description of both her sister's and mother's relationships with men.

Characteristics of Family Members

Blanche D'Niale: Blanche is a white woman 29 years of age. She evidenced mild to severe deficits on all assessment measures. Her intellectual ability fell in the borderline to mentally retarded range. On the Beck Depression Inventory, Blanche's score of 27 placed her in the moderate to severe range for depression. She has no job skills and has been living on welfare since the birth of her first child.

Blanche was easily engaged in the assessment process, and she talked freely about the problems in her family and marriage. In our Family of Origin Interview Blanche reported that she was born and has lived all of her life within several blocks of her current apartment. Shortly after Blanche's birth her mother abandoned her to the care of her maternal grandmother, where she lived for 5 years until her grandmother overdosed on drugs. She remembers those 5 years as the happiest of her life. In the subsequent years of her childhood she was shuffled from one home to another as family members proved unable to provide adequate care for her. The descriptions of her early experiences seem split between reports of horrendous abuse and neglect and reminiscences of idealized family relationships.

At the time of the assessment, Blanche had minimum social support and much consequent stress. Her current relationship was physically violent and occasionally life-threatening to both parties. She reported major conflicts over childrearing and was awaiting the beginning of her husband's jail sentence. On the Locke-Wallace Marital Satisfaction Scale, Blanche's score of 56 is over 2 standard deviations below average. She indicated that she wished she hadn't married and that she was "very unhappy" in her marriage.

There were noticeable skill deficits in Blanche's parenting. She consistently placed age-inappropriate expectations on her children's behavior, at times infantilizing them and at times expecting them to act like adults. She told her 2-year-old son to go into the kitchen and get some juice and a plate of cookies for her guests, and then later reprimanded her 5-year-old for drinking out of a glass and not a spill-proof plastic cup. She stated that Sonny Jr. helped with the housework because even at the age of 2 he realized it was too much work for her to do alone. Blanche seemed to possess little understanding of the developmental needs of children, especially those needs that are related to healthy social and psychological development. Despite constant interruptions, Blanche answered all of our questions without hesitation. However, her responses indicated a severe lack of integration and an almost total absence of reflective thought. She repeatedly contradicted herself, denying the obvious and producing answers that were inconsistent. The most striking example of this was her response when asked how she would raise her children differently than she was raised. She answered that she would not abuse her children as she had been abused, while simultaneously making threatening gestures with a lit cigarette to Sonny Jr., who was attempting to climb into her lap. Although she was not able to identify any sources of satisfaction in her parenting role or any strengths in her relationships with her children, Blanche claimed that she enjoys being a parent and "loves children." She is currently trying to conceive another child.

Sonny D'Niale: Sonny is a chronic alcoholic who suffers from alcohol-related seizures and episodes of violent acting-out. One month prior to our visit, upon discovering there was no cold beer in the apartment, he dragged the refrigerator onto the back porch and sent it plunging into the alley four floors below. At the time of the assessment he was unemployed, had just been convicted on charges of breaking and entering, and was awaiting sentencing. We were able to obtain little information on his family of origin other than the fact that his father was an alcoholic and his brother had recently overdosed on narcotics. Although Blanche had little positive to say about her husband, she did emphasize that he is an involved father and has good relationships with both of her sons.

Sonny Jr.: Sonny Jr., just over 2 years of age, has a small but solid stature similar to his father's. He was in constant movement for the 4 hours that we were present, engaging in continual limit-testing and oppositional behavior. The toys in the house bore testimony to his destructiveness, for all of the toy cars were without windows or wheels, and there was an extensive collection of dolls and stuffed animals with missing ears or limbs. He constantly bullied his older brother and continually punched, kicked, and poked both members of the assessment team. For some reason, Sonny Jr. seemed to be favored by his mother, and despite overwhelming evidence to the contrary, she proudly exclaimed that he is the brightest and best behaved of her children.

Joey: Joey is Blanche's 5-year-old son. He is a severely withdrawn child who shies away from interaction with both family and strangers. His development is markedly delayed, and since infancy he has been involved in various developmental intervention programs. However, his attendance has been poor and his progress has been limited. His protective service records contain numerous complaints by service providers that

Blanche neglects to follow through on recommendations and fails to take Joey to scheduled appointments. While Blanche seems to appreciate the involvement of agency staff in her life during periods of crisis, she seems committed to keeping the attention focused upon herself, and actively sabotages attempts to address Joey's needs.

Joey has experienced much early trauma in his home. Not only was he physically abused by his mother, his grandmother, and his younger brother, but in addition, he witnessed the battering of his mother by his stepfather, the rape of his mother by a neighbor, and the death of a child care provider, and he was burned out of his home by arsonists. After we were there for several hours, Joey did cautiously approach us and happily played with the drawing materials we provided. His quiet gentleness provided a stark contrast to the constant acting-out of his little brother.

When assessed at school, Joey obtained an IQ of 91 on the Wechsler Preschool and Primary Scale Intelligence Test, which placed him at the bottom end of the average range of functioning. His readiness skills were assessed with the Woodcock-Johnson Tests of Academic Achievement, in which he scored in the low average range. On the Perceived Self Competence Teacher Form, Joey's teacher rated him very low on peer acceptance and low on the cognitive competence scale. On the Child Behavior Checklist (CBC) his ratings placed him in the clinical range on the internalizing scale. His scores were above the 98th percentile on the anxious, socially withdrawn, and obsessive compulsive subscales. On the CBC the teacher also reported that Joey was less hardworking, behaved less appropriately, seemed less happy, and learned less than his special education peers. The teacher's comments about Joey reflect her ratings on the various scales. She wrote: "Joey is a very passive little boy who shows very little emotion. He communicates through whispers and physical gestures. He plays alone or next to peers. He has a tendency to observe other children at play and he tunes out others at group time."

Francine: At age 8, Francine is Blanche's oldest child. When Francine was 5 months old, an anonymous report that Blanche was leaving her child unsupervised for long periods of time was filed through the Child Abuse Hotline. During the investigation the social worker reported that she witnessed Blanche yelling at the infant in an abusive fashion and that the child was not receiving adequate physical care. Blanche agreed to relinquish custody of Francine to her mother (Beatrice). The neglect and abuse continued under the custody of Beatrice. Early in 1983, charges of neglect were substantiated when a local hospital reported that Francine had received emergency services for the ingestion of toxic substances three times in as many months. Then, in 1985, charges of physical abuse were substantiated against Beatrice when Francine appeared at school with a bruised face.

Affirming her continued involvement in her daughter's life, Blanche explained that she is often recruited to help with the disciplining of Francine, who acts like a "juvenile delinquent." Describing a recent incident in which Francine ran away from her grandmother's home, Blanche stated:

"That was no way to treat my mother. I hunted her down and beat her. I only hope she has learned something." Although we were unable to obtain any information from Francine's school, it is documented that she received special education services and that the school has filed complaints of educational neglect.

Psychological Maltreatment in the D'Niale Family

Spurning was clearly evidenced in the D'Niale family. Blanche continually belittled her children, calling Joey a sissy, a baby, "stupid," and an assortment of other degrading names. She referred to Sonny Jr., who spent the 4 hours of our visit in a soiled diaper, as "stinker" and "my little shit." Blanche's lack of knowledge of child development and unrealistic expectations of her children continually created opportunities for disappointment and frustration, which she would then angrily vent upon her children. Joey's anxiety and low self-esteem and Sonny Jr.'s angry acting-out are clearly related to Blanche's repeated verbal attacks.

Terrorizing seemed to be one of the D'Niale family's most frequently used means of asserting control and power. The use of corporal punishment is an unquestioned aspect of parenting for Blanche. She claimed: "Even my social worker says it's all right to hit your kids as long as you use your bare hand. I never use my fist, and when I kick them I always use the side of my foot, never the front."

During the assessment Blanche used threats of physical punishment that bordered on brutality. When Sonny Jr. spilled a glass of milk, a not uncommon occurrence for a 2-year-old child, Blanche responded with the threat "Clean that up or I'll break your fingers." She repeatedly threatened to break bones and noses, to burn with her cigarette, and to put Joey out with the garbage.

There appears to be a clear causal relationship between Joey's social withdrawal, Sonny Jr.'s hypervigilance, Francine's habitual running away, and the climate of terror that is created by the verbal and physical assaults that family members inflict upon one another. Since this situation is supplemented with experiences of rape, death, fire, and homelessness, it is easy to understand how the D'Niale children exhibit various patterns of maladaption and psychological distress.

The D'Niale family exhibited several isolating behaviors. Blanche listed her mother, her sister, and her sister-in-law as her three best friends, and commented that the family tends not to socialize with outsiders. Frequent conflicts with their neighbors is the norm. Blanche never lets her children play with other children in the neighborhood and has been cited repeatedly for keeping her children home from school. Several times during the assessment she advised us to ignore the children, and made unsuccessful attempts to confine the children in their bedroom. The deficits in social competence that all of the children display are related to this extensive restriction of opportunities to interact with peers and adults outside the family.

Exploiting and corrupting behavior was seen in Sonny Sr.'s models of criminal behavior, alcohol abuse, and violent acting-out. Blanche used threats and extortion to control her children's behavior, reported keeping the children home from school when she wanted company, and used the children for protection when Sonny was drunk and abusive. In the D'Niale family, the multigenerational pattern of chronic unmet needs and crisis addiction, coupled with extremely limited emotional, financial, and intellectual resources, has led to both overt and unintentional exploitation of others.

The chronic omission of appropriate emotional responses in the D'Niale family constituted extreme denied emotional responsiveness. Reflecting her depression, Blanche generally exhibited a flat affect, with an occasional outburst of hostility that seemed more related to her internal processes than an appropriate response to ongoing interactions. A startling example of her denied emotional response, with an element of corruption, occurred during our visit. Joey had been attempting to draw at the coffee table, but Sonny Jr. kept tearing up the paper Joey was working on. Without protest, Joey moved his paper to the sill of the open window, where he could draw while shielding the paper from his little brother. Sonny Jr. responded by going over and slamming the window sash down upon Joey's hands. Joey turned toward Blanche, crying. She shot him an annoyed glance and admonished him, "You are three years older, you have to learn to hit back."

With so much loss, pain, and anger in Blanche's relationships, it is understandable that she does not possess the necessary emotional resources to respond adequately to the needs of her children. However, the extent of her emotional neglect of her children almost certainly places them at risk for serious psychological maladaption. While there are undeniably strong bonds in the D'Niale family, it is a family that is devoid of healthy attachments, and the qualities of care and protection that are so essential to human development are noticeably absent. Without extensive therapeutic interventions these maladaptive patterns of attachment will most likely persist, creating problems and disruptions in relationships throughout the D'Niale children's lives. In addition, their disorganized and problematic patterns of attachment jeopardize the establishment of future relationships that can provide corrective experiences.

Medical Issues

Psychological maltreatment as a separate form of maltreatment is not usually associated with medical problems, nor is it typically identified by medical professionals unless it co-occurs with failure to thrive, medical neglect, or accidents resulting from poor supervision. However, Blanche D'Niale had been reported to CPS on charges of medical neglect for not attending to Joey's ear infections.

Legal Issues

Psychological maltreatment is a relatively new legal concept in family law (see Corson & Davidson, 1987; Melton & Corson, 1987). The federal Child Abuse Prevention and Treatment Act of 1974 included a "mental injury" category in its definition but left further definition to the states (see Corson & Davidson, 1987, for a review). State statutes vary dramatically in the degree to which the term *mental injury* is specified, with most delegating the drafting of regulations to child protective services. When CPS does not assume this role, social workers are left to their own devices in deciding whether psychological maltreatment is serious enough to warrant state intervention.

Even where states have clear guidelines, state welfare supervisors have indicated that although caseworker understanding of the concept has improved, there is little increase in the number of cases identified. However, where cases are identified, there is more willingness to investigate them and they are more consistently handled (M. Fuller, personal communication, September 9, 1985; J. Tondrowski, personal communication, September 12, 1985; cited in Melton & Corson, 1987).

We have found CPS reluctant to pursue psychological maltreatment cases unless it cooccurs with another form of abuse and neglect. Agency action in the D'Niale case is typical. The department was concerned about medical neglect, educational neglect, physical abuse, and lack of adequate supervision. When each of these issues had been successfully dealt with, the CPS case was closed despite awareness of continuing psychological abuse and neglect.

Social and Family Issues

Much research has been done on the social influences and family characteristics associated with child maltreatment in its various forms (Brassard *et al.*, 1987; Gil, 1970; Wolfe, 1987). Unfortunately, we know very little about families where maltreatment occurs but that do not come to the attention of child protective services. Our own research and the clinical observations of others indicate that many of the factors related to other forms of maltreatment are also associated with psychological maltreatment. However, patterns of these factors unique to psychological maltreatment have yet to be identified. The combination of poverty, substance abuse, maternal depression, marital violence and instability, and the absence of adequate problem-solving and parenting skills in the D'Niale family constitute a cluster of problems that is quite typical in families where child maltreatment occurs and is likely to be identified.

Assessment of Psychopathology

The assessment of psychological maltreatment has proven difficult since its conceptualization as a unique category of abuse and neglect. As part of a 3-year federal grant from the National Center on Child Abuse and Neglect, we found that psychological maltreatment can be differentiated into the five distinct subtypes described earlier. We also found that it is possible to distinguish between maltreatment and appropriate parenting through the use of a multidimensional scaling of parenting practices. Maltreating mothers of preschool and school-aged children can be discriminated from carefully matched control mothers using ratings of psychological maltreatment displayed during videotaped parent–child interactions on age-appropriate tasks. These video scale observation measures were significantly related to child interpersonal competence and successfully identified 93% of the children rated by their teachers as having unusually poor peer relationships (Hart & Brassard, 1989).

Blanche obtained moderate scores on all five of the psychological maltreatment subscales, combining to give her a high total scale score. She did not obtain a single point on our good parent scales, which measure prosocial and prodevelopment behavior of the mother exhibited during the videotaped session.

Using Belsky's (1984) model of the determinants of parenting, we assumed that Blanche's ability to parent would be determined by (a) her personal resources (history of care and development in childhood, personality, competencies, and presence and degree of psychopathology); (b) the social support available to her and stress she has to contend with (marital satisfaction, life stress and hassles, and family/community support for her childrearing efforts); and (c) the ease or difficulty involved in rearing her particular children (a function of constitutional factors and behavioral shaping of interactional patterns over time inferred from current developmental status and case records). Therefore, these were the variables we examined in order to assess prognosis for treatment and to attempt to understand the extent of family dysfunction we observed.

Treatment Options

Much of the treatment research and clinical experience with maltreating families suggests that they are very difficult to work with and that often our efforts are unsuccessful (Cohn & Daro, 1987). In working with psychologically maltreating families, we have been developing a comprehensive treatment model derived from a combination of ecological/ systemic theory, psychoanalytically influenced organizational theory, and social learning theory.

The pattern of isolation and limited openness to new information from the environment that exists in the D'Niale family is common in maltreating families. Absence of exposure to other models of parenting maintains the belief that abusive behavior is appropriate and that acts of abuse are ultimately the fault of the child (Kaufman, 1988: Spinetta & Rigler, 1972). It not only allows maltreatment to occur undetected but also weakens the social supports necessary to mediate family stresses and increases the likelihood that abusive and maladaptive problem-solving strategies will be employed (Garbarino, 1977; Polansky, Chalmers, Buttenweiser, & Williams, 1981; Wahler, 1980).

Owing to this pattern of isolation from social supports and inadequate problem-solving skills, the D'Niales, like other multiproblem families, are caught in cycles of "perpetual crisis" (Kagan & Schlosberg, 1989). Continual experiences of abandonment, trauma, and anxious arousal divert the family from productive problem solving and reinforce chaotic behavioral patterns of violent acting-out, denial, projection, and hopelessness.

Because multiproblem families are often less resistant to outside intervention during crisis periods, within our treatment model each crisis is used as an opportunity to build a supportive, consistent relationship with the family. As we work with the family to deal with the crisis on the concrete level, we not only demonstrate and teach appropriate problem-solving skills but also present more rewarding models of interpersonal relationships and provide opportunities for family members to come to terms with past traumas.

Critical to engaging the D'Niale family in treatment is establishing a relationship with Blanche. As with other parents, Blanche's unresolved issues from her own childhood have enormous impact on her own parenting. In maltreating families, the unmet psychological needs of the adults prohibit their empathizing with and protecting their children (Erickson, 1988; Fraiberg, 1983). Parents abused as children need assistance in learning new models of relating to and communicating with others. They must have an opportunity to work through, cognitively and affectively, the painful experiences of childhood trauma that prevent them from forming nurturing relationships with their children. Whether conceptualized as transference issues (Fraiberg, 1983), dysfunctional representational working models of relationships (Bretherton, 1985; Sroufe & Fleeson, 1986), unresolved issues in parents' families of origin (Bowen, 1978), or a cognitive developmental immaturity (Ivey, 1987; Newberger, 1980), many maltreating parents are not psychologically able to assume the role of adult and parent because of unmet needs and concomitant delays in their own cognitive and emotional development.

In many maltreating families, including the D'Niale family, parents often need extensive individual attention and nurturance before interventions with other family members can occur. As the therapeutic relationship with Blanche is developed and stabilized, this individual attention will be balanced by attempts to reach out and engage Sonny in the treatment process. Not only are marital issues an important part of the treatment of maltreating families, but the existence of drug or alcohol problems in families greatly impedes all interventions to improve family functioning and eliminate abuse (Daro, 1988).

A lack of skills for solving both interpersonal and concrete problems exacerbates the psychological neediness and social isolation that these families experience. The treatment provider needs to offer parents assistance in acquiring specific skills, such as (a) parenting (child management, knowledge of child development and how to facilitate it); (b) relationship forming and maintaining (communication, social skills, problem solving, perspective taking); (c) anger management; and (d) basic life skills and empowerment (money management, assertiveness with institutions such as welfare, hospitals, schools). Behavior therapists have demonstrated the effectiveness of their interventions with maltreating parents in these areas (Goldstein, Keller, & Erne, 1985; Lutzker, 1983; Wolfe, 1987).

Because child maltreatment is usually seen as a symptom of parental dysfunction, most interventions have focused on changing the parents or the home environment rather than on direct treatment of children (cases where a child is removed from the home and provided with treatment would be the exception). This approach rarely relieves the children's emotional response to the maltreatment and leaves them vulnerable to repeating problematic patterns of relating in all of their relationships, most notably in relationships with their own children (Mann & McDermott, 1983).

Therapeutic work with children in general is still in its infancy (Kazdin, 1988), but there are promising models and research findings that suggest that this is a fruitful area for exploration. Play therapy (Mann & McDermott, 1983), developmental therapy (Ivey, 1987), and group therapy for children (Steward, Farquhar, Dicharry, Glick, & Martin, 1986) are several models that merit further evaluation.

Both Sonny Jr. and Joey have been referred to therapists who specialize in work with abused and neglected children. As with their parents, interventions will focus on the working through of traumas, the development of corrective relationships, and skill development in the areas of interpersonal relations, affect modulation, and behavior control.

The problems and crisis of the D'Niale family are so numerous and severe that it is quite easy for professionals dealing with this type of family to become as overwhelmed and hopeless as the family members are themselves. It is a vital aspect of the treatment process to realize the family resources that are available and personal strengths of its members (Karpel, 1986). These strengths are not always readily apparent, yet they must be identified, actively validated, and used as building blocks.

Summary and Conclusions

There is growing agreement that psychological maltreatment is the core issue in child maltreatment. We have demonstrated that the strength of this argument rests on the widely supported assumptions that (a) psychological maltreatment is inherent in all forms of child maltreatment; (b) the negative consequences of child maltreatment are generally psychological in nature, affecting the victim's sense of self, interpersonal relationships, and world view; and (c) the concept clarifies and unifies the dynamics that underlie the destructive power of all forms of child abuse and neglect. We further articulated the five subtypes of child maltreatment with concrete examples from a case study and have offered suggestions for appropriate interventions in these cases.

Acknowledgments

The authors would like to thank Carey Dimmitt for her comments on an earlier draft of this manuscript, the Massachusetts Department of Social Services for their ongoing assistance in our work, and the "D'Niale" family for their willingness to share their experiences with us.

References

American Humane Association. (1988). *Highlights of official child neglect and abuse reporting 1986.* Denver: Author.
American Humane Association. (1989). *Highlights of official child neglect and abuse reporting 1987.* Denver: Author.
Baily, F. T., & Baily, W. H. (1986). *Operational definitions of child emotional maltreatment.* Augusta, ME: Maine Department of Social Services.
Belsky, J. (1984). The determinants of parenting: A process model. *Child Development, 55,* 83–96.
Bowen, M. (1978). *Family therapy in clinical practice.* New York: Jason Aronson.
Brassard, M. R., & Gelardo, M. S. (1987). Psychological maltreatment: The unifying construct in child abuse and neglect. *School Psychology Review, 16,* ·127–136.
Brassard, M. R., & McNeill, L. (1987). Child sexual abuse. In M. R. Brassard, R. Germain, & S. N. Hart (Eds.), *Psychological maltreatment of children and youth* (pp. 69–88). New York: Pergamon.
Brassard, M. R., Germain, R., & Hart, S. N. (1987). *Psychological maltreatment of children and youth.* New York: Pergamon.

Bretherton, I. (1985). Attachment theory: Retrospect and prospect. In I. Bretherton & E. Waters (Eds.), *Growing points in attachment theory and research: Monographs of the Society for Research in Child Development, 50*(1–2, Serial No. 209). Chicago: University of Chicago Press.

Broadhurst, D. D. (1984). *The educator's role in the prevention and treatment of child abuse and neglect.* Washington, DC: National Center on Child Abuse and Neglect, U.S. Department of Health and Human Services.

Cohn, A. H., & Daro, D. (1987). Is treatment too late: What ten years of evaluative research tell us. *Child Abuse and Neglect, 11*, 433–442.

Corson, J., & Davidson, H. (1987). Emotional abuse and the law. In M. R. Brassard, R. Germain, & S. N. Hart (Eds.), *Psychological maltreatment of children and youth* (pp. 185–202). New York: Pergamon.

Crittenden, P. (1989, March). Oral presentation to the NCCAN Research Grantees Meeting, Washington, DC.

Daro, D. (1988). *Confronting child abuse.* New York: Free Press.

Egeland, B., & Erickson, M. F. (1987). Psychologically unavailable caregiving. In M. R. Brassard, R. Germain, & S. N. Hart (Eds.), *Psychological maltreatment of children and youth* (pp. 110–120). New York: Pergamon.

Egeland, B., Sroufe, L. A., & Erickson, M. (1983). The developmental consequences of different patterns of maltreatment. *Child Abuse and Neglect, 7*, 459–469.

Erickson, M. F. (1988). *School psychology in preschool settings.* Paper presented at the annual meeting of the National Association of School Psychologists, Chicago.

Erickson, M. F., & Egeland, B. (1987). A developmental view of the psychological consequences of maltreatment. *School Psychology Review, 16*, 156–168.

Farber, E. A., & Egeland, B. (1987). Invulnerability among abused and neglected children. In E. J. Anthony & B. C. Cohler (Eds.), *The invulnerable child* (pp. 253–288). New York: Guilford Press.

Fraiberg, S. (Ed.). (1983). *Clinical studies in infant mental health: The first year of life.* New York: Basic Books.

Garbarino, J. (1977). The human ecology of child maltreatment: A conceptual model for research. *Journal of Marriage and the Family, 39*, 721–735.

Garbarino, J., Guttman, E., & Seeley, J. (1986). *The psychologically battered child: Strategies for identification, assessment, and intervention.* San Francisco: Jossey-Bass.

Gil, D. B. (1970). *Violence against children: Physical child abuse in the United States.* Cambridge, MA: Harvard University Press.

Goldstein, A. P., Keller, H., & Erne, D. (1985). *Changing the abusive parent.* Champaign, IL: Research Press.

Hart, S. N., & Brassard, M. R. (1987). A major threat to children's mental health: Psychological maltreatment. *American Psychologist, 42*, 160–165.

Hart, S. N., & Brassard, M. R. (1989). *Developing and validating operationally defined measures of emotional maltreatment* (NCCAN Research Grant Final Report). Unpublished.

Hart, S. N., Germain, R., & Brassard, M. R. (1987). The challenge: To better understand and combat psychological maltreatment of children and youth. In M. R. Brassard, R. Germain, & S. N. Hart (Eds.), *Psychological maltreatment of children and youth* (pp. 3–24). New York: Pergamon.

Ivey, A. (1987). *Developmental therapy.* San Francisco: Jossey-Bass.

Kagan, R., & Scholsberg, S. (1989). *Families in perpetual crisis.* New York: W. W. Norton.

Karpel, M. (Ed.). (1986). *Family resources: The hidden partner in family therapy.* New York: Guilford Press.

Kaufman, K. (1988). *Child abuse assessment from a systems perspective.* Unpublished paper. Obtainable from the author at Children's Hospital, Department of Pediatrics, Ohio State University, Columbus, OH 43210.

Kazdin, A. (1988). *Child psychotherapy.* New York: Pergamon.

Lutzker, J. R. (1983). Project 12-Ways: Treating child abuse and neglect from an eco-behavioral perspective. In R. F. Dangel & R. A. Polster (Eds.), *Parent training* (pp. 260–297). New York: Guilford Press.

Mann, E., & McDermott, J. F., Jr. (1983). Play therapy for victims of child abuse and neglect. In C. Schaefer & K. O'Connor (Eds.), *Handbook of play therapy* (pp. 283–307). New York: Wiley.

Melton, G. B., & Corson, J. (1987). Psychological maltreatment and the schools: Problems of law and professional responsibility. *School Psychology Review, 16,* 188–194.

Newberger, C. M. (1980). The cognitive structure of parenthood: The development of a descriptive measure. In R. Selman & R. Yando (Eds.), *New directions of child development: Clinical developmental research.* San Francisco: Jossey-Bass.

Polansky, N. A., Chalmers, M., Buttenweiser, E., & Williams, D. (1981). *Damaged parents: An anatomy of child neglect.* Chicago: University of Chicago Press.

Spinetta, J. J., & Rigler, D. (1972). The child abusing parent: A psychological review. *Psychological Bulletin, 77,* 296–304.

Sroufe, L. A., & Fleeson, J. (1986). Attachment and the construction of relationships. In W. W. Hartup & Z. Rubin (Eds.), *Relationships and development* (pp. 51–72). Hillsdale, NJ: Erlbaum.

Steward, M. S., Farquhar, L. C., Dicharry, D. C., Glick, D. R., & Martin, P. W. (1986). Group therapy: A treatment of choice for victims of child abuse. *International Journal of Group Psychotherapy, 36,* 261–269.

United States Department of Health and Human Services. (1988). *Study findings: Study of national incidence and prevalence of child abuse and neglect: 1988.* Washington, DC: National Clearinghouse on Child Abuse and Neglect.

Wahler, R. G. (1980). The insular mother: Her problems in parent-child treatment. *Journal of Applied Behavioral Analysis, 13,* 207–219.

Wald, M. (1961). *Protective services and emotional neglect.* Denver: American Humane Association.

Wolfe, D. A. (1987). *Child abuse: Implications for child development and psychopathology.* Beverly Hills: Sage.

III

Violence toward Adults

16

Wife Battering

Edward W. Gondolf and Ellen R. Fisher

Description of the Problem

Wife battering has been described as the social problem of the past decade. According to a 1976 national survey, it had reached "epidemic" proportions (Straus, Gelles, & Steinmetz, 1980): nearly 2 million women battered a year. At least one act of violence occurs per year in 16% of all married couples. Nearly one-third of all married couples experience physical abuse at some point. Some researchers estimate that actually over one-half of all wives will be assaulted sometime during their marriage (Walker, 1979). One-fifth of all homicides are committed by family members (FBI, 1988), and the vast majority of these are related to a long history of wife battering (Browne, 1987), as is discussed in Chapter 20.

According to a more recent national survey, the incidence of battering may have decreased as much as 20% since the mid-1970s (Straus & Gelles, 1986). This alleged reduction is most likely related to increased public awareness of battering, the advent of women's shelter programs, and more decisive intervention from the criminal justice system. At the same time, local social services, particularly battered women shelters, have been overwhelmed by requests for assistance. The women requesting services have needs far more acute and complex than in the past. Consequently, a wider range of social service staff is encountering wife

Edward W. Gondolf • Western Psychiatric Institute and Clinic, University of Pittsburgh School of Medicine, Pittsburgh, Pennsylvania 15213; and Department of Sociology, Indiana University of Pennsylvania, Indiana, Pennsylvania 15705.   **Ellen R. Fisher** • La Casa de las Madres, San Francisco, California 94103.

battering firsthand or is being called upon to assist in wife battering cases.

Despite these alarming trends, wife battering has a long history as a deep-seated social phenomenon. Several social historians have documented the informal and formal sanctions that have encouraged wife battering (Davidson, 1978; Martin, 1976; Pleck, 1987). In early 19th-century America, a husband was permitted to discipline his wife physically without prosecution for assault and battery. The legendary "rule of thumb" law derived from English common law eventually restricted the instrument of wife beatings to a stick no thicker than the man's thumb. Only in the last 15 years have courts finally considered wife battering to be a criminal offense. These historical circumstances led several social scientists to explain that men batter women basically because they are permitted and encouraged to do so (Gelles, 1983).

Such "selective inattention," as it has been called (Pleck, Pleck, Grossman, & Bart, 1978), has important social implications. It was not until the women's movement in the 1970s identified and responded to wife battering that it emerged as a "social problem" (Tierney, 1982). Social scientists, physicians, social workers, psychologists, and clergy had virtually overlooked and even denied that wife battering existed prior to this time. This markedly contrasted to extensive professional involvement in the issue of child battering (Finkelhor, 1983).

Feminists concluded that such negligence was a symptom of the sexist attitudes that pervade our society and contribute to wife battering (Martin, 1976). According to the feminist analysis, wife battering is merely an extension of the low status imposed on women. It is a part of the rape, sexual harassment, incest, and pornography to which women are disproportionately subjected (see Russell, 1984; Stanko, 1985). To address this problem and compensate for what other social services and the criminal justice system had largely shunned, nearly 1000 women's shelters were established across the country, largely through the grassroots efforts of the women's movement of the 1970s (Schechter, 1982).

More recently, the efforts to deal with wife battering have been increasingly "professionalized." Grassroots activists have been replaced by trained clinicians and social workers at many shelters. Family service and mental health agencies have increasingly developed programs for battered women and for batterers. In the process, the explanations and treatments for wife battering have become increasingly psychological in emphasis (David, 1987). The popularity of family systems theory, in particular, has led to interpretation of wife battering as an interactive dysfunction between two individuals. The women may, in this light, be equally involved as perpetrators or provocators.

This shift of emphasis has brought a heated debate among researchers, clinicians, and shelter advocates, as is documented in the recent exchange in *Social Work* (see Saunders, 1988). The feminist opposition has objected to what it refers to as "victim blaming" implied by the family systems theorists and practitioners. According to feminists, the social sanctions for wife battering and the control and subjugation imposed on battered women warrant a different picture. If women are violent, it is largely in retaliation or defense against their secondary status in and outside the home (Saunders, 1986). And whatever the woman's part, it does not typically have the same impact as a man's (Pagelow, 1985).

While differences remain over the definition of battering and its dynamics, there is consensus that social services have inadequately responded to the problem. Clergy have been accused of promoting compliance and submission to the abusive man (Horton & Williamson, 1988); physicians have tended to identify battered women as "troublesome" (Kurz, 1987); police have, for the most part, accepted a "hands-off" approach (Dolon, Hendricks, & Meagher, 1986); psychiatric staff are inclined to overmedicate battered women and return them to their spouses (Gondolf, 1990).

These deficiencies are reflected in the observations of battered women. A survey of formerly battered women rated women's shelters to be the "most effective" in helping to end the violence. Lawyers were the next most helpful. The other forms of social service were, on the whole, rated as less than satisfactory (Bowker, 1983, 1986).

In sum, professional social service workers are faced with a difficult challenge with regard to wife battering. They must first address the systemic oversight or neglect of the problem inherent in their profession. Second, they must confront the resistance in themselves to deal with what is an uncomfortable and unwieldy problem in itself. Third, they must assess what has been a controversial and oftentimes inconclusive field (see Gondolf & Fisher, 1988).

To assist in this important and necessary endeavor, we attempt to summarize some of the leading issues facing social service professionals. We accept the assertion of domestic violence experts that wife battering is a distinct behavioral syndrome (Walker, 1984), which may be compounded by psychological disorders or substance abuse but not explained by them. "Wife battering" here refers to the physical assault of women by their husbands or partners that is accompanied by a constellation of psychological abuse, marital rape, child abuse, and even threats of homicide that make for an abusive relationship—that is, a "reign of terror." The varied aspects of abuse are discussed more specifically in the following chapters. Our effort is to identify the prevailing and most current treatment considerations, but our recommendations tend to reflect the feminist approach, to which we subscribe. In sum, we address "wife battering" primarily as a power dynamic between victim and perpetrator. We draw on the findings of our recent study of nearly 6000 battered women from Texas shelters (Gondolf & Fisher, 1988), as well as the following case study.

Case Description

Barbara, like so many other battered women, has led two lives for many years. There is the "business" Barbara, who appears competent, professional, and tremendously conscientious in her secretarial duties. There is also a side of Barbara that very few people, and until recently virtually nobody, know about—the battered Barbara. Barbara at 26 years old has been severely shoved, hit, and threatened at least monthly during the 3 years of her relationship with boyfriend Mark.

The recent developments in Barbara's life serve to illustrate the clinical issues that confront professionals in dealing with wife battering. Barbara is not typical of the battered women in shelters. The majority of these women have children, have little or no income of their own, and lack a high school diploma (Gondolf & Fisher, 1988). Barbara represents the unmarried battered women who are often reluctant to seek out social service assistance and who especially resist shelter care. They have access to resources and, more important, tend to resist identifying themselves as battered women. It is these women that social service professionals are more likely to overlook but are in an ideal position to assist.

Barbara had told no one about "her problems," as she referred to the battering. She later explained that she could not talk to her family about it. Both her adoptive parents had been dead for several years. Her older sister was married to a fundamentalist minister who Barbara feared would scold her and force her back to her boyfriend, Mark. "Everyone expected Mark and me to be together," she said. She was concerned, too, that if her employer found out about the battering, her job might be jeopardized. Furthermore, she relented on repeated occasions, "Some of it is my fault anyway." She blamed herself not only for some of the battering but also for not doing anything about it.

She liked the attention and companionship that her boyfriend initially offered her after their meeting at a church social several years ago. The two of them took college night classes together and spent more and more of their free time together. Barbara began to cook for Mark and spent most of her weekends at his apartment. She noticed his imposing jealousy and rigid opinions early on, but assumed she could change those in time. There were, too, those "occasional fights" in which Mark would get furious about something. She would talk back to him, and Mark would start yelling and would shove her if she questioned him further. Mark was particularly violent when he had been drinking and slapped, punched, and even kicked her on occasion.

Then Mark moved to a nearby community to attend college fulltime. He expected Barbara to move in with him, but Barbara insisted that she could not leave her job and schoolwork. Also, she did not *want* to leave town or live with Mark. The "fights" intensified. Mark called Barbara a "whore" when she opposed him and threatened to "get her." In an effort to settle him down, Barbara would agree to his demands, including his wishes for sex. She even arranged to have her college grade card altered so Mark would not expect that she was enrolled in social service courses— something that might anger him. But the violence became more frequent and more severe, as it tends to in wife-battering cases, and Barbara began to fear for her life.

Barbara's first call for help, however, was a faint one. She made a passing reference to her abusive relationship in an essay exam in the college course she was taking. She knew much about battering from a sociology course that she had previously taken and had an analytical understanding of her abusive relationship, even though she was reluctant to take decisive action about it. In a visit to her professor's office after the exam, Barbara did not mention the problem until the professor questioned her about the remarks in her essay about being abused.

Very cautiously she revealed some of the situation. With prompting, she explained how she mentally separated herself from the battering in order to escape the fear and pain. She repeatedly turned the conversation about the abuse to questions about how to prevent it from happening— quickly and easily: "What can *I* do to stop it?" She dismissed each suggestion as impractical or too dangerous. "I don't want to involve the police. That will just cause more problems." "I don't belong in a shelter. My friends will ask too many questions if I'm not around." Finally, Barbara relented enough to refuse to see Mark that weekend. She would begin to tell him on the phone what she was feeling.

Mark blew up on the phone and began to threaten her. Barbara, after talking to a shelter crisis line, felt more determined not to see him. She continued her phone objections and received threats of suicide, then threats of retaliation. Mark arrived late one night drunk, kicked her apartment door in, and attacked her. The apartment supervisor heard the commotion and intervened. He managed to chase off the boyfriend, but only after receiving a broken arm. The police were notified but charges were not filed.

Barbara moved to a different address with an unlisted phone. Then she began receiving threatening and disruptive phone calls at work. She eventually notified the community police about the threats and started spending nights at the shelter. Then one afternoon Mark arrived at her new apartment. Before she could call the police he grabbed her. In the scuffle that followed, Mark threw a bottle of rubbing alcohol, which had been sitting on the counter, into Barbara's eyes. Mark evidently fled during Barbara's screams, leaving Barbara to find her way several blocks to the hospital.

"I knew then that he didn't really love me. I also finally realized that it was never going to get better. Even though I hoped he would change, I wasn't going to be the one to do it." With that Barbara filed for an "order of protection" to keep Mark away from her. He retaliated with more threats and attempted another visit. This time he was arrested and eventually ordered to counseling. Mark has not seen or talked with Barbara since the arrest, but he has made his contempt for her known through a few of his friends.

Barbara, consequently, still fears for her life. But what were formerly "two lives" are now more like one. She continues to make public the private battered side. In return, she is receiving the support to make her life whole again.

Medical Issues

The very nature of wife battering includes assault that often injures. In our study of Texas shelter women, we found that nearly half of the battered women who had contacted a shelter reported head injuries, 13% had bones broken by their batterers, 42% had sought medical care for battering injuries sometime during their relationship, and 10% required hospitalization. Another study estimates that as many as 20% of the trauma cases in a hospital emergency room injuries are related to wife battering (Stark, Flitcraft, & Frazier, 1979).

Because of battered women's fear of retaliation, her self-doubts and suspicion, and the batterer's surveillance of the woman, battered women are generally reluctant to visit an emergency ward or a physician. The battered woman often tries her best to take care of herself, until the injury is too serious to be ignored. Batterers will frequently strike where bruises will not show, and excuses are made to friends who notice a black eye or a limp: "I bumped into a door" or "I fell down the steps."

If battered women do come to a hospital emergency room, they come out of desperation. Barbara, for instance, sought medical help only when her eyesight was severely endangered. And typically she gave a misleading account of the circumstances. Furthermore, battered women that arrive at an emergency room are usually in a crisis state. Their main concern is alleviating the immediate pain, as is that of the medical staff. Therefore, information about the battering relationship is not likely to be readily disclosed.

A recent study of several hospital emergency rooms revealed that hospital staff tend to view battered women's unwillingness to talk as "unresponsiveness" or "evasiveness." Prevention, referral, and priority are not given to these cases. In fact, battered women cases are typically viewed by hospital personnel as "dirty work"—that is, detracting from the "real" emergencies. These cases also have complicated social dimensions that demand involvement that hospital staff feel unequipped to address (Kurz, 1987).

These sorts of oversights can be offset in the following ways, according to the recommendations of several reports on the subject (see Campbell & Humphreys, 1984). First, battered women need to be identified as such. Details about the circumstances of the injury need to be routinely requested. Several screening devices are now available to assist in this sort of questioning (Lewis, 1985).

Second, careful documentation of the injuries and their suspected cause can serve as vital court evidence and aid in obtaining needed referral assistance. Some emergency rooms have begun to keep a special file of all suspected battered women, which enables prompt response to inquiries and recognition of repeat cases.

Third, identified battered women need to be referred to specialized domestic violence programs that can help address the emotional and social issues facing the patient (Rich & Burgess, 1986). Some emergency rooms present a card to the battered woman indicating the hotline of a women shelter, and staff outline other social service and criminal justice options that may help in establishing safety.

Legal Issues

Many battered women do not initially consider their battering to be a crime and consequently have little contact with the legal system. Some women may have a vague sense that if their injury were severe enough, they could press charges. Other battered women (e.g., Barbara) expect that the police will do little except complicate matters. Police, in turn, often believe that battered women and/or their batterers will attack intruding police and eventually drop the charges if arrests are made (Bolton & Bolton, 1986; Thyfault, Bennett, & Hirschhorn, 1987).

These notions are gradually changing as proarrest policies are established across the country. About 50% of the nation's "large" police departments now implement such a policy in which the batterer is arrested if "probable cause" exists and is prosecuted by the state. Proarrest has markedly decreased battering recidivism (Sherman & Berk, 1984) and lowered domestic homicide rates (Bureau of Justice, 1986). Court prosecutions and convictions are similarly being increased in the process (Erez, 1986).

Helping a women to secure the legislated police action and court response is a service that many women shelters offer or coordinate. An increasing number of women are beginning to call the police and press charges on their own, in response to the increased public awareness and improved police response. Over half of the women (64%) in our Texas study had previously contacted the police on at least one occasion; one-fifth (19%) had previously taken legal action.

The most common legal action sought by battered women is an "order of protection." This court injunction, which goes under a variety of names in different states, is separate from filing criminal charges that attempt to bring about punishment. The court injunction prohibits the batterer from a designated proximity of the woman for up to 2 years. If the batterer violates this specification, he may be subject to immediate arrest and prosecution, as was Mark in our case study. However, it is still questionable how long the batterer will stay in jail or what his sentence will be.

These court orders may be useful in communicating a decisive message to the batterer, especially if he is likely to be intimidated by the judicial system. The police or court action is often an essential step in convincing the batterer that he has a problem, as well as a necessary means of interrupting an otherwise escalating situation (Gondolf, 1987b). They also provide the battered women with some leverage against the batterer, if she does eventually return to the relationship.

There are, of course, some serious shortcomings to "court orders." One is that they are particularly difficult to enforce. Consequently, the order may give a woman an illusion of safety when none yet exists. The orders also seldom resolve an abusive relationship without further intervention or separation. Most importantly, an order of protection may initially incite the batterer with what he considers to be retaliation, as was the case with Barbara's boyfriend, Mark.

Ideally, the legal measures of arrest, persecution, and orders of protection need to be coordinated with other social services. In most communities, shelter advocates are available to help women negotiate with the legal system to try to get the most protection from it. While reform of the criminal justice system remains uneven, it does provide an essential first step in ending wife battering.

Family Issues

Wife battering, like other forms of family violence, raises a variety of family issues. But unlike child and elder abuse, it threatens the very foundation of the family structure—the marriage (or partnership) between a man and woman. The most crucial family issue, therefore, is whether the family is to exist or continue. Given the tendency of wife battering to escalate and denial of the problem to persist, most in the field strongly recommend separating the batterer from the battered women and children.

This can be achieved temporarily through an "order of protection," discussed above, which orders the man from the home. Also, separation is frequently obtained through shelter residence, in which the woman and children leave home for safety and support. Ultimately, it may mean a legal separation and divorce. We saw that Barbara attempted to separate from her violent boyfriend by all of these means in a progression of attempts to keep away the batterer.

A combination of separations usually occurs over a period of time. Studies of battered women show that they tend to pass through a number of different kinds of separations prior to either terminating the relationship completely or experiencing a cessation of the violence (Okum, 1988). (In fact, as many as one-third of shelter women return to their batterer upon leaving the shelter.) The separation offers a time to gain support, recover from emotional and physical injuries, and clearly weigh one's options. It also gives the women some leverage over the man in what might otherwise be a gross imbalance of power and control. Saying "I'll leave again" may prove to be a kind of defense (Bowker & Maurer, 1985).

The consequences of leaving, even temporarily, weigh heavy in the balance. For many battered women, separating from a violent man means a loss of income, housing, and transportation—the essentials of survival (Strube, 1988). The majority must care for children, as well, with little or no assistance. No matter how threatening and violent the relationship, it still provides women with a sense of economic security. Children may long for the father, and women, too, may feel attachments as a result of their long emotional investment. In other words, they experience a kind of "psychological entrapment" (Brockner & Rubin, 1985).

A separation, moreover, brings with it complicated custody problems and property rights. These can often incite conflicts and impose couple contact in a way that puts the woman further at risk. Often an advocate is essential in negotiating these issues and assisting in child visits or the dividing of property.

Perhaps the most neglected family issue is the impact of family violence on the children (Roy, 1988). The children are first and foremost affected by the violence they see between their parents. The battering presents a role model, especially for the boys, but it also creates a state of terror and insecurity among both sexes. A substantial portion of children who witness wife battering also are abused themselves (Kalmuss, 1984). As much as half of our Texas sample of battered women reported child abuse.

The violence affects children differently at different developmental stages. It nonetheless has a uniform emotional disruption on children not unlike that on children brought up in war-torn countries (Roy, 1988). The boys in particular tend to act out aggressively, and the girls characteristically fall into a state of suspicion and distrust.

The children are affected not only by the violence but also by the separations and the moves that accompany the effort to gain safety. Leaving their home, changing schools, and fleeing under cover deprive children of social support and stability. For this reason, these children have been referred to as "yo-yo" children—dangling at the end of a string (NSPCC, 1977).

One of the most frequently asserted explanations for family violence is "intergenerational transmission" (Kalmuss, 1984). That is, children from violent homes are very likely to be in violent homes as adults. While there remains some debate over whether women might be prone toward victimization in this way, men overwhelmingly have violent backgrounds. A range of studies shows that from 60 to 80% of the batterers come from violent homes.

Helping children who have witnessed wife abuse is essential in order to improve the child's adjustment as a child and to help prevent that child from reexperiencing battering as an adult. A variety of curriculum and counseling techniques have been and are being developed to help children, first, to identify their emotional struggles and, second, to learn alternatives to the violence that has so encompassed them (see Roy, 1988).

Assessment of Psychopathology

There are those who claim that psychopathology has been sorely neglected in a field that is so strongly influenced by sociological and criminal justice perspectives (Hamberger & Lohr, 1989). The efforts to establish some typifying characteristics or "profile" of battered women and battering men have been in vain. The diversity of both the battered and the batterers leads us to conclude that at best we might identify a typology of batterers and perhaps battered women in which only a small portion have major psychiatric disorders.

The most common concern in assessment is the presence of alcohol abuse, especially since a disproportionate percentage of wife-battering cases includes alcohol abuse. Experts in the field, however, view alcohol abuse as a compounding factor, and often a symptom of the battering. It provides an excuse for the violence but is not its cause (Gelles, 1974). Alcoholic batterers have been shown to batter as much as 40% of the time without being under the influence of alcohol. The battering and injury it causes tend to be more severe after drinking (Kantor & Straus, 1987; Roberts, 1988; Van Hasselt, Morrison, & Bellack, 1985). There is an open debate, however, as to whether battered women should be considered "codependent" as opposed to entrapped and coping the best they can (Bograd, 1988).

Profile of Battered Women

The diagnosed psychopathology of battered women does not conform to any particular pattern. In a recent study of psychiatric patients, the self-identified battered women arriving in a psychiatric emergency room had a diversity of diagnoses (Gondolf, 1990), whereas the diagnoses of other kinds of victims were relatively similar. Interestingly, the battering was not specifically addressed in any of the psychiatric cases. No referrals were made, safety was not evaluated, nor was the women informed of her options. Those women who were not currently suicidal, delusional, or threatening counterattack were released to return to their batterers.

Preliminary clinical observation and personality testing, nevertheless, have typified battered women as fearful, overwhelmed, and depressed (Rosewater, 1988; Walker, 1979). (Fourteen percent of the Texas shelter women reported having attempted suicide in response to the battering.) Other clinicians have linked wife battering to a kind of masochism (Kleckner, 1978; Shainess, 1979).

At first glance, battered women might therefore appear to have personality disorders or even schizophrenic tendencies. Experienced clinicians in the field explain, however, that the "symptoms" are reactive states rather than character traits. MMPI test results, for instance, reflect the battering and the terror that accompanies it—they suggest the "symptoms" of battering rather than of a mental disorder (Rosewater, 1988). They reflect the life of isolation, put-downs, and threats, as well.

The popularized notion of "learned helplessness" has also been used to explain the reactive symptoms (Walker, 1979). The abuse and battering "condition" the battered women to feel helpless. They become pessimistic and passive, and even blame themselves for the violence. Research efforts to document this profile, however, have not been able to establish that battered women as a group are any more depressed or passive than nonbattered women (Launius & Lindquist, 1988; Walker, 1984).

In our study of Texas women, we found battered women that were active help-seekers despite the severity and duration of their abuse. A more active profile based on the coping and help-seeking may be that of a "survivor." Barbara, for instance, was clearly depressed and over-whelmed by the battering she experienced and the threat of further violence. She nevertheless attempted, in a variety of creative ways, to stem the battering herself.

Another research finding of significance is that formerly battered women contact a diversity of help sources to stop the violence. No one strategy or series of strategies appears as the "most" successful (Bowker, 1983, 1986). Social services staff might, therefore, see their initial, and perhaps primary function as facilitating and furthering this process: encouraging and aiding the women's involvement with a variety of informal and formal help sources and assuring the appropriate response of the helpers.

Profile of Men Who Batter

The diagnosed psychopathology of batterers is shown to be less diversified than that of battered women. The research with psychiatric patients identified as batterers shows them to be disproportionately diagnosed as having personality disorders (Gondolf, 1990). A series of studies using the MCMI have suggested that the vast majority of batterers in counseling programs show symptoms of a variety of personality disorders, but that no overriding profile exists (Hamberger & Hastings, 1986).

Men in treatment programs may also appear clinically depressed or paranoid. These states are more likely to be reactions to the consequences of his battering—arrest, loss of family, and facing punishment. Batterers may even threaten suicide in response to the depression and, in part, as a means of manipulation—to get their wives or partners back.

Clinicians and researchers alike have characterized battering men as less communicative, more impulsive, lower in self-esteem, and more rigid in sex-role expectations (Maiuro, Cahn, & Vitaliano, 1986; see Dutton, 1988, for an overview). They are also more likely to have come from a violent home, as mentioned, and to be involved in substance abuse (see Hotaling & Sugarman, 1986). One shortcoming of such a profile is that it does not substantially differentiate batterers from other sorts of offenders, such as rapists, robbers, or molesters.

The "characteristics" may represent merely an extension of a normative process that might be called the "failed macho complex" (Gondolf & Hanneken, 1987). A qualitative study of batterers suggests that their battering is an overcompensation for a distorted male ideal that they feel obliged to fulfill. Their distortions are in part the result of the role models of their fathers or of media heroes. Batterers are not so much super "macho" men as much as they feel they fall short of what they are "supposed" to be as "a man." Their low self-concept may be related to the abuse they witnessed or received while growing up.

We have to differentiate batterers to account for the sometimes contradictory or inconclusive efforts to formulate a batterer profile. One empirical study based on behavioral descriptions of batterers established a typology of batterers that suggests a continuum of violence (Gondolf, 1988a). Those identified as "sporadic" batterers were those who were less frequently abusive and were more likely to apologize and regret their battering. The "chronic" batterers battered more frequently and severely, and were more likely also to be abusive to the children.

Another group of batterers were generally "antisocial" in that they were violent outside the home as well as in it. They were more likely as well to be heavily abusing alcohol and to use weapons in their battering. Finally, a small group of batterers appeared to be "sociopathic" and probably had serious psychiatric disorders. These batterers had extensive criminal records and histories of severe drug and alcohol abuse. The generally violent antisocial and sociopathic batterers notably had caused more serious injury to their wives and children.

Barbara's boyfriend, Mark, rapidly developed into what might be a chronic batterer. While some of his behavior might suggest a narcissistic personality disorder, Mark's battering may be part of a larger continuum of normative male control and dominance. His psychological problems warrant attention, but they should be viewed more as compounding the battering rather than causing it. Primarily, the battering needs to be interrupted and addressed. Further, the batterer's distorted expectations for himself and women need to be replaced with a more accepting and supportive self-image.

Treatment Options

As mentioned at the beginning, two specialized treatment options have been developed to deal with wife battering: battered women's shelters and batterer programs. These emerged, in large part, in response to the neglect or oversight of the professionalized social services to address the problem (Schechter, 1982). More recently, a variety of social services and family agencies have also developed treatment programs of their own for wife-abuse cases. Their philosophy and approach often differ from the domestic violence programs. They are more likely to adopt existing family systems practices or cognitive-behavioral therapy in the treatment of wife abuse (see Adams, 1988; Gondolf, 1985).

The fundamental objective of treatment, in any case, should be to bring about a cessation of the battering. This means assuring interruption of the current battering and addressing the chronic nature of the battering syndrome. This generally is accomplished by separate group sessions for women, often convened at a shelter, and separate group sessions for batterers. Couples counseling, which has become a controversial format in this field, is generally discouraged at least until battering has been stopped for 6 months to a year, and after some period of separation (Bograd, 1984).

The counseling process for both men and women needs initially to confront denial and minimalization (Gondolf, 1985). Helping the women and men to recognize the nature and dynamics of abuse helps, in itself, to develop precautions. This entails identifying the kinds of abuse that occur, and their frequency, and establishing in this way that battering is not a series of isolated incidents but part of a controlling pattern of behavior. Several inventories are available to help identify emotional, financial, sexual, and child abuse accompanied by male privilege, intimidation, isolation, and threats (see Pence, 1989). After defining battering, there is a need to clarify the options to battering and advantages associated with them.

Treatment for Battered Women

A variety of counseling approaches have been proposed for battered women in recent years. Grieving, existential, and shame therapy, for instance, are some of them being proposed (e.g., Turner, & Shapiro, 1986). But fundamental to the counseling efforts should be a design to move the battered woman from status as a "victim" to that of a "survivor" (Rieker & Carmen, 1986). It is this shift in self-perception that is most associated with safety and recovery (see Gondolf & Fisher, 1988).

According to several victimization studies, battered women tend to move through several phases in response to abuse (Ferraro & Johnson, 1983; Mills, 1985). These phases are distinguished by an attributional shift on the woman's part. In essence, she begins to perceive that the battering was not "all her fault" but largely due to her husband. It is not up to her to change the batterer; in fact, it is not likely that he will change. She is capable of taking care of herself, with the support and assistance she deserves from others.

The objective in counseling might, therefore, be to reinforce and encourage this realization. Many shelters subscribe to an "empowerment" mode of counseling to achieve this end. The feminist approach is directed toward helping the woman realize her options and choices and begin to make decisions that assure her worth, integrity, and determination (Bograd, 1988). As mentioned, a previous study of formerly battered women rated this sort of counseling to be the most effective in stopping the violence (Bowker, 1983).

Our study of Texas shelter women raises an additional objective: resource allocation. What seems to contribute most to a women's move toward safety is obtaining an income of her own, transportation, child care, and housing. Having mobility not only enables a women to leave the violence but also helps "equalize" the relationship. These essential resources are, however, particularly problematic in wife-abuse cases. As mentioned, the majority of the Texas shelter women have little education, few job skills, and young children.

Barbara's situation illustrates the role of this sort of counseling. The first step was to help her see the nature of the battering as more than a few arguments that she could somehow "fix." As this occurred, Barbara became more responsive to the options presented to her and eventually decisively asserted herself. One of the factors facilitating the process was certainly her mobility, owing to her not being formally married and to having an income of her own. Typically, her boyfriend was intent on having her give up her job and schooling—the things that assisted her in leaving him.

Treatment for the Batterer

The treatment of batterers has similarly seen a proliferation of approaches and with it increased debate (see Adams, 1988). The leading programs are characterized by a group process that prompts men to take responsibility for their abuse, to exercise alternatives to the violence, and to restructure their sex-role perceptions (Gondolf, 1987a). There is a questionable trend, however, toward short-term anger-control treatment that unwittingly reinforces the batterer's penchant for control (Gondolf & Russell, 1986b).

The research on cessation suggests that batterers who do reform their behavior pass through a series of developmental stages (Fagan, 1987; Gondolf, 1987b). The change process begins with "realization." The egocentric batterer acknowledges the consequences of his abuse and that it may be in his own self-interest to contain it. Gradually, batterers become more "other-oriented" and begin to make some "behavioral changes" to improve relationships or at least avoid totally destroying them. Some men eventually begin to think more in terms of values and principles and integrate these into a change of self-concept. A number of the leading batterer programs consequently employ a phased approach that moves batterers from didactic sessions of accountability and consequence to social support groups with a focus on service (see Gondolf, 1985).

The most outstanding challenges, besides the high dropout rates, are collusion, self-pity, and self-congratulations. There is a tendency for batterers and even male counselors to "collude" with one another. They sometimes very subtly acknowledge one another's excuses or fail to challenge them. They begin to pity themselves for the consequences of their battering that add to bad experiences they encountered growing up. In simply attending a program, batterers feel some congratulations and trust is due them from their spouse and often cannot understand why she does not come running back. All these diversions from change can, of course, be challenged and turned into lessons about rationalization (see Gondolf & Russell, 1986a).

The most pressing question about batterer programs is: How "successful" are they? (Gondolf, 1987c). This is a difficult question to answer, given how one defines success. Shelter workers have noted that batterers after counseling may become "nonviolent terrorists." They cease their battering but heighten their psychological abuse and other controlling behaviors. Those who do stop their abuse and violence are likely to do so as a result of a constellation of interventions (Bowker, 1983). The counseling in and of itself does not stop the battering, but counseling, along with police action, women's leaving, divorce suit, and Alcoholics Anonymous, may be an incentive. It may be, as suggested previously, that certain types of batterers are poor candidates for counseling and need comprehensive residential psychiatric and substance-abuse treatment, along with the batterer counseling (Gondolf, 1988a). It is important to emphasize, however, that there is good evidence that these treatments *alone* are not sufficient.

It is particularly important that batterer programs be carefully coordinated with, and accountable to, shelter services and women's counseling. Some shelter workers, in fact, have outlined a rationale and plan for "monitoring" batterer programs (Hart, 1987). This is critical for two immediate reasons. One is because of the variety and uncertainty of batterer counseling at this juncture. The other is because of the effect batterer counseling has on women. The batterer's participation in a counseling program is the most influential factor in a woman's returning to him and putting herself at risk (Gondolf, 1988b). Yet it is the woman's separation that is the prime motivator for a man's attending counseling in the first place. Once batterers "get her back," they are much more likely to drop out of counseling—and batter again.

Summary and Conclusions

Increasingly there is a call to recognize wife battering as a complex social problem that warrants decisive and comprehensive intervention. Singular-focused treatment has historically been ineffective for the victims and frustrating for the practitioners. First, wife battering needs to be recognized as a chronic syndrome of control as well as violence. Second, decisive interruption of the violence and safety for the victims needs to be assured through legal and shelter options. Third, the survivor process in victims and the cessation process in batterers may be reinforced by group counseling that establishes the responsibility for battering, its consequences, and alternatives to it. Fourth, battered women especially need substantial resources, as well as emotional support, to assure their mobility. Batterers contrarily need to be made accountable to a reference group that offers them an alternative role model and nonviolent values.

Model wife-abuse programs are distinguished by their integrated interventions (Brygger & Edleson, 1987; Pence, 1989). While this ideal is far from a reality in most communities, at least better referral and coordination is possible. In sum, no professional should feel he or she can do it alone. The most valuable contribution may be to bring the wife-abuse case to a diversity of services. This makes the problem not the battered woman's but the community's problem as well.

References

Adams, D. (1988). Treatment models of men who batter: A profeminist analysis. In K. Yllo & M. Bograd (Eds.), *Feminist perspectives on wife abuse*. Newbury Park, CA: Sage.

Bograd, M. (1984). Family systems approaches to wife battering: A feminist critique. *American Journal of Orthopsychiatry, 54*, 558–568.

Bograd, M. (1988). Feminist perspectives on wife abuse: An introduction. In K. Yllo & M. Bograd (Eds.), *Feminist perspectives on wife abuse*. Newbury Park, CA: Sage.

Bolton, F., & Bolton, S. (1986). *Working with the violent family*. Newbury Park, CA: Sage.

Bowker, L. (1983). *Beating wife beating*. Lexington, MA: Lexington Books.

Bowker, L. (1986). *Ending the violence: A guidebook based on the experiences of 1,000 battered wives*. Holmes Beach, FL: Learning Publications.

Bowker, L., & Maurer, L. (1985). The importance of sheltering in the lives of battered women. *Response, 8*, 2–8.

Brockner, J., & Rubin, J. (1985). *Entrapment in escalating conflicts: A social psychological analysis*. New York: Springer-Verlag.

Browne, A. (1987). *When battered women kill*. New York: Free Press.

Brygger, M. P. & Edleson, J. (1987). The domestic abuse project: A multi-systems intervention in woman battering. *Journal of Interpersonal Violence, 2*, 324–333.

Bureau of Justice Statistics. (1986). *Preventing domestic violence against women*. Washington, DC: U.S. Department of Justice.

Campbell, J., & Humphreys, J. (1984). *Nursing care of victims of family violence*. Reston, VA: Reston Publishing.

Davidson, T. (1978). *Conjugal crime: Understanding and changing the wifebeating problem*. New York: Hawthorn.

Davis, L. (1987). Battered women: The transformation of a social problem. *Social Work, 32*, 306–311.

Dolon, R., Hendricks, J., & Meagher, M. (1986). Police practices and attitudes toward domestic violence. *Journal of Police Science and Administration, 14*, 187–192.

Dutton, D. (1988). Profiling of wife assaulters: Preliminary evidence for trimodal analysis. *Violence and Victims, 3,* 5–30.

Erez, E. (1986). Intimacy, violence, and the police. *Human Relations, 39,* 265–281.

Fagan, J. (1987). Cessation of family violence: Deterrence and dissuasion. In L. Ohlin & M. Tonry (Eds.), *Crime and justice: An annual review of research.* Chicago: University of Chicago Press.

Federal Bureau of Investigation. (1988). *Uniform crime reports—1987: Crime in the United States.* Washington, DC: U.S. Department of Justice.

Ferraro, K., & Johnson, J. (1983). How women experiencing battering: The process of victimization. *Social Problems, 30,* 325–339.

Finkelhor, D. (1983). Common features of family abuse. In D. Finkelhor, R. Gelles, G. Hotaling, & M. Straus (Eds.), *The dark side of families: Current family violence research.* Newbury Park, CA: Sage.

Gelles, R. (1974). *The violent home: A study of physical aggression between husbands and wives.* Newbury Park, CA: Sage.

Gelles, R. (1983). An exchange/social control theory. In D. Finkelhor, R. Gelles, G. Hotaling, & M. Straus (Eds.), *The dark side of families: Current family violence research.* Newbury Park, CA: Sage.

Gondolf, E. W. (1985). *Men who batter: An integrated approach to stopping wife abuse.* Holmes Beach, FL: Learning Publications.

Gondolf, E. W. (1987a). Evaluating programs for men who batter: Problems and prospects. *Journal of Family Violence, 2,* 95–108.

Gondolf, E. W. (1987b). Changing men who batter: A developmental model of integrated interventions. *Journal of Family Violence, 2,* 345–369.

Gondolf, E. W. (1987c). Seeing through smoke and mirrors: A guide to batterer program evaluations. *Response, 10,* 16–19.

Gondolf, E. W. (1988a). Who are those guys? Toward a behavioral typology of batterers. *Violence and Victims, 3,* 187–204.

Gondolf, E. W. (1988b). The effect of batterer counseling on shelter outcome. *Journal of Interpersonal Violence, 3,* 275–289.

Gondolf, E. W. (1990). *Psychiatric response to family violence: Identifying and confronting neglected danger.* Lexington, MA: Lexington Books.

Gondolf, E. W., & Fisher, E. R. (1988). *Battered women as survivors: An alternative to treating learned helplessness.* Lexington, MA: Lexington Books.

Gondolf, E., & Hanneken, J. (1987). The gender warrior: Reformed batterers on abuse, treatment, and change. *Journal of Family Violence, 2,* 177–191.

Gondolf, E. W., & Russell, D. M. (1986a). *Man to man: A guide for men in abusive relationships.* Bradenton, FL: Human Services Institute.

Gondolf, E. W., & Russell, D. M. (1986b). The case against anger control treatment programs for batterers. *Response, 9,* 2–5.

Hamberger, L. K., & Hastings, J. E. (1986). Personality correlates of men who abuse their partners: A cross-validation study. *Journal of Family Violence, 1,* 323–341.

Hamberger, L. K. & Lohr, J. (1989). Proximal causes of spouse abuse: A theoretical analysis for cognitive-behavioral interventions. In P. L. Caeser & L. K. Hamberger (Eds.), *Treating men who batter.* New York: Springer.

Hart, B. (1987). *Safety for women: Monitoring batterer's programs.* Harrisburg, PA: Pennsylvania Coalition Against Domestic Violence.

Horton, A., & Williamson, J. (Eds.). (1988). *Abuse and religion: When praying isn't enough.* Lexington, MA: Lexington Books.

Hotaling, G., & Sugarman, D. (1986). An analysis of risk markers in husband to wife violence: The current state of knowledge. *Violence and Victims, 1,* 101–124.

Kalmuss, D. (1984). The intergenerational transmission of marital aggression. *Journal of Marriage and the Family, 47*, 11–19.

Kantor, G. K., & Straus, M. A., (1987). The drunken bum theory of wife beating. *Social Problems, 34*, 213–229.

Kleckner J. (1978). Wife beaters and beaten wives: Co-conspirators in crimes of violence. *Psychology, 15*, 54–56.

Kurz, D. (1987). Emergency department responses to battered women: Resistance to medicalization. *Social Problems, 34*, 69–81.

Launius, M., & Lindquist, C. (1988). Learned helplessness, external locus of control, and passivity in battered women. *Journal of Interpersonal Violence, 3*, 307–318.

Lewis, B. (1985). The wife abuse inventory: A screening device for the identification of abused women. *Social Work, 20*, 32–35.

Maiuro, R., Cahn, T. & Vitaliano, P. (1986). Assertiveness deficits and hostility in domestically violent men. *Violence and Victims, 1*, 279–289.

Martin, D. (1976). *Battered wives*. New York: Pocket Books.

Mills, T. (1985). The assault on the self: Stages in coping with battering husbands. *Qualitative Sociology, 8*, 103–123.

NSPCC School of Social Work. (1977). Yo-yo children: A study of two violent matrimonial cases. In M. Roy (Ed.), *Battered Women*. New York: Van Nostrand Reinhold.

Okum, L. (1988). Termination or resumption of cohabitation in woman battering relationships: A statistical study. In G. Hotaling, D. Finkelhor, J. Kirkpatrick, & M. Straus (Eds.), *Coping with family violence*. Newbury Park, CA: Sage.

Pagelow, M. (1985). The battered husband syndrome: Social problem or much ado about little? In N. Johnson (Ed.), *Marital violence*. Boston: Routledge & Kegan Paul.

Pence, E. (1989). Batterers programs: Shifting from community collusion to community confrontation. In P. L. Caesar & L. K. Hamberger (Eds.), *Therapeutic interventions with batterers*. New York: Springer.

Pleck, E. (1987). *Domestic tyranny: The making of American social policy against family violence from colonial times to the present*. New York: Oxford University Press.

Pleck, E., Pleck, J., Grossman, M., & Bart, P. (1978). The battered data syndrome: A reply to Steinmetz. *Victimology, 2*, 680–683.

Rich, R., & Burgess, A. W. (1986). NIMH report: Panel recommends comprehensive program for victims of violent crime. *Hospital and Community Psychiatry, 37*, 437–439.

Rieker, P., & Carmen, E. H. (1986). The victim-to-patient process: The disconfirmation and transformation of abuse. *American Journal of Orthopsychiatry, 56*, 360–370.

Roberts, A. (1988). Substance abuse among men who batter their mates: The dangerous mix. *Journal of Substance Abuse Treatment, 5*, 83–87.

Rosewater, L. (1988). Battered or schizophrenic? Psychological tests can't tell. In K. Yllo & M. Bograd (Eds.), *Feminist perspectives on wife abuse*. Newbury Park, CA: Sage.

Roy, M. (1988). *Children in the crossfire: Violence in the home—How does it affect our children?* Deerfield Beach, FL: Health Communications.

Russell, D. E. (1984). *Sexual exploitation: Rape, child sexual abuse, and workplace harassment*. Newbury Park, CA: Sage.

Saunders, D. (1986). When battered women use violence: Husband-abuse and self-defense. *Violence and Victims, 1*, 47–60.

Saunders, D. (1988). Other "truths" about domestic violence: A reply to Mcneely and Robinson-Simpson. *Social Work, 32*, 179–183.

Schechter, S. (1982). *Women and male violence: The visions and struggles of the battered women's movement*. Boston: South End Press.

Shainess, N. (1979). Vulnerability to violence: Masochism as a process. *American Journal of Psychotherapy, 33*, 174–189.

Sherman, L., & Berk, R. (1984). The deterrent effects of arrest for domestic assault. *American Sociological Review, 49,* 261–272.

Stanko, E. A. (1985). *Intimate intrusions: Women's experience of male violence.* Boston: Routledge & Kegan Paul.

Stark, E., Flitcraft, A., & Frazier, W. (1979). Medicine and patriarchal violence: The social construction of a "private" event. *International Journal of Health Services, 9,* 461–493.

Straus, M., & Gelles, R. (1986). Societal change and change in family violence from 1975 to 1985 as revealed by two national surveys. *Journal of Marriage and the Family, 48,* 465–479.

Straus, M., Gelles, R., & Steinmetz, S. (1980). *Behind closed doors: Violence in the American family.* New York: Anchor/Doubleday.

Strube, M. (1988). The decision to leave an abusive relationship: Empirical evidence and theoretical issues. *Psychological Bulletin, 104,* 236–250.

Thyfault, R., Bennett, C., & Hirschhorn, R. (1987). Battered women in court: Jury and trial consultants and expert witnesses. In D. Sonkin (Ed.), *Domestic violence on trial.* New York: Springer.

Tierney, K. J. (1982). The battered women movement and the creation of the wife beating problem. *Social Problems, 29,* 207–220.

Turner, W., & Shapiro, C. H. (1986). Battered women: Mourning the death of a relationship. *Social Work, 31,* 372–376.

Van Hasselt, V. V., Morrison, R. L., & Bellack, A. S. (1985). Alcohol abuse in wife abusers and their spouses. *Addictive Behaviors, 10,* 127–135.

Walker, L. (1979). *The battered woman.* New York: Harper.

Walker, L. (1984). *The battered woman syndrome.* New York: Springer.

17

Psychological Maltreatment of Spouses

Susan M. Andersen, Teresa Ramirez Boulette, and Amy H. Schwartz

Abusive behavior in the context of intimate relationships can take many forms, ranging from intense psychological intimidation and threats of violence to life-threatening episodes of physical assault. In virtually all cases of physical violence, however, some form of psychological maltreatment is also present. Psychological maltreatment, in fact, can quite reasonably be considered a common denominator in ongoing interpersonal relationships that are violent.

In this chapter, we describe a particular constellation of patterns that are frequently involved in the psychological maltreatment of spouses in the context of violent relationships. In so doing, we use the terms *spouse, wife, husband,* and *marriage,* but wish to target all married or unmarried couples in which the woman has shown "evidence of physical abuse on at least one occasion at the hands of an intimate male partner" (Rounsaville & Weissman, 1978).[1] Although it is true that these

---

[1]Although we recognize that some serious husband battering does take place, it is not a social problem of the same proportions as is wife battering (Ptacek, 1988). It often emerges in self-defense, is usually not physical, and when it is physical, is less severe (e.g., Ptacek, 1988; Saunders, 1986). We focus here on spousal abuse when husbands are the aggressors and battered women the victims. It should be noted, however, that the patterns of psychological maltreatment we describe could, in principle, be perpetrated by members of either sex.

Susan M. Andersen and Amy H. Schwartz • Department of Psychology, New York University, New York, New York 10003.   **Teresa Ramirez Boulette** • Santa Barbara County Mental Health Care Services, Santa Barbara, California 93110.

patterns of psychological maltreatment may be present in intimate relations when actual physical violence is not, viewing these patterns as risk factors for violent behavior is likely to be of value in understanding the psychosocial forces operating in the relationships of violent couples.

The psychosocial climate within which wife battering takes place often involves subtle manipulation—a form of "mind control" or "brainwashing" perpetrated by the battering husband—including the use of very potent strategies of manipulation (Boulette & Andersen, 1985). Elsewhere termed "the marital brainwashing syndrome" (Boulette, 1981) and "traumatic bonding" (Dutton & Painter, 1981), this familial pattern is characterized by many of the features of psychological coercion and deception that are found in religious or political cults and that distinguish them from other tightly knit social systems in society (Andersen, 1985; Andersen & Zimbardo, 1980). Further research is necessary to determine the prevalence and limiting conditions of this form of psychological maltreatment in disturbed relationships.

Description of the Problem

Mind Control and Battering

Over the last decade increasing attention has been directed toward the phenomenon of "wife battering," a syndrome that appears to transcend both social class and ethnicity (Berk, Berk, Loseke, & Rauma, 1983; Dobash & Dobash, 1979; Gelles, 1974, 1976; Hilberman, 1980; Martin, 1976; Steinmetz, 1977; although, see Fagan, Stewart, & Hansen, 1983; Snyder & Fruchtman, 1981). The hypothesized association between wife battering and mind control has been suggested by a number of investigators (Andersen, 1985; Boulette, 1981; Boulette & Andersen, 1985; Dutton & Painter, 1981; Hilberman, 1980) who have identified some of the manipulative techniques battering men may use against their wives (Steinmetz, 1977; Walker, 1978, 1979). These include isolation and the provocation of fear; the alternation of kindness and threats which produces disequilibrium; and the induction of guilt, self-blame, dependency, and learned helplessness (cf. Seligman, 1975). Members of extremist cults report similar experiences in the form of dissociation from all that is familiar, prohibitions against free expression and dissent, the mobilization of fear and guilt, and the establishment of an omnipotent master who demands self-sacrifice (Andersen & Zimbardo, 1980; Enroth, 1977; Singer, 1979).

Interpersonal systems, whether they are two-person relationships

**Table 1. Features of a Prototypic Pattern of
Psychological Maltreatment (Termed Psychological
Coercion) That the Battering Male Perpetrates in
Violent Intimate Relationships**

Early verbal and/or physical dominance
Isolation/imprisonment to various degrees
Guilt induction to promote victim self-blame
Hope-instilling behaviors via contingent expressions
  of love
Fear arousal, maintenance, and escalation to terror
Promotion of powerlessness and helplessness
Pathological expressions of jealousy
Required secrecy
Enforced loyalty and self-denunciation

If the battered woman attempts to leave the relationship:
  Cocky disbelief
  Confused searching
  Bargaining
  Pleading
  Threatening
  Seeking revenge

or larger social groups, have the potential to become totalistic in nature, in that they may exercise exceptional controls over the individual freedoms of their members (Andersen, 1985). The presence of this kind of totalism can be identified based on the *degree* to which such controls are present in the system. On the most simplistic level, this can be accomplished simply by counting the number and severity of the features of psychological coercion (e.g., social isolation, threat of harm, confusion and guilt, love that is strictly contingent on self-sacrifice and self-denunciation) and deception (e.g., direct misrepresentation or lying, distortion of individual options) present in the system (Andersen, 1985). Those intimate relationships that involve psychological coercion or "mind control" typically possess a significant number of these features (Boulette, 1981; Boulette & Andersen, 1985), which are presented in Table 1.

From a philosophical point of view, these features are likely to constitute a "fuzzy set" or prototype representing the overall pattern of psychological coercion found in battering relationships (cf. Cantor & Mischel, 1979; Rosch, 1978). Hence, a given case will vary in terms of the number of these features it possesses, as well as in their severity and duration. The relevant question to be asked is whether a couple manifests a significant constellation of these features (Andersen, 1985). If so, psychological coercion is probably present.

Early Verbal and/or Physical Dominance. During the courtship or early marriage the man typically establishes his role as "boss" and "master" by using acts of verbal or physical dominance. The woman may misinterpret this behavior as love and commitment offered by a "strong" man.

Isolation/Imprisonment to Various Degrees. The male frequently isolates the woman from her friends and relatives, both geographically and emotionally. In this way, he weakens her support system, produces a more influenceable spouse, and prevents her escape. Cultural notions of male and female roles are typically used to legitimize and reinforce the male's control.

Guilt Induction to Promote Victim Self-Blame. The battering male may induce guilt in his victim by blaming *her* for the abuse until she comes to blame herself. Blaming the victim is frequently used to justify the use of coercive power (Kipnis, 1976); self-blame is also found among rape victims (Janoff-Bulman, 1979; Libow & Doty, 1979).

Hope-Instilling Behaviors via Contingent Expressions of Love. The battered woman is usually provided with periodic hope that somehow her mistreatment and abuse will end if she pleads, cries, prays, endures, or sacrifices long enough. The man offers occasional hope-instilling behaviors in the form of contingent expressions of love that provide powerful intermittent reinforcements, prompting further self-sacrifice (Dutton & Painter, 1981; Steinmetz, 1977; Walker, 1979).

Fear Arousal, Maintenance, and Escalation to Terror. The battering man arouses fear in his spouse by frightening verbalizations, including threats of abandonment and of physical violence, and by actual physical abuse of varying severity. Over time, the woman usually builds tolerance and may thus fail to respond in expected ways, resulting in escalated terrorizing behaviors by the man. He may push her out of the car, hold her hostage for hours at knife-point, rape her, or threaten to burn the house down.

Promotion of Powerlessness and Helplessness. The unpredictable and pervasive abuse eventually debilitates the battered woman, promoting her feelings of powerlessness and helplessness. Her failure to predict or control her abuse engenders learned helplessness (Seligman, 1975) her husband's control over available monies impoverishes her and the victim-blaming postures of helpers who believe in a just-world hypothesis

(Lerner, 1970) promote further self-blame and powerlessness (Boulette & Andersen, 1985; Dutton & Painter, 1981; Walker, 1979).

Pathological Expressions of Jealousy. The battered woman may be repeatedly accused of infidelity by the man, who may express a pathological, potentially psychotic jealousy and yet brag about his own infidelity.

Required Secrecy. Secrecy is intimately a part of abusive relationships, which are characterized by dominance and often by child abuse, incest, and rape. The woman's support system has been destroyed so that contacts with individuals who might observe her bruises and encourage disclosure are nonexistent. Her secrecy is further prompted by his vigilance and by her shame and bewilderment.

Enforced Loyalty and Self-Denunciation. The woman has been debilitated by living in a closed system and being completely isolated from other people's opinions. Hence, she may come to believe in his "worldview" and excuse his oppressiveness, romanticize his desirable characteristics, and even show a missionary zeal about rescuing him from his vulnerability, temper, or alcoholism (Hilberman, 1980). Often she believes that only she can understand and rescue him. Similarly, debilitated prisoners of war often come to feel intense loyalty to their captors (as in the Stockholm syndrome, Ochberg, 1971), expressing an attachment based on the experience of terror and gratefulness for not being further damaged or killed (Boulette & Andersen, 1985; Dutton & Painter, 1981; Libow & Doty, 1979; Zimbardo, Ebbesen, & Maslach, 1977; see also Freire, 1984).

Interestingly, the set of factors described above is uncannily similar to the criteria for psychological torture applied by Amnesty International (cited by Walker, 1988), as shown in Table 2.

Table 2. Amnesty International's Definition of Psychological Torture[a]

Isolation
Induced debility (sleep and food deprivation)
Monopolizing of perceptions
Verbal degradation (denial of powers, humiliation)
Hypnosis
Drugs
Threats to kill
Occasional indulgences

[a]Adapted from Walker (1988).

Risks Associated with Escape

Upon leaving her husband, the battered woman frequently experiences insecurity, lethargy, and fear similar to that described by defecting cult members (Singer, 1979), but exacerbated by the husband's active recapture behaviors. Thus, the woman's own symptoms (including self-blame, guilt, self-denunciation, and loyalty) may cause her to repeatedly leave and then return to the victimizing situation or to fail to leave in the first place. Additionally, her husband's separation reaction serves as a powerful recapture maneuver.

Battering men have been found to exhibit a number of responses, as a separation reaction, to the battered woman's departure (Boulette, 1981; Boulette & Andersen, 1985), which can expose the woman to even greater danger.

Cocky Disbelief. At the outset, the battering man typically responds with cocky, self-assured, and contemptuous comments about his wife, such as "She'll come crawling back."

Confused Searching. The next stage of the husband's reaction typically involves aimless, pressured searching for his wife's whereabouts, which may be accompanied by symptoms of panic and agitation.

Bargaining. Next, the man may begin a bargaining process, by attempting to send messages to his wife, promising to change, and/or professing love and commitment.

Pleading. If the husband's bargaining is unsuccessful, he may cry unconsolably and plead for another chance. These behaviors can debilitate the woman, who may be convinced that he has finally changed.

Threatening. If the preceding four stages have not resulted in the wife's return, the husband now threatens to kill her, to kidnap the children, and/or to terrorize her family and friends until she does so. The woman's fear that these threats may be carried out provides a strong incentive for her return.

Seeking Revenge. Finally, the threats are likely to intensify and the husband may make specific plans to harm his wife or her "accomplices," which may include her family, friends, and therapist. Indeed, these plans can often be successful.

Case Description

Mary Elizabeth is a frail, 35-year-old white woman who presented for treatment because she couldn't sleep, was very anxious, "numb," and felt she "just couldn't cope." Married for 15 years, with two children, Mary Elizabeth is a college graduate of above-average intelligence and is currently unemployed. She expressed strong ambivalence about entering treatment and canceled two appointments before coming in for her first session, during which she appeared tired, frightened, and depressed. She attempted to conceal the bruises on her neck and face with makeup.

During the first month of treatment, Mary Elizabeth was often tearful and confused. She complained of tensions with her husband that she felt she had caused, and expressed guilt about her "failures" as a wife and mother. When asked about the nature of her failures, she was unable to be specific about how she had failed and was evasive about the details of her home life. She needed continual reassurance from the therapist that participating in therapy was likely to be good for her, and that therapy was completely confidential. Gradually, over the course of several months, Mary Elizabeth described her background and the development of her complex and destructive marriage.

Mary Elizabeth is the oldest daughter in a family of four children. She described her father as stern, domineering, and critical, and her mother as sickly, passive, and possibly depressed. During her childhood, Mary Elizabeth's role in the family was one of caretaker—both to her bedridden mother and to her younger siblings. Mary Elizabeth was an excellent student and worked hard to achieve the high grades her father demanded. As an adolescent, she never dated, and she had a limited social life. She did, however, win a scholarship to study pharmacology in college, where she excelled academically while remaining socially isolated.

During her last year of college Mary Elizabeth was befriended by her future husband, Robert. He too was a pharmacy student, but he was struggling academically and Mary Elizabeth took on the task of helping him along, letting her own grades slide in the process. In spite of her efforts, Robert did not complete the program, but Mary Elizabeth graduated with her degree. The couple then married. Mary Elizabeth believed she could help Robert to return to school and finish his training. However, Robert never completed his education and instead took a job as a lab technician.

Robert's abusive behavior began soon after the couple married and then escalated progressively over the course of the relationship. Often the abusive behavior was provoked by seemingly arbitrary struggles for control. Mary Elizabeth remembers a disturbing incident during their honeymoon when Robert insisted that she drink milk even though she had always been allergic to it. Mary Elizabeth remembers almost believing Robert's assertion that the allergy was "in her head." She drank the milk, became sick, and vomited. Mary Elizabeth remembers her deep sense of humiliation and Robert's anger at her for defying him and "faking sick."

Over the years, Robert exercised increasing control over Mary Elizabeth's life. He prohibited visits and phone calls from her family and friends. He criticized her for spending time away from home and constantly accused her of infidelity. He routinely searched her purse, pockets, and car for evidence of her "cheating," although she was always faithful to him. He also regularly devalued her, telling her she was ugly, plain, and worthless, and criticized and alienated her co-workers, neighbors, and family. He controlled the finances in the family (even though Mary Elizabeth worked full time) and could therefore leave Mary Elizabeth virtually penniless.

Mary Elizabeth's reactions to Robert's behavior were complicated and ambivalent. In spite of her fear of him, Mary Elizabeth excused her husband's behavior and minimized it. She felt he was a bright man who had not gotten his proper due from the world, and so he became angry from time to time. Mary Elizabeth also felt that she was often to blame for his rage. She felt she provoked him because she was "slow" and "forgetful." Mary Elizabeth's decision to seek therapy was based on the escalating pattern of her husband's abuse. She was in constant fear of Robert. He was completely unpredictable and would fly into a rage over trivial incidents, forcing her out of the car and leaving her on the side of the highway or locking her out of the house at night. He threatened her at work, called her supervisor, and accused him of being Mary Elizabeth's lover. He threatened to kill her or leave her.

Although she eventually acknowledged that Robert was physically violent with her, showing the therapist the bruises and scars on her torso and upper body, Mary Elizabeth consistently minimized the physical aspects of Robert's abuse. She reported that the attacks occurred only three or four times a year, and that during an episode Robert would "try not to" hurt her too badly, indicating that she got facial bruises only when she "got scared and moved so he hit my head."

Another factor contributing to Mary Elizabeth's decision to seek treatment was her increasing fear for the safety of her children. Robert's unpredictable behavior had been occurring more and more frequently in front of the children, as opposed to the earlier years of their marriage, when Robert confined these episodes to the couple's private hours. Recently, the police were called by neighbors on three separate occasions. Each time Robert was calm when the police arrived, and explained that he and his wife were having a "small family problem." On each occasion, Mary Elizabeth backed up Robert's story and declined to file a complaint or press charges against her husband.

In the months leading up to her decision to begin treatment, Mary Elizabeth began to buckle under the stress of the relationship and became afraid that she might "go crazy." She developed insomnia and began to feel strangely detached. She was chronically tired and anxious.

Mary Elizabeth's treatment proceeded slowly and in total secrecy. She was fearful that if Robert knew she was in treatment, he might confront or physically harm the therapist. Over the course of her treatment, Mary

Elizabeth gradually revealed her husband's pervasive and sadistic psychological coercion. After 9 months of treatment, Mary Elizabeth decided to divorce Robert. She felt strongly that she had to leave him "before he kills me physically or spiritually." She frequently spoke of the many ways in which he had "killed her spirit." Mary Elizabeth hired a lawyer, obtained a restraining order, and moved her belongings and those of her children out of the house while Robert was at work. Robert continued to badger Mary Elizabeth, begging, pleading, and threatening her in person and on the phone. Although weakened physically and emotionally, Mary Elizabeth held onto her resolve and pressed for the divorce.

Medical Issues

Certain types of injuries may be diagnostic of spousal abuse—in particular, injuries to the head, neck, upper abdomen, and upper extremities (Goodstein, 1987; Goodstein & Page, 1981). In the present case, the patient sustained injuries to her face, neck, and upper torso, which she tried to hide with makeup. The patient's initial evasiveness and refusal to acknowledge the battering are also typical of first encounters with battered women (Hilberman, 1980). This poses a serious obstacle to appropriate psychological treatment, as well as to the recognition and reporting of abuse by medical professionals, who may be the providers of first resort.

Research has suggested that the staff in hospital emergency rooms rarely ask patients about cause of their injuries and readily accept seemingly plausible stories of accidental misfortunes (Dutton, 1983; Kurz, 1987; Stark Flitcraft, & Frazier, 1979). In fact, one survey of 1000 battered women (solicited by advertisement) indicated that they sought help from medical professionals more frequently than from other professionals, and yet were less satisfied with the physician's response (Bowker & Maurer, 1987).

Part of the problem in services provided by medical personnel may be that these professionals are unable to accurately identify the factors associated with battering. The extent to which psychiatric problems can be accurately identified by primary care physicians has recently been the subject of empirical research (e.g., Andersen & Harthorn, 1989), and further work is needed to ascertain their capacity to identify battering per se and the more elusive psychological aspects of battering as well.

On another level, physicians may often consider battering a possibility but are unaware of the appropriate referral responses. Even though some efforts have been made to educate physicians about the needs of battered women (Walker, 1987), more research and applied programs are sorely needed to teach primary care physicians and nurses to accurately identify the signs of suspected battering and to serve as a liaison in referring battered women to the appropriate mental health and social service professionals in the community. Comparable research has recently been undertaken to educate physicians about psychiatric disorders more generally (Andersen and Harthorn, 1989).

Finally, it should be noted that the psychological concomitants of battering are likely to be even more difficult for primary care physicians and nurses to detect than are the causes of their multiple injuries. The woman's psychological damage can range dramatically in severity, depending upon the degree to which the abuse has escalated. Hence, it is only by attending to relatively subtle cues that are not necessarily medical in nature that the medical professional may be able to recognize and identify psychological coercion as a concomitant of, or risk factor for, battering. The appropriate action when such abuse is identified is referral to a mental health professional equipped to handle serious dysfunction, since the pathology can vary greatly for both the husband and the wife.

Legal Issues

One of the most serious legal considerations surrounding wife battering is that responses from criminal justice systems vary widely across different states. In many states, spousal abuse has a privileged status among violent crimes, in terms of the likelihood both of arrest and of prosecution. In these states, the perpetrator is arrested and tried for assault only if the victim signs a complaint and is willing to press charges in court. This requirement makes it difficult to take legal action to stop spousal abuse. In the present case, the battered woman would not issue a complaint against her husband or press charges when the police had been summoned by neighbors. Hence, no legal action was taken, because all parties concurred that the assaultive behavior was a "family problem" that did not warrant outside intervention. It was only after Mary Elizabeth filed for divorce that she had the strength and resolve to press for a restraining order, which Robert largely ignored.

It has been suggested that if physical assault between a man and a woman in an intimate relationship were simply treated in the same manner as physical assault between strangers, progress would be made in the justice system response to battering (Emery, 1989). Research on the efficacy of using the criminal justice system to respond to cases of wife assault supports the notion that arrest, prosecution, and treatment of offenders may be effective in reducing recidivism (Dutton, 1987). In one study, for example, police officers were randomly assigned to respond to domestic calls either by attempting to mediate the dispute informally, by ordering the assailant to leave the premises, or by arresting him. A 6 month follow-up indicated that only 10% of the men in the arrest group repeated the violence, in contrast to 19% in the informal-mediation group and 24% in the leave-the-premises group (Sherman & Berk, 1984).

Unfortunately, many factors other than the requirement to sign a complaint and press charges seem to conspire to make the use of the criminal justice system unlikely in cases of spousal abuse. One factor has to do with the attitudes of medical and mental health professionals, who often appear to believe that spousal assault is best dealt with within the family (Saunders & Size, 1986), and that efforts should be made to keep the family together (Emery, 1989). Hence, law enforcement and legal professionals often fail to make appropriate referrals. Interestingly, when police officers have made it a policy to bring criminal charges against husbands who beat their wives, surveys of the battered wives indicate a higher level of satisfaction with police services, although police officers report more negative attitudes about the policy (Jaffe, Wolfe, Telford, & Austin, 1986). Similarly, when battered women have been compared with police officers, the majority of the victims preferred arrest, while very few of the police officers viewed arrest as the best solution (Saunders & Size, 1986; see also Bowker, 1983). Victim-blaming among police officers was also found to be positively correlated with their having traditional attitudes about women's roles (Saunders & Size, 1986).

Further education is thus needed to make police officers and legal professionals aware of the special problems of battered women and of their own legal and ethical responsibilities in cases of suspected spousal abuse. Failure to properly educate these professionals may, in fact, lead to unfair judiciary decisions toward these women, who may romanticize and lie to protect their husbands.

It has been suggested that a two-tiered approach to family violence is now developing, in which the first tier is distinctly legal and involves arresting perpetrators of violent acts if these acts would lead to arrest and prosecution among strangers (Attorney General's Task Force, 1984, cited in Emery, 1989). The second tier concerns social services and mental health (Emery, 1989). More emergency services are sorely needed, of course, so that once a case is filed, the battered woman is no longer risking her life by having reported the abuse (Ryback & Bassuk, 1986). Hence, the alleviation of family violence requires increases in the state and federal allocation of resources to shelters, child care, and educational/vocational assistance for the victims of family violence.

It should also be noted that children may be complexly interwoven into the legal system's procedures in cases of spousal abuse, because they are often called upon as witnesses in court proceedings (Ryback & Bassuk, 1986). This poses a number of problems for the child, who is often asked to testify against a parent. Systematizing the legal procedures for use with children in such cases would be very valuable not only in reducing child stress but also in eliciting accurate testimony (Emery, 1989).

Social and Family Issues

It has been argued that "battering" is not only a societal problem but one that has largely social origins (Davis, 1987; Ferraro, 1988; Walker, 1979). Historically, husbands in Western society were legally and morally responsible for their wives' actions, and the use of physical force was acceptable for certain offenses, so long as it did not cause serious physical injuries (Walker, 1979, 1981). In fact, it was legal for a man to physically chastise his wife less than 100 years ago (Davidson, 1978; Ptacek, 1988). Recent data from a national sample of over 5000 families suggests, in fact, that men who agree with the normative question "Are there situations you can imagine in which you would approve of a husband slugging his wife?" are more likely to abuse their wives (Kantor & Straus, 1987). Furthermore, within the context of sex-role socialization, men are taught that their role is to be intelligent, strong, and the economic provider in a marriage, and that their wife's role is to take care of their emotional needs. He may also learn that "controlling" his wife, making her adhere to his desires, is his "right," a belief that may serve to legitimize violence (Ponzetti, Cate, & Koval, 1982). When his wife fails to meet his emotional needs, he may then act out aggressively, at which point "the difference between a slap in the name of discipline and one occurring out of frustration may become an issue of semantics" (Walker, 1981, p. 82; see also Ferraro, 1988).[2]

In the present case, the battered woman and her spouse agreed about the role of the wife in the family unit, believing she should be a selfless caretaker and, ultimately, a passive victim. Further, she was nearly powerless within her marriage, in that she was isolated from

---

[2]In spite of the beliefs about male/female roles in our society that may facilitate spousal violence, it should be noted that it is a misconception to consider wife battering a social norm, since the incidence of wife assault is less than 10% when assault is defined as any case in which a man kicks or bites a women, hits her with his fist or with an object, beats her up, threatens her with a weapon or actually uses one (Dutton, 1983).

outside contacts, denied access to resources, and plagued by the responsibility of making the relationship work.

Sex-role socialization, in general, tends to support the notion that the success or failure of intimate relationships is the woman's responsibility, and this may lead some women to make great efforts to stay in intimate relationships, even after episodes of abuse, to show their commitment to their partner and to weathering the "difficult times" together (Dutton & Painter, 1981; Strube, 1988). In addition, when an abusive event occurs, the woman may presume it will not recur, and so "try to make the relationship work under the belief that if she tries hard enough her efforts will succeed" (Strube, 1988, p. 24).

Traumatic Bonding. In cases of wife assault, the aggressor usually uses violence in part to create and sustain a power advantage in the relationship (Dutton *et al.*, 1982). Creating a power advantage can be accomplished using various forms of psychological abuse ranging from complete control of a woman's use of her time, her social contacts, and her capacity to view herself as a worthwhile person. It need not be (and usually is not) limited to physical violence. The battering often starts early in the relationship (Dutton, 1983; Gelles, 1976; Rounsaville, 1978) and may therefore be perceived by the woman as an aberration, something that will not recur. Furthermore, it is often followed by a period of relative calm, creating a cycle including (a) the building of tension, (b) the eruption of violence, and (c) a relative calm (Walker, 1979). This intermittent reinforcement, the strongest schedule for the development of emotional attachments known to research psychology (Dutton, 1983; Dutton & Painter, 1981; see also Rajecki, Lamb, & Obsmacher, 1978; Suomi & Harlow, 1977), creates a traumatic bonding effect in which the victim becomes progressively more desperately attached to the batterer and intent on trying to mollify him (Dutton, 1987; Dutton & Painter, 1981; Walker, 1979).

Psychological Entrapment. Along these lines, it has been argued that a kind of psychological entrapment exists in battering relationships (Strube, 1988). The woman begins the relationship with her partner with the goal of making it work and later encounters obstacles that she tries to disregard, making a greater investment (trying harder) to reach her goal of relationship harmony (cf. Brockner & Rubin, 1985). As further incident of abuse occurs, she is likely to feel conflicted about staying but may still feel there is some chance that she can make the relationship work. In this view, it is the woman's choice to stay or leave the relationship (Strube, 1988), but the extent of initial investments militates against her leaving because she feels personally responsible for the success of the relationship (Staw, 1976; Strube, 1988). To increase the success of entrapment, the male may seek out a partner who can be easily victimized, by being willing to take responsibility for the maintenance of the relationship and to take on a traditionally passive and self-sacrificing female role.

Social Isolation. In battering relationships the woman is virtually always isolated from outside sources of social support (Boulette & Andersen, 1985; Ponzetti *et al.*, 1982; Straus, Gelles, & Steinmetz, 1980), which is also a central feature of being in a "cult" (Andersen & Zimbardo, 1980; Singer, 1979). Since she rarely encounters anyone else, the battered woman's world is limited to the battering man, and her judgment may therefore be compromised. A lack of social support is clearly associated with greater severity in abuse (Mitchell & Hodson, 1983).

Economic Stress. People in battering relationships are often financially burdened, usually owing to unemployment (Straus *et al.*, 1980). When a woman has few personal resources, this is associated with greater severity in violence (Mitchell & Hodson, 1983), and it is much more difficult to leave the relationship (Kalmuss & Straus, 1982; Walker, 1979). Hence, although battering cuts across class lines (Straus *et al.*, 1980), some battered women and their children are at risk for becoming homeless (Ryback & Bassuk, 1986).

Alcohol Abuse. The literature clearly indicates a strong relationship between alcohol use and marital violence (Eisenberg & Micklow, 1977; Gayford, 1975; Gelles, 1974; Kantor & Straus, 1987; Ponzetti *et al.*, 1982; Rosenbaum & O'Leary, 1981; Roy, 1977; Walker, 1979, 1988). Battering husbands often abuse alcohol, and this may have a disinhibiting effect on their violent behavior. Abusive men are significantly more alcoholic than are nonabusive men, even when both are in discordant marriages (Van Hasselt, Morrison, & Bellack, 1985). Hence, it is possible that alcohol is associated with the actual eruption of spousal violence, rather than only with psychological coercion.

Power Imbalance in the Relationship. Power-imbalanced relationships are associated with spousal abuse, especially when the imbalance threatens the male's power. Research based on a random sample of over 1000 married women (Harris and Associates, 1979) showed a greater risk for wife battering, including both life-threatening violence (i.e., with a weapon) and psychological abuse, in couples in which the woman's occupational status exceeded her education to a greater degree than did her husband's (i.e., when she was, relatively speaking, an overachiever) (Hornung, McCullough, & Sugimoto, 1981). More generally, this type of status inconsistency is related to high levels of marital dissatisfaction among men. Overachievement on the part of men (i.e., when their occupational status exceeded their education) appears to be associated with greater satisfaction among men (Hornung & McCullough, 1981) and with less spousal violence (Hornung et al., 1981). When women are less educated than their spouses, this is also associated with increased spousal violence (Hornung et al., 1981), suggesting that education in women is positively related to their not being abused, not simply because the uneducated nonprofessional woman is abused, but also because the woman who achieves more professionally than her education would predict is also abused (Hornung et al., 1981). Furthermore, equalitarian couples have a lower rate of conflict and violence than do couples in which one partner is dominant (Coleman & Straus, 1986), among whom conflict is more positively correlated with violent behavior (Coleman & Straus, 1986).

Intergenerational Transmission. It has been argued that wife abuse is a learned behavior that can be acquired on the basis of modeling, which might account for its transmission from generation to generation. The empirical literature on wife battering demonstrates that it does tend to be learned in the home and to be passed down between generations (Carlson, 1977; Gayford, 1975; Gelles, 1974; Hilberman & Munson, 1978; Roy, 1977; Straus et al., 1980). In particular, a large percentage of battering men sampled either observed or experienced violence as children (Rosenbaum & O'Leary, 1981). Hence, the importance in spousal abuse of the perpetrator's own familial upbringing has been stressed (e.g., Belsky, 1980; Egeland, Jacobvitz, & Sroufe, in press; Kalmuss, 1984).

Ecological models of family violence, typically based on social learning theory, are largely supported in the literature, which shows that social learning theory nicely explains how family members are socialized into becoming abusive (Dutton & Browning, 1988; Emery, 1989), although the literature is fraught with methodological problems. To understand how violent behavior is learned among battering husbands, it is instructive to consider how all aggressive behavior is learned. The origins of aggression can be traced to observing violence in the family of origin, in one's subculture, or on television, and to being reinforced for violent acts (Bandura, 1973; Dutton & Browning, 1988). The instigation of aggression can be either aversive experiences (insults), incentive expectancies (expecting some reward from the act), or delusional (having bizarre beliefs about the act; Dutton & Browning, 1988). The function of aggression in this sense is to gain inroads for the aggressor, for example, in terms of gaining power in the situation or terminating an experience perceived as aversive. If a person learns as a child that violent or abusive behavior is appropriate when angry or frustrated, he may be more likely to use violence as a reaction to stress later in life (Rouse, 1988).

Family systems models have also been utilized to explain intergenerational transmission. In such models, children react to parental conflict in three phases (Emery, 1989). In the first, the child experiences the conflict as an aversive event. In the second, the child reacts emotionally, instrumentally, or presumably both, in an attempt to alleviate distress. In the third, the reaction the child used to reduce distress (or that the parents used) is negatively reinforced by an actual reduction in distress (in the child or in the family). The emotional or instrumental patterns learned in this way are likely to be maintained and to contribute, later in life, to how the individual copes with his/her own marital distress. Hence, inadequacies in the working model or cognitive script for interpersonal relationships may be learned. A recent longitudinal study spanning 22 years has shown, in fact, that aggression is found to be very stable across generations within a family, when measured at comparable ages (Huesmann, Eron, Lefkowitz, & Walder, 1984), supporting the idea of intergenerational transmission.

Assessment of Psychopathology

The Battering Man

In the present case, the battering man was both controlling and impulsive, trying to order the battered woman's life, taking charge of all responsibilities, and yet being highly reactive and explosive. He appeared to need the security of controlling his wife, keeping her at home, and jealously guarding her from any outside influences. His urgent need for control and inability to tolerate any threat to his dominance is typical among battering men, as are rigidly traditional concepts of masculinity and fragile self-esteem.

Although available research demonstrates that men and boys engage in more physical violence than do women and girls (Gove, 1979; Maccoby & Jacklin, 1974), little is known about how these factors influence the phenomenon of wife battering. The battering husband has rarely been studied in empirical research, and what is "known" is based largely on theoretical considerations and clinical experience (Ptacek, 1988). A list of factors that typically describe battering men is presented in Table 3.

**Table 3. Prototypic Features
Characterizing the Battering Male**

Personality disorder (usually antisocial or bor-
 derline; common quality: lack of empathy)
Easily threatened masculinity
Low self-esteem
Lack of assertiveness
Excessive, hostile attachment to wife
Need for power/control over wife
Pathological jealousy
Alcohol/drug abuse
Violence in his family of origin
Coping by minimizing abusiveness

Personality Disorders. Many investigators assume that identifiable psychopathology exists among battering husbands (Ptacek, 1988), and particularly that battering men may often suffer from various personality disorders. For example, battering men have been described as passive-aggressive, obsessive, compulsive, paranoid, and sadistic (Shainess, 1977). They have also been characterized as passive-dependent (Faulk, 1974). Bolstering these clinical assumptions, a recent study indicated that of nearly 100 abusive men only 13% showed *no* evidence of personality disorder (on the Millon Inventory). The remaining 87% tended to score as one of three personality types: (a) schizoidal/borderline, (b) narcissistic/antisocial, and (c) passive-dependent/compulsive (Hamberger & Hastings, 1986).

It may be valuable to note that two of these personality disorders directly involve abusive behavior. That is, violence and lawlessness characterize antisocial personality while explosiveness, exploitativeness, and self-destructiveness characterize borderline personality. Pertinent to this, 80% of the battering males in another study (Walker, 1984) were found to be violent with people other than their wives, such as their children (including incest), parents, pets, and objects (Walker, 1988). More batterers than nonbatterers in this study had also been arrested (71% vs. 34%) and convicted (34% vs. 19%).

In terms of assessment, it should be noted that these personality disorders are severe and carry a negative prognosis. They imply either a lack of expression of emotion or a lack of emotional empathy for the feelings of others.

Easily Threatened Masculinity. It has been shown that abusive husbands have more traditional views of women than do nonabusive husbands (Rosenbaum & O'Leary, 1981; Walker, 1979, 1988). Sex-role socialization is instrumental in defining the attitudes men have about violence and their perceptions of the appropriate power balance in marital relationships. Some have strongly argued that violence tends to erupt when there is a clash of ideologies between traditional, conservative, patriarchal husbands and nontraditional, liberated wives (Whitehurst, 1984). In a recent study, in fact, reformed abusers attributed their past violent behavior to their stereotypic images of manhood, which they felt had somehow been challenged (Gondolf & Hanneken, 1987). Compared with nonviolent men (even in discordant marriages), battering men also score lower on masculinity based on standardized measures, and lower on psychological androgyny (Rosenbaum, 1986), supporting the notion that they may be highly sensitive to issues around their own masculinity (although see Johnston, 1988; Rouse, 1988). Hence, the battering male may easily have his masculinity threatened and may seem brittle concerning his capacity to be adequate as a man.

Low Self-Esteem. It has also been suggested (Boyd, 1978; Gayford, 1975; Labell, 1979; Martin, 1976) that batterers tend to have low self-esteem and to use violence to compensate for these feelings (Johnston, 1988). Research has generally supported this notion (Gelles, 1974; Hilberman & Munson, 1978; Johnston, 1988; Roy, 1982), perhaps because violence can be a vehicle for achieving a more positive attitude toward the self if the individual has experienced its being subtly condoned (Johnston, 1988; Kaplan, 1972).

Lack of Assertiveness. Battering men have been shown to lack assertiveness (i.e, the skills to communicate their emotions and needs in interpersonal relationships; Rosenbaum & O'Leary, 1981). Similarly, men who lack communication skills have been found to be more likely to respond to their own anger as a cue to aggression (Dutton & Browning, 1988; Rule & Nesdale, 1976).

Excessive, Hostile Attachment to Wife. Theories of attachment and loss suggest other interesting hypotheses about the excessive attachment battering men often have to their mates (Bowlby, 1969, 1973, 1980). Specifically, individuals who make very strong demands on others and respond with anger and anxiety when these demands are not met may have experienced, at one time, a loss or a threatened loss of a mothering figure early in life. Such adults may then come to have not only excessive dependency needs and fears of abandonment but also underlying feelings of hostility and anger which may later be directed toward a spouse.

Need for Power/Control over Wife. Trait-type descriptions can go only so far in detailing the actual responses of battering men in their relationships. Studies of actual arousal responses among abusive males have shown that these men respond with more arousal and anger than do nonabusive males to an argument between a man and a woman (Dutton & Browning, 1988). It has been suggested that for battering men, the argument signifies threat of abandonment and loss of power over the woman (Dutton & Browning, 1988; Walker, 1988), and hence any hint of this in the woman may serve as a situational trigger for violence. Similarly, when the woman seeks more intimacy from the man, this may threaten his power and trigger violence by invading the emotional distance he attempts to maintain (Dutton & Browning, 1988).

Delusional Jealousy. As indicated, the battering male may ultimately demand absolute loyalty from his wife, accuse her of disregarding him, and require constant reassurance and attention (Ferraro, 1988).

Alcohol/Drug Abuse. Again as indicated, battering men often have a drug or alcohol dependency (cf. Kantor & Straus, 1987; Ponzetti *et al.*, 1982; Rosenbaum & O'Leary, 1981; Walker, 1979, 1988).

Violence in His Family of Origin. Social learning theory (Bandura, 1973) provides a theoretical backdrop for understanding the correlation between a reportedly violent family background and becoming a victim or a perpetrator of abuse (Fleming, 1979; Gayford, 1975; Kipnis, 1976). Past family violence may contribute to the learning of these patterns and of pathological sex-role behaviors (Frieze, Parsons, Johnson, Ruble, & Zellman, 1978). Reports of being abused as a child and of witnessing parental spousal abuse are both associated with battering later in life (Rosenbaum & O'Leary, 1981). Moreover, men who observe their mother enduring this type of suffering may become desensitized as adults to observing manifestation of pain and suffering in women, which might otherwise have an inhibitory effect (Baron & Byrne, 1977).

The social learning model assumes that the battering male is violent with his wife in order to control her behavior (to get rid of what he sees as aversive in her behavior or to get her to behave as he wishes). Despite the power of the theory in accounting for wife battering, the applications of the model have also been limited by failing to deal directly with "internal" maintaining conditions for violent marital behaviors (thoughts, feelings, wishes that may provoke and/or maintain the behavior beyond wanting to control the wife; Emery, 1989). Instead, the literature has focused rather exclusively on "external" contingencies (Emery, 1989), which is problematic because the goal of aggressive behavior is often to inflict pain, rather than to attain some external, instrumental end (Berkowitz, 1983; Emery, 1989). Hence, it may be valuable to distinguish, in assessing spousal abuse, between violent behavior that emerges because of an *attempt to control* the victim and that which emerges because of an *attempt to harm* the victim (Emery, 1989).

Coping by Minimizing His Own Abusiveness. Battering men typically conceptualize and describe assaultive behavior in a manner that makes it seem less reprehensible (Dutton & Browning, 1988). They minimize the extent of the damage they have done and the frequency of the episodes. They are also likely to use euphemisms to refer to the episodes and to attribute them to alcohol, so as to deflect blame (Dutton & Browning, 1988).

The Battered Woman

It is difficult to identify the battered woman and to separate her individual characteristics from those of the pathological system in which she is ensnared. In the present case, the battered woman came for treatment in a state of depression, was evasive about her injuries, rationalized her husband's treatment of her, felt guilty for failing as a wife and mother, and generally showed signs of learned helplessness. There was little evidence of pathology in her history, although she described her mother as docile and was apparently content to relinquish power in her own marriage to her strong, dominant husband. Hence, Mary Elizabeth may have learned some victim behaviors in her family of origin.

The most obvious cues to identifying the battered woman in most cases will be physical. In the present case, although explicit questions were asked about the incidents causing the injuries, the victim nonetheless responded in vague, evasive terms, and her descriptions lacked detail and plausibility. There will, however, be cases in which no obvious physical damage can be detected; in these cases, and in those that show obvious signs of violence, it usually will be possible to identify other patterns that are associated with psychological abuse—in this case, psychological coercion.

The effects of psychological coercion and battering can best be described in terms of three aversive psychological states: debility, dependency, and dread, all of which typically are suffered by victims of brainwashing (Hilberman & Munson, 1978; West, 1963). Battered women experience paralyzing terror, constant anxiety, apprehension, vigilance, and feelings of impending doom (Walker, 1988). As the oppression and fear continue and perhaps escalate, these women may also come to feel fatigued, passive, and unable to act, exhibiting concrete thinking and poor memory (Dutton & Painter, 1981; Strube, 1988; Walker, 1979; see also West, 1963). Clinically, these victimized women often appear detached and smiling when describing their frightening experiences, separating their affective responses (e.g., terror, humiliation) from their description. They rarely express anger over their plight and typically report multiple somatic and other symptoms that fit within the diagnostic categories of panic disorder, recurrent major depression, dysthymic disorder, or somatization disorder (American Psychiatric Association, 1980, 1987).

The literature on spousal abuse suggests that battered women have a distinguishable pattern of symptoms, which has been termed the battered woman syndrome and is a version of posttraumatic stress disorder described in DSM-III and DSM-III-R (American Psychiatric Association, 1980, 1987). The symptoms overlap both with affective and anxiety disorders, but they contain other features as well, such as dissociation, memory loss, reexperiencing of the traumatic event, disruption of interpersonal relationships, and associated psychophysiological responses (Walker, 1988).

On a different note, some investigators have assumed that if a woman is in an abusive relationship, she must be psychologically disturbed, and that an identifiable disorder of personality would account for her behavior (Shainess, 1977). In particular, some writers have suggested that battered women suffer from a masochistic personality disorder (Shainess, 1977). In this view, the battered woman *likes* being beaten— that is, she derives gratification from the abuse, where "gratification is connected with suffering or physical or mental pain at the hands of the sexual object" (Freud, 1938, pp. 569, cited in Dutton, 1983). On the other hand, a review of studies of masochism—both in behavior and in traits—has provided no support for the notion that women cause their own victimization, even by verbal provocation (Saunders, 1986). Hence, there was considerable controversy over the inclusion of this type of diagnostic category in DSM-III-R (American Psychiatric Association, 1987), and it was ultimately relegated to an appendix.

As an alternative, it has been argued that the battered woman is in a kind of "social trap" (Platt, 1973) in which an immediate payoff (a momentary reprieve and some kindness) obscures the violent events that precede it. In this process, the relationship alternates unpredictably from periods of violence to periods of relative peace, thereby creating hope that things could be made to be alright if the woman can just keep things running smoothly (Dutton & Browning, 1988; Dutton & Painter, 1981). This kind of attachment, in which escape rarely occurs without an ultimate return, develops in all higher-order primates when intermittent abuse occurs (Dutton, 1983; Rajecki et al., 1978; Suomi & Harlow, 1977),

Table 4. Prototypic Features
Characterizing the Battered Woman

Traumatic bonding to the battering man
Fear and terror
Learned helplessness
   Cognitive deficits (to learn that there is a
     way out)
   Motivational deficits (to try a way out)
   Affective deficits (depressive affect)
Guilt and self-blame
Low self-esteem
(Violence in her family of origin?)
Coping by minimizing her abuse

and in many human relationships characterized by extreme power imbalances (e.g., Bettelheim, 1943). Since this pattern of bonding is not particular to the battered woman, it should not be attributed to defects in her "masochistic personality" (Dutton, 1983).

Factors typical of battered women are depicted in Table 4 and described below.

Traumatic Bonding and Entrapment. As indicated, for most battered women the battering, traumatic bonding, and entrapment begin early in the relationship (Rosenbaum & O'Leary, 1981) and are followed by periods of relative calm, in which the woman hopes that her husband will get through this "rough time" and that the humiliation, manipulation, and violence will not recur (Dutton & Browning, 1988; Strube, 1988; Walker, 1988). By the time it is repeated, and is repeated again, often with escalating severity (Dutton, 1983; Dutton & Painter, 1981), the battered woman feels she has invested too much to leave the relationship or to stop trying within it, leading her to justify staying and to deny the frequency or intensity of her abuse (Brockner & Rubin, 1985; Strube, 1988). In fact, because psychological entrapment is particularly likely when the goal (in this case, relationship maintenance) is very valuable (Brochner & Rubin, 1985) and socially appropriate (Brockner, Rubin, & Lang, 1981; Strube, 1988), women who give exclusive value to their marriages or love relationships over and above other aspects of their lives may be at risk for battering.

Fear and Terror. The battered woman is likely to respond with great fear to her husband's threats of violence and unpredictable punishments (such as locking her out of the house at night). She may show constant apprehension and vigilance in preventing these episodes (Boulette &

Andersen, 1985; Dutton & Painter, 1981; Strube, 1988; Walker, 1979, 1988) but, over time, may give up on attempting to prevent the abuse (Strube, 1988; Walker, 1988).

Learned Helplessness. Battered women may often suffer from learned helplessness (Boulette & Andersen, 1985; Walker, 1979, 1983), in that they come to expect that no relationship exists between their actions and the outcomes. After trying and failing to prevent abuse, she may give up and become unable to learn that there is a way out of the situation (a cognitive deficit) and unable to try new responses (a motivational deficit). In addition, learned helplessness is more likely when the victim of abuse attributes the abuse to internal, stable, and global causes (Abramson, Seligman, & Teasdale, 1978), such as to her own stable characteristics. To the extent that battered women believe that future abuse is inevitable, they are likely to give up and experience learned helplessness and depressive affect (Andersen & Lyon, 1987). The psychological sequelae of battering may thus occur in two stages, beginning with entrapment and followed by learned helplessness (Strube, 1988). Research confirms the notion that depressive affect and symptoms are more likely in battered women as violence increases and also as social isolation and economic stress increase (Mitchell & Hodson, 1983).

Guilt and Self-Blame. Once intermittent abuse has occurred, the battered woman attempts to cope with her situation and, in so doing, develops a sense of self-blame (Dutton *et al.*, 1982), as do most victims of uncontrollable violence who feel powerless to control it (Bettelheim, 1943; see also Wortman, 1976). Outside observers to incidents of spousal abuse, if unaware of the powerful forces operating in battering situations, may tend to attribute it to the battered woman's internal dispositions, thereby blaming her for her victimization (Jones & Nisbett, 1972) and encouraging her to blame herself. This error, termed the "fundamental attribution error" (Nisbett & Ross, 1980), is likely to be incorrect, mainly because powerful situations of abuse produce similar patterns in other people besides battered women and in other species as well. Nonetheless, self-blame is common in battered women, who invest more and more effort in the relationship to make it work, and blame themselves for the failure.

Low Self-Esteem. Many investigators have argued that battering should produce low self-esteem in women exposed to it. In support of this assumption, research has shown that increased violence is associated with lower self-esteem among battered women (Mitchell & Hodson, 1983).

Violence in Her Family of Origin? As is the case with the battering male, it has been suggested that a woman's willingness to remain in an abusive marital relationship is based on her own learning history in her family (Schulman, 1979; Snyder & Fruchtman, 1981; Straus, 1977; although see Geiles, 1976; Rosenbaum & O'Leary, 1981). This general hypothesis can be conceptualized in terms of learning theory, attachment theory, or family systems theory, but the common element is that women exposed to violence may have a predisposition to get into abusive relationships. In fact, besides getting involved with a violent man, women exposed to violence in their family of origin may also have a learned tendency to startle, cower, placate, and plead (from being beaten themselves as children or from having watched their mother being beaten), which may actually trigger the previously learned aggressive responses in the battering man, based on his own socialization, if he is sufficiently aroused and these external cues were previously associated with aggression (Berkowitz, 1974, 1983).

Although the frequency of personally experienced violence in a woman's family of origin is associated with increased violence in her own marriage (Dutton, 1983; Schulman, 1979; Straus, 1977), battered and nonbattered women do not always differ in whether or not they witnessed parental spousal abuse or experienced child abuse in their families of origin (Rosenbaum & O'Leary, 1981). Hence, neither witnessing violence in one's own parents nor being the target of it is a necessary or sufficient condition for being a battered woman later in life. Even if the abuse in the child's home is mainly psychological, however, she may learn important victim characteristics, such as passivity, self-sacrifice, and tolerance for psychological abuse, and may ultimately be attracted to insecure, domineering men.

It is important to note, however, that from a social-psychological standpoint, it is quite possible that a marital situation could be constructed in which the features of psychological coercion and mind control were of sufficient magnitude (cf. Andersen, 1985; Boulette & Andersen, 1984) that women from any number of different backgrounds might be retained within it.

Coping by Minimizing Her Abuse. Battered women specifically resist the notion that they should leave their battering husbands (Walker, 1979), a fact consistent with the definition of psychological entrapment in which one's efforts to attain a desired goal (i.e., making a relationship work) are so strong that one must justify the effort by still greater commitment (Strube, 1988). In one recent paper, some of the reasons battered wives offer for remaining in their abusive relationships were identified (Ferraro, & Johnson, 1983), and these are presented in Table 5.

Table 5. Typical Coping Statements Battered Women May Use to Minimize Their Injuries and Justify Staying in a Violent Relationship[a]

Desire to care for (save) the battering man
I'm the only one who can "save" him.
He needs me, so I have to stay.
If I can just do the right thing, all this will stop.
Desire to be loyal to the battering man
I want to be loyal to him and to be a good wife.
I promised to be true to him.
He is the primary person in my life "until death do us part."
Deny the extent/frequency of the beatings
He doesn't really hit me that often.
I know he tries not to hit me in the face.
Fortunately, he gets over it fairly quickly.
Deny the battering man's responsibility for the beatings
He doesn't want to hurt me; he just loses control.
It's not his fault; it's his drinking.
The stress in his life gets to be too much for him.
Denying her option to leave the relationship
No one else will have me and I can't be alone.
I can't face life without him.
I just don't know what else to do.

[a]Adapted from Ferraro and Johnson (1983).

First, battered women may believe that they can "save" their man, and that it is their mission to do so, especially if he's a substance abuser. Second, they may want to be loyal to the battering male and/or to their religious values and vows. Third, they may deny their injuries and tolerate a wide range of abuse before defining it as assault. Fourth, they may deny that the battering male intends to harm them, blaming the abuse on events beyond the control of both spouses and denying his responsibility (Ferraro & Johnson, 1983). Finally, they may deny that they have emotional options ("I can't live without him") and practical options (calling for emergency assistance) in the situation.

Treatment Options

One major challenge in the treatment of spousal abuse is that the treatment for either partner is likely to be unsuccessful while the couple remains together, because otherwise the abuse is unlikely to end. Although some have argued for a family systems approach, most interventions in spousal abuse focus on individual family members (Emery,

1989). Treatments directed at the abusive husband may be most appropriate, especially at the beginning of therapy, since in this case changing the individual changes the cycle of abuse (Emery, 1989).

Unfortunately, helping to effect a separation is, perhaps, the most difficult challenge. The husband's psychological coercion may have rendered the wife too helpless to escape, and the husband remains inaccessible to treatment because he denies any problems and projects all blame onto his wife (Boulette & Andersen, 1985; Steinmetz, 1977; Straus *et al.*, 1980; Walker, 1979, 1988). His vulnerability to a therapeutic intervention is likely to develop only when his wife's escape ultimately triggers intense feelings of abandonment, anger, and despair. Prior to this stage, he is likely to forbid, prevent, or sabotage treatment because his wife's improvement would signal a decrease in his power, aggravating his feeling of insecurity and his fear of abandonment (Boulette & Andersen, 1985). If treatment is sought, conjoint assessment and marital therapy are likely to increase the abuse because the process is likely to empower the woman and make the husband feel more insecure.

The irony for the battered woman is that separation is necessary for treatment and ultimately for survival, and yet when she leaves her husband, she exposes herself to an ever-increasing risk of violence. The husband is likely to have strong feelings of rage associated with the shame of exposing his vulnerability associated with her leaving, and the punishments for this transgression are likely to involve increased dictatorial control, oppression, and abuse. Thus, the wife must not be encouraged to leave her husband until she has the resources to stay away either permanently or long enough to facilitate significant change in the husband's behavior. Further, if the husband has a severe personality disorder, change is unlikely. In any event, separation is the first treatment of choice.

Treating the Battering Man

The therapeutic issue of most importance in treating the battering male is the sense of safety he feels when he has power over the thoughts and actions of his wife (Walker, 1981) and the lack of it he feels upon entering therapy and separating from her. Therefore, the battering man is likely to be suspicious of the therapist and to make pressured attempts to somehow resume the relationship in its previous form (Walker, 1981). He may also be at risk for suicide and homicide, and must be carefully evaluated to rule out a need for involuntary hospitalization and for a Tarasoff warning. Helping the battering male to learn to cope more functionally with his feelings of insecurity is a central treatment issue, as is helping him to deal more appropriately with separation and anger.

Assessment and treatment of the battering man must initially focus on evaluating and reducing his potential for further violence. After this early effort, grief therapy (Worden, 1982) is usually needed to assist with the sorrow, anger, and guilt associated with the temporary or permanent loss of his mate. After some degree of symptom reduction, therapy can then proceed toward identifying and resolving the conflicts and early losses that are associated with needing hostile and excessively dependent marital unions. If a personality disorder such as borderline or antisocial is present (Hamberger & Hastings, 1986), the therapeutic task is much more difficult. Treatment may also need to focus on alcohol or drug abuse, since violent behavior is related to alcohol abuse (Van Hasselt et al., 1985), although it is neither a necessary nor a sufficient cause of spousal abuse (Kantor & Straus, 1987).

Overall, the most relevant treatment issues for the battering male can be identified only on the basis of a comprehensive assessment. If the individual has an antisocial personality or borderline personality disorder, the prognosis is poor. If he has a severe identity disorder characterized by low self-esteem and easily threatened masculinity, treatment is likely to be long-term. If he is abusing alcohol or other substances, proper referral is obviously needed. For an intermittent impulse control disorder, referral to a psychiatrist may be appropriate, since medication can be helpful. With relatively minor disorders characterized by poor anger management and interpersonal skills, as well as with the more severe disorders, the individual may benefit (within the limitations of his pathology) from learning how to (a) control anger and physical aggression, (b) handle separation/abandonment, (c) to treat his partner with respect rather than trying to control her, (d) to value relationships built on equal partnership, (e) to admit mistakes and personal foibles, and (f) become more empathic with others (i.e., more sensitive to their feelings) (Walker, 1981).

Also relevant to treatment is the fact that as many as 58% of the battered women in one sample reported having been raped by their batterer (Walker, 1981). Both researchers and clinicians have noted that violent men may have trouble distinguishing anger from sexual arousal cues (cf. Malamuth, Feshback, & Jaffee, 1977, for rapists), suggesting the importance of developing treatment techniques that focus on this problem (Walker, 1981).

Thus far, treatment programs for spousal abuse have been based on cognitive-behavioral therapy approaches to stress management, parenting, and controlling anger and aggression (Ptacek, 1988). Group therapy with abusive men has also been employed in anger and aggression management (Emery, 1989).

Interestingly, one study of abusive men who had reformed in treatment indicated that they attributed their successful treatment to learning to accept responsibility for their problems, learning to become more empathetic, and learning to redefine their conceptions of their own manhood (Gondolf & Hanneken, 1987). Other interventions have also focused on the reduction of stereotypic sex-role expectations among abusive males and on teachings effective interpersonal skills as an alternative to explosive, violent outbursts (Ponzetti *et al.*, 1982). Even though there is debate about the effectiveness of court-mandated treatment program for offenders, recent research has begun to suggest that even mandated cognitive-behavioral intervention strategies can be effective (Emery, 1989).

Treating the Battered Female

In dealing with the female in a battering relationship, it is critical to assess not only her symptoms and the level of her impairment, but also her potential for being hurt or killed. In addition, battered, debilitated, helpless women have been known to kill their aggressors. This risk *must* be evaluated. Depending on the degree of danger and debility, the therapist may initially need to allow the woman considerable dependence on her therapist, while she is provided with information, support, and direction aimed at reducing the violence and facilitating escape. The availability of supportive neighbors, of police intervention, and of shelters must be discussed at this time. If the woman remains in the home, her treatment may need to be kept hidden from her husband because of the danger of treatment sabotage and danger to the therapist.

At the outset, the biggest problem in treating the battered woman is that she may minimize her psychological and physical abuse. She may even succeed in convincing the therapist that she has the situation under control. That is, she may believe that if she just does everything the batterer wants, she will have nothing to fear (Walker, 1981).

Once a separation has been effected, the battered woman will experience extreme anxiety, since she has been exposed to psychological maltreatment that has damaged her self-confidence, self-esteem, and coping abilities. Therapists must also watch for the emergence of their own anger toward the female client, who may attempt to return to a dangerous and oppressive situation. The client's loyalty to the aggressor is likely to lead to guilt over the legal ordeals he may face. Initially, treatment should focus on reducing risk of harm, facilitating escape and resettlement, ultimately dealing with any posttraumatic stress sequelae, helping her to work through the loss of the relationship, and helping her to recognize her own worth and value.

Furthermore, treatment should also focus heavily on deprogramming or identifying and correcting the distorted social and personal beliefs that have helped establish and maintain the battering relationship. Does the woman believe she will save the batterer, that her injuries are unimportant, that she will get him to stop, and that the beatings are her own fault? She must be encouraged to understand and to change her self-destructive ways of construing the relationship by redirecting her efforts from placating her husband to rescuing and improving herself. When the woman leaves the relationship, she must clearly understand the danger of the manipulative efforts her husband will utilize to recapture her, so that she can predict and resist her husband's persistent recapture behaviors. Ultimately, the battered woman's own conflicts about vulnerability, power, and control must also be explored so as to discourage her from repeating the same pattern with other abusive men. As she improves, this may be reinforced by changing her role from victim to rescuer in a different context, by participating in social support groups for similarly victimized women. Participation in such groups, however, should be encouraged only after considerable progress has been made.

Beyond this, when the woman is much healthier, she is likely to express anger, resentment, and rage toward her batterer (Walker, 1981). Helping the battered woman learn to accurately distinguish angry feelings from others she may have, to recognize their appropriate target, and to express them without dire consequences is of considerable therapeutic importance (Walker, 1981).

Battered women have also been shown to be less likely than nonbattered women to use active problem-solving behavior to cope with stress felt within their marriages and are more likely to use passive strategies (Finn, 1985). In fact, while the woman remains in the home, passivity is likely to lower the risk of being injured or killed. Hence, passivity should not be discouraged until a separation has been effected. Once this has occurred, however, the treatment of battered women could involve direct problem-solving approaches to therapy. Community, family-system, and individual interventions that empower women and encourage both men and women to value equal partnership in a marital relationships may be important in reducing spousal abuse and in preventing the development of marital conflict and pathological family ties (Coleman & Straus, 1986).

Finally, as with victims of incest, battered women often experience a dissociation from their own bodies, a separation between body and self due to their experience of violence (Walker, 1981). Bodily sensations and sensual experiences can be reintegrated with the battered woman's sense of self after long and successful therapy (Walker, 1981).

On a different note, children in the familial situation, especially if abused themselves, should also become involved in some form of treatment, which should be directed toward working through repeated parental separations and exposure to dysfunctional and violent parenting. Otherwise, developmental delays, symptoms of anxiety and depression, or indications of a conduct disorder may emerge for these children, who are at risk to become victims or perpetrators of violence themselves.

Summary and Conclusions

Although the precise methodology for identifying psychological maltreatment in relationships, especially in battering relationships, awaits further empirical research, any relationship that involves covert strategies of psychological coercion or regulation over individual freedoms is maladaptive (Andersen, 1985; Boulette & Andersen, 1985). By definition, the battering male in such relationships makes use of psychological coercion, oppression, and degradation to get his partner to adhere to his needs (Boulette & Andersen, 1985; Dutton & Painter, 1981; Walker, 1979). All human relationships involve some manipulation, compromise, and pain. But psychological coercion, which should be conceptualized as a matter of degree (Andersen, 1985), is present when one individual loses the will to be self-determining (Enroth, 1977) and the ability both to recognize and to avoid abuse. Such relationships may be totalistic and, as a result, increase the probability that pathological and degrading interactions will transpire within them. If physicians, nurses, police officers, legal professionals, community workers, and mental health professionals can learn to identify this syndrome with its developing signs, and to make the appropriate referrals when such abuse is suspected, a dent might be made in the human tragedy of spousal abuse.

References

Abramson, L. Y., Seligman, M. E. P., & Teasdale, J. (1978). Learned helplessness in humans: Critique and reformulation. *Journal of Abnormal Psychology, 87,* 49–74.

American Psychiatric Association. (1980). *Diagnostic and statistical manual of mental disorders* (3rd ed.). Washington, DC: Author.

American Psychiatric Association. (1987). *Diagnostic and statistical manual of mental disorders* (3rd ed., rev.). Washington, DC: Author.

Andersen, S. M. (1985). Identifying coercion and deception in social systems. In B. Kilbourne (Ed.), *Divergent perspectives on the new religions* (pp. 12–23). Washington, DC: American Association for the Advancement of Science.

Andersen, S. M. (in press). The inevitability of future suffering: The role of depressive predictive certainty in depression. *Social Cognition*.

Andersen, S. M., & Harthorn, B. H. (1989). The recognition, diagnosis, and treatment of mental disorders by primary care physicians. *Medical Care, 27*, 869–886.

Andersen, S. M., & Harthorn, B. H. (1990). *Changing the psychiatric knowledge of primary care physicians: The effects of a brief intervention on clinical diagnosis and treatment. General Hospital Psychiatry, 12*, 177–190.

Andersen, S. M. & Lyon, J. E. (1987). Anticipating undesired outcomes: The role of outcome certainty in the onset of depressive affect. *Journal of Experimental Social Psychology, 23*, 428–443.

Andersen, S. M., & Zimbardo, P. G. (1980). Resisting mind control. *USA Today, 109*, 44–47.

Attorney General's Task Force on Family Violence. (1984). *Final report*. Washington, DC: U.S. Government Printing Office.

Bandura, A. (1973). *Aggression: A social learning analysis*. Englewood Cliffs, NJ: Prentice-Hall.

Baron, R., & Byrne, D. (1977). *Social psychology*. Boston: Allyn and Bacon.

Belsky, J. (1980). Child maltreatment: An ecological integration. *American Psychologist, 35*, 320–335.

Berk, R. A., Berk, S. F., Loseke, D. R., & Rauma, D. (1983). Mutual combat and other family violence myths. In D. Finkelhor, R. J. Gelles, G. Hotaling, & M. A. Straus (Eds.), *The dark side of families* (pp. 197–212). Beverly Hills, CA: Sage.

Berkowitz, L. (1974). Some detriments of impulsive aggression: The role of mediated associations with reinforcements for aggression. *Psychological Review, 81*, 165–176.

Berkowitz, L. (1983). Aversively stimulated aggression: Some parallels and differences in research with animals and humans. *American Psychologist, 38*, 1135–1144.

Bettelheim, B. (1943). Individual and mass behavior in extreme situations. *Journal of Abnormal and Social Psychology, 38*, 417–452.

Boulette, T. R. (1981, August). *The marital brainwashing syndrome*. Paper presented at the American Psychological Association Convention, Los Angeles.

Boulette, T. R., & Andersen, S. M. (1985). "Mind control" and the battering of women. *Community Mental Health Journal, 21*, 109–117.

Bowker, L. H. (1983). Battered wives, lawyers, and district attorneys: An examination of law in action. *Journal of Criminal Justice, 11*, 403–412.

Bowker, L. H., & Maurer, L. (1987). The medical treatment of battered wives. *Women and Health, 12*, 25–45.

Bowlby, J. (1969). *Attachment and loss* (Vol. 1). New York: Basic Books.

Bowlby, J. (1973). *Attachment and loss* (Vol. 2). New York: Basic Books.

Bowlby, J. (1980). *Attachment and loss* (Vol. 3). New York: Basic Books.

Boyd, V. D. (1978, September). *Domestic violence: Treatment alternatives for the male batterers*. Paper presented at the annual meeting of the American Psychological Association, Toronto.

Brockner, J., & Rubin, J. Z. (1985). *Entrapment in escalating conflicts: A social psychological analysis*. New York: Springer-Verlag.

Brockner, J., Rubin, J. Z., & Lang, E. (1981). Face-saving and entrapment. *Journal of Experimental Social Psychology, 17*, 68–79.

Cantor, N., & Mischel, W. (1979). Prototypes in person perception. In L. Berkowitz (Ed.), *Advances in Experimental Social Psychology, 12*, 3–52.

Carlson, B. E. (1977). Battered women and their assailants. *Social Work, 22*, 455–465.

Coleman, D. H., & Straus, M. A. (1986). Marital power, conflict, and violence in a nationally representative sample of American couples. *Violence and Victims, 12*, 141–157.

Davidson, T. (1978). *Conjugal crime: Understanding and changing the wife beating pattern.* New York: Hawthorn.

Davis, L. V. (1987). Battered women: The transformation of a social problem. *Social Work, 32,* 306–311.

Dobash, R. E., & Dobash, R. (1979). *Violence against wives.* New York: Free Press.

Dutton, D. G. (1983, April). *Masochism as an explanation for traumatic bonding: An example of the "fundamental attribution error."* Paper presented at the American Orthopsychiatric Association Convention, Boston.

Dutton, D. G. (1987). Wife assault: Social psychological contributions to criminal justice policy. *Applied Social Psychology Annual, 7,* 238–261.

Dutton, D. G., & Browning, J. J. (1988). Concern for power, fear of intimacy, and aversive stimuli for wife assault. In G. T. Hotaling, D. Finkelhor, J. T. Kirkpatrick, & M. A. Straus (Eds.), *Family abuse and its consequences* (pp. 163–175). Beverly Hills, CA: Sage.

Dutton, D. G., & Painter, S. L. (1981). Traumatic bonding: The development of emotional attachments in battered women and other relationships of intermittent abuse. *Victimology: An International Journal, 1,* 139–155.

Dutton, D. G., Fehr, B., & McEwen, H. (1982). Severe wife battering as deindividuated violence. *Victimology, 7,* 13–23.

Egeland, B., Jacobvitz, D., & Sroufe, L. A. (in press). Breaking the cycle of abuse: Relationship predictors. *Child Development.*

Eisenberg, S. E. & Micklow, P. L. (1977). The assaulted wife: Catch-22 revisited. *Women's Rights Law Reporter, 58,* 138–161.

Emery, R. E. (1988). *Marriage, divorce and children's adjustment.* Beverly Hills, CA: Sage.

Emery, R. E. (1989). Family violence. *American Psychologist, 44,* 321–328.

Enroth, R. (1977). *Youth, brainwashing and the extremist cults.* Ann Arbor, MI: Zondervan.

Fagan, J. A., Stewart, D. K., & Hansen, K. V. (1983). Violent men or violent husbands? In D. Finkelhor, R. Gelles, G. Hotaling, & M. Straus (Eds.), *The dark side of families* (pp. 49–68). Beverly Hills, CA: Sage.

Faulk, M. (1974). Men who assault their wives. *Medicine, Science, and Law, 14,* 180–183.

Ferraro, K. J. (1988). An existential approach to battering. In G. T. Hotaling, D. Finkelhor, J. T. Kirkpatrick, & M. A. Straus (Eds.), *Family abuse and its consequences* (pp. 126–138). Newbury Park, CA: Sage.

Ferraro, K. J., & Johnson, J. M. (1983). How women experience battering. *Social Problems, 30,* 325–339.

Finn, J. (1985). The stresses and coping behavior of battered women. *Social Casework, 66,* 341–349.

Fleming, J. B. (1979). *Stopping wife abuse.* Garden City, NY: Anchor Books.

Freire, P. (1984). *Pedagogy of the oppressed.* New York: Continuum.

Freud, S. (1938). Three contributions to the theory of sex. In A. A. Brill (Ed.), *The basic writings of Sigmund Freud.* New York: Random House.

Frieze, I. J., Parsons, J., Johnson, P., Ruble, D. N., & Zellman, G. L. (1978). *Women and sex roles: A social psychological perspective.* New York: W. W. Norton.

Gayford, J. J. (1975). Wife battering: A preliminary study of 100 cases. *British Medical Journal, 1,* 194–197.

Gelles, R. (1974). *The violent home: A study of physical aggression between husbands and wives.* Beverly Hills, CA: Sage.

Gelles, R. (1976). Abused wives: Why do they stay? *Journal of Marriage and the Family, 38,* 659–668.

Gondolf, E. W., & Hanneken, J. (1987). The gender warrior: Reformed batterers on abusers, treatment, and change. *Journal of Family Violence, 2,* 177–191.

Goodstein, R. K. (1987). Violence in the home: I. The battered spouse syndrome. *Carrier Foundation Letter, 125,* 1–4.

Goodstein, R. K., & Page, A. W. (1981). Battered wife syndrome: Overview of dynamics and treatment. *American Journal of Psychiatry, 138,* 1036–1044.

Gove, W. (1979). Sex differences in the epidemiology of mental disorder: Evidence and explanations. In E. S. Gomberg & V. F. Brunner (Eds.), *Gender and disordered behavior* (pp. 23–68). New York: Mazel.

Hamberger, L. K., & Hastings, J. E. (1986). Personality correlates of men who abuse their partners: A cross-validation study. *Journal of Family Violence, 1,* 323–341.

Harris, L., and Associates (1979). *A survey of spousal violence against women in Kentucky.* Report prepared for the Kentucky Commission on Women.

Hilberman, E. (1980). Overview: The wife beater's wife considered. *American Journal of Psychiatry, 137,* 1336–1347.

Hilberman, E., & Munson, M. (1978). Sixty battered women. *Victimology: An International Journal, 2,* 460–471.

Hornung, C. A., McCullough, B. C., & Sugimoto, T. (1981). Status relationships in marriage: Risk factors in spouse abuse. *Journal of Marriage and the Family, 43,* 675–692.

Huesmann, L. R., Eron, L. D., Lefkowitz, M. M., & Walder, L. O. (1984). Stability of aggression over time and generations. *Developmental Psychology, 20,* 1120–1134.

Jaffe, P., Wolfe, D. A., Telford, D. A., & Austin, G. (1986). The impact of police charges in incidents of wife abuse. *Journal of Family Violence, 1,* 37–49.

Janoff-Bulman, R. (1979). Characterological versus behavioral self-blame: Inquiries into depression and rape. *Journal of Personality and Social Psychology, 37,* 1798–1809.

Johnston, M. E. (1988). Correlates of early violence experience among men who are abusive toward female mates. In G. T. Hotaling, D. Finkelhor, J. T. Kirkpatrick, & M. A. Straus (Eds.), *Family abuse and its consequences* (pp. 192–202). Beverly Hills, CA: Sage.

Jones, E. E., & Nisbett, R. (1972). *The actor and observer: Divergent perceptions of the causes of behavior.* Morristown, NJ: General Learning Press.

Kalmuss, D. (1984). The intergenerational transmission of marital aggression. *Journal of Marriage and Family, 47,* 11–19.

Kalmuss, D., & Straus, M. A. (1982). Wife's marital dependency and wife abuse. *Journal of Marriage and the Family, 44,* 277–286.

Kantor, G. K., & Straus, M. A. (1987). The "drunken bum" theory of wife beating. *Social Problems, 34,* 213–230.

Kaplan, H. B. (1972). Toward a general theory of psychosocial deviance: The case of aggressive behavior. *Social Science and Medicine, 6,* 593–617.

Kipnis, D. (1976). *The powerholders.* Chicago: University of Chicago Press.

Kurz, D. (1987). Emergency department responses to battered women: Resistance to medicalization. *Social Problems, 34,* 69–81.

Labell, L. S. (1979). Wife abuse: A sociological study of battered women and their mates. *Victimology, 4,* 258–267.

Lerner, M. J. (1970). The desire for justice and reactions to victims. In J. McCauley & L. Berkowitz (Eds.), *Altruism and helping behaviors: Social psychological studies of some antecedents and consequences.* New York: Academic Press.

Libow, J., & Doty, D. (1979). An exploratory approach to self blame and self derogation by rape victims. *American Journal of Orthopsychiatry, 49,* 670–679.

Maccoby, E., & Jacklin, C. (1974). *The psychology of sex differences* (Vol. 1). Stanford, CA: Stanford University Press.

Malamuth, N. Feshback, S., & Jaffee, Y. (1977). Sexual arousal and aggression: Recent experiments and theoretical issues. *Journal of Social Issues, 22,* 110–113.

Margolin, G. (1988). Interpersonal and intrapersonal factors associated with marital violence. In G. T. Hotaling, D. Finkelhor, J. T. Kirkpatrick, & M. A. Straus (Eds.), *Family abuse and its consequences* (pp. 203–217). Beverly Hills, CA: Sage.

Martin, D. (1976). *Battered wives.* San Francisco: Glide.

Mitchell, R. E., & Hodson, C. A. (1983). Coping with domestic violence: Social support and psychological health among battered women. *American Journal of Community Psychology, 11,* 629–654.

Nisbett, R., & Ross, L. (1980). *Human inference: Strategies and shortcomings of social judgment.* Englewood Cliffs, NJ: Appleton-Century-Crofts.

Ochberg, F. M. (1971). Victims of terrorism. *Journal of Clinical Psychiatry, 41,* 73–74.

Platt, J. (1973). Social traps. *American Psychologist, 28,* 641–651.

Ponzetti, J. J., Cate, R. M., & Koval, J. E. (1982). Violence between couples: Profiling the male abuser. *Personnel and Guidance Journal, 61,* 222–224.

Ptacek, J. (1988). The clinical literature on men who batter: A review and critique. In G. T. Hotaling, D. Finkelhor, J. T. Kirkpatrick, & M. A. Straus (Eds.), *Family abuse and its consequences* (pp. 149–162). Beverly Hills, CA: Sage.

Rajecki, P., Lamb, M., & Obsmacher, P. (1978). Toward a general theory of infantile attachment: A comparative review of aspects of the social bond. *Behavioral and Brain Sciences, 3,* 417–464.

Rosch, E. (1978). Principles of categorization. In E. Rosch & B. B. Lloyd (Eds.), *Cognition and categorization* (pp. 27–48). Hillsdale, NJ: Erlbaum.

Rosenbaum, A. (1986). Of men, macho, and marital violence. *Journal of Family Violence, 1,* 121–129.

Rosenbaum, A., & O'Leary, K. D. (1981). Marital violence: Characteristics of abusive couples. *Journal of Consulting and Clinical Psychology, 41,* 63–71.

Rounsaville, B. (1978). Theories of marital violence: Evidence from a study of battered women. *Victimology, 3,* 11–31.

Rounsaville, B., & Weissman, M. M. (1978). Battered women: A medical problem requiring detection. *International Journal of Psychiatry and Medicine, 67,* 760–761.

Rouse, L. P. (1988). Conflict tactics used by men in marital disputes. In G. T. Hotaling, D. Finkelhor, J. T. Kirkpatrick, & M. A. Straus (Eds.), *Family abuse and its consequences* (pp. 176–191). Beverly Hills, CA: Sage.

Roy, M. (Ed.). (1977). *Battered women: A psychosocial study of domestic violence.* New York: Van Nostrand Reinhold.

Roy, M. (Ed.). (1982). *The abrasive partner: An analysis of domestic violence.* New York: Van Nostrand Reinhold.

Rule, B. G., & Nesdale, A. R. (1976). Emotional arousal and aggressive behavior. *Psychological Bulletin, 83,* 851–863.

Ryback, R. F., & Bassuk, E. L. (1986). Homeless battered women and their shelter network. *New Directions for Mental Health Services, 30,* 55–61.

Saunders, D. G. (1986). When battered women use violence: Husband-abuse or self-defense? *Violence and Victims, 1,* 47–60.

Saunders, D. G., & Size, P. B. (1986). Attitudes about woman abuse among police officers, victims, and victim advocates. *Journal of Interpersonal Violence, 1,* 25–42.

Schulman, M. (1979). *A survey of spousal violence against women in Kentucky.* Washington, DC: U.S. Department of Justice, Law Enforcement Assistance Administration.

Seligman, M. E. P. (1975). *Helplessness: On depression, development and death.* San Francisco: W. H. Freeman.

Shainess, N. (1977). Psychological aspects of wife-battering. In M. Roy (Ed.), *Battered women: A psychosocial study of domestic violence.* New York: Van Nostrand Reinhold.

Sherman, L. W., & Berk, R. A. (1984). *The Minneapolis domestic violence experiment.* Washington, DC: Police Foundation.

Singer, T. (1979, January). Coming out of cults. *Psychology Today, 72–82.*

Snyder, D. K., & Fruchtman, L. A. (1981). Differential patterns of wife abuse: A data-based typology. *Journal of Consulting and Clinical Psychology, 49,* 878–885.

Stark, E., Flitcraft, A. & Frazier, W. (1979). Medicine and patriarchal violence: The social construction of a private event. *International Journal of Health and Services, 9,* 461–493.

Staw, B. M. (1976). Knee deep in the big muddy: A study of escalating commitment to a chosen course of action. *Organizational Behavior and Human Performance, 16,* 27–42.

Steinmetz, S. K. (1977). *The cycle of violence: Assertive, aggressive and violent family interaction.* New York: Praeger.

Straus, M. A. (1977). Sociological perspective on the prevention and treatment of wife beating. In M. Roy (Ed.), *Battered women: A psychosocial study of domestic violence.* New York: Van Nostrand Reinhold.

Straus, M. A., Gelles, R. J., & Steinmetz, S. K. (1980). *Behind closed doors: Violence in the American family.* Garden City, NY: Anchor Books.

Strube, M. J. (1988). The decision to leave an abusive relationship: Empirical evidence and theoretical issues. *Psychological Bulletin, 104,* 236–250.

Suomi, S. J., & Harlow, H. (1977). Production and alleviation of depressive behavior in monkeys. In J. D. Masser & M. E. P. Seligman (Eds.), *Psychopathology: Experimental models* (pp. 131–173). New York: Academic Press.

Van Hasselt, V. B., Morrison, R. L., & Bellack, A. S. (1985). Alcohol use in wife abusers and their spouses. *Addictive Behaviors, 10,* 127–135.

Walker, L. E. (1978). Battered women and learned helplessness. *Victimology, 2,* 525–534.

Walker, L. E. (1979). *The battered woman.* New York: Harper & Row.

Walker, L. E. (1981). Battered women: Sex roles and clinical issues. *Professional Psychology, 12,* 81–91.

Walker, L. E. (1983). *Battered women in the correctional system.* Paper presented at the American Correctional Association Annual Congress, Chicago.

Walker, L. E. (1984). *The battered women syndrome.* New York: Springer.

Walker, L. E. (1987). Identifying the wife at risk of battering. *Medical Aspects of Human Sexuality, 21,* 107–114.

Walker, L. E. (1988). The battered woman syndrome. In G. T. Hotaling, D. Finkelhor, J. T. Kirkpatrick, & M. A. Straus (Eds.), *Family abuse and its consequences* (pp. 139–148). Beverly Hills, CA: Sage.

West, L. J. (1963). Brainwashing. In A. Deutsch (Ed.), *The encyclopedia of mental health* (Vol. 1). New York: Franklin Watts.

Whitehurst, R. N. (1984). Violence in husband-wife interaction. In S. R. Steinmetz & M. A. Straus (Eds.), *Violence in the family.* New York: Dodd Mead.

Wolfe, D. A., Jaffe, P., Wilson, S. K., & Zak, L. (1988). A multivariate investigation of children's adjustment to family violence. In G. T. Hotaling, D. Finkelhor, J. T. Kirkpatrick, & M. A. Straus (Eds.), *Family abuse and its consequences* (pp. 228–239). Beverly Hills, CA: Sage.

Worden, W. (1982). *Grief counseling and grief therapy.* New York: Springer.

Zimbardo, P. G., Ebbesen, E. B., & Maslach, C. (1977). *Influencing attitudes and changing behavior.* Reading, MA: Addison-Wesley.

18

Marital Rape

Heidi S. Resnick, Dean G. Kilpatrick, Catherine Walsh, and Lois J. Veronen

Description of the Problem

Recognition of marital rape as a crime with serious and long-term consequences for victims, as well as an important topic of research within the area of domestic violence, has been relatively recent. As Kilpatrick, Best, Saunders, and Veronen (1988) noted, marital rape victims suffer from both legal and attitudinal discrimination that may be based upon underestimates of the scope or prevalence of the problem, the assumption that marital rape is a less serious crime than stranger rape in terms of the levels of violence and perceived threat that may be experienced by the victim, and a lack of awareness of the potential mental health impact on the victim.

Kilpatrick *et al.* (1988) designed a study that allowed for a test of these assumptions in a representative community sample of 391 women. Of this sample, 91 (23.3%) had been victims of at least one completed rape (defined as completed vaginal, anal, or oral penetration occurring without the victim's consent, and involving force or threat of force) and 10 had experienced two rapes. Data on the prevalence of different types of rape indicated that marital rape occurred more frequently than stranger rape, occurring in 24 (23.8%) of the 101 rape cases,

Heidi S. Resnick and Dean G. Kilpatrick • Department of Psychiatry and Behavioral Sciences, Crime Victims Research and Treatment Center, Medical University of South Carolina, Charleston, South Carolina 29425. **Catherine Walsh** • Private Practice, Mt. Pleasant, South Carolina 29464. **Lois J. Veronen** • Human Development Center, Rock Hill, South Carolina 29730.

versus 21 (21.8%) in which the perpetrator was a stranger. Date rape occurred in 16.8% of the cases. Comparisons made between the three rape victim groups in terms of physical injury sustained and presence of perceived threat of loss of life or serious injury indicated that there were no significant differences on these measures designed to assess objective and subjective aspects of dangerousness. Physical injuries were sustained in 45.8, 46.7, and 38.1% of marital, date, and stranger rapes, respectively. Perceived life threat or fear of serious injury was reportedly present during 41.6, 53.3, and 38.1%, of the marital, date, and stranger rapes. Finally, the first data available from marital rape victims in a representative community sample, using a structured diagnostic interview schedule, indicated that there were no significant differences across the three victim groups in terms of current presence of major psychiatric disorders (including major depression, social phobia, obsessive-compulsive disorder, or sexual dysfunction). With the exception of obsessive-compulsive disorder, all of the diagnoses were currently present at significantly higher rates in the combined rape victim group than those observed in a comparison group of 96 women who had not experienced any crime. In addition, the fact that the rapes had occurred on average 17 years prior to the study indicated that the mental health impact may be of a long-term nature.

Kilpatrick *et al.* (1988) concluded that these data on the prevalence, level of dangerousness, and effects of marital rape directly contradict major assumptions that are the foundation of the lack of societal and legal recognition of the significance of the problem of marital rape.

This section of the chapter contains a review of the literature related to prevalence of marital rape, victim characteristics, and psychological and behavioral indices associated with marital rape.

Prevalence

As several authors have noted (Hanneke & Shields, 1985; Kilpatrick *et al.* 1988, Koss, 1983; Russell, 1982), there are inherent difficulties in accurate assessment of the prevalence rates of marital rape, or rape in general. These problems include underestimates of rates in legal statistics of rape in general, because of failure to use sufficiently sensitive screening questions that ask about specific behaviors rather than single global questions about occurrence of "rape." In addition, of course, marital rape has no legal status in many states. It has also been pointed out by these authors that asking nonlabelled screening questions is an important methodological component of assessment studies, because victims themselves may hold biases about what constitutes rape that reflect general societal attitudes. For example, Koss (1983) found that victims of rape (defined on a strictly behavioral level as intercourse without consent through threat of force or actual force) were less likely to acknowledge the acts of rape if they knew their perpetrator. None of the unacknowledged victims reported the incidents to the police. These factors may be even more important in the assessment of marital rape, where the ambiguous legal status and the nature of the relationship with the perpetrator may lead to perceptual and reporting biases. In support of this notion, Frieze (1980) found that a subset of women, of a group of 137 women in violent relationships, described threats associated with sexual behavior in their relationships that would objectively be defined as rape but were not subjectively labeled as such by these women.

An additional issue that has been raised in the marital rape literature is the question of whether rape occurs apart from general violence. Hanneke, Shields, and McCall (1986) have suggested that the strong associations observed in several studies may indicate that similar processes underly both types of behavior, that both may be expressions of violence or control, or, finally, that the low frequencies of rape observed apart from other violence may reflect perceptual biases. In regard to the latter possibility, Koss (1983), in reference to victims of rape in general, suggested that presence of higher levels of physical force may be a stereotype about rape that affects victims' conceptualizations. Shields and Hanneke (1987) also suggested that an additional factor in nonacknowledgment may be the dissonance of this recognition for the woman in terms of traditional views of the romantic and marital relationship. A related issue raised by Finkelhor and Yllo (1983) is that thus far only the presence of physical force or threat of physical force has been included to formulate the definitions of rape, while there may be other very real threats aside from physical force involved in marital rape. They suggested that other types of coercion may be important to assess within the context of a marital relationship, including threats of loss of social or financial support, and memories of the occurrence of physical force following resistance. Finally, as Hanneke and Shields (1985) noted, because of their relationship and continued contact with the perpetrator, victims of marital rape may have difficulty disclosing the rape for fear of retribution from the partner.

Hanneke et al. (1986) reviewed results of studies of the prevalence of marital rape in community samples as well as in more select samples identified for the presence of general marital violence. They concluded that the average frequency of occurrence observed in studies of less select samples was about 10% overall. For example, Russell (1982), in a survey of rape in the San Francisco area, found that 12% of 644 women who had been married or had cohabitated had experienced marital rape.

Finkelhor and Yllo (1983) reported the results of a study of 326 women in the Boston area that indicated a 10% rate of partner rape in the subgroup of women who had been in a marital or cohabiting relationship. As was observed in the Kilpatrick *et al.* (1988) study, both studies found marital rape to be more frequent than stranger rape.

Within more select samples identified because of the presence of domestic violence, Hanneke *et al.* noted that marital rape occurred in at least one-third to one-half of the samples across several studies. Frieze (1983) found that 34% of a group of 137 battered women were acknowledged rape victims, while only 6% of a matched control group that had also experienced marital violence (battered control) identified themselves as rape victims. In a comparison group of nonbattered women, the rate was 1%. For the combined control groups the rate was 3%, which Frieze suggested might be representative of a general population rate. Reports of having been pressured to have sex were much higher, however, occurring in 73, 60, and 37% of the battered, battered control, and nonbattered groups, respectively.

Shields and Hanneke (1983) observed a rate of 46% for occurrence of marital rape within a group of wives who had husbands who were violent within the family. In an attempt to obtain a larger number of women who had experienced marital rape without violence, Hanneke *et al.* (1986) used a questionnaire strategy to obtain a less select sample. However, as they acknowledged, the final sample was in fact fairly select, obtained mainly from a family planning agency. Of 307 final cases, 69% had not experienced any violence, 1% had experienced rape only, while 7.8% had experienced rape and battery, and 22.1% had experienced battery only. The authors suggested that the lower rates of sexual and nonsexual violence observed might reflect sampling differences.

In terms of the relationship between frequency of co-occurrence of marital rape and battery, Hanneke *et al.* (1986) summarized the findings across studies in subgroup terms. They noted that the observed occurrence of rape within nonbattering relationships ranged between about 1% and 4%, while the figures for rape occurring within battering relationships ranged between 30 and 59%. As previously noted, the authors raised various hypotheses about the observed relationships between the two types of violence, including the possibility of perceptual biases that may affect victim's perceptions of sexually abusive/nonabusive behavior. For example, they suggested that presence of other violence may be necessary to sensitize the women to identify behavior as forced sex or rape.

In summary, for the reasons discussed at the beginning of this section, these prevalence rates are likely to be underestimates of the actual occurrence of marital rape. These data indicate that marital rape occurs more frequently, or is reported at a higher rate, in cases where nonsexual battering is also present. However, the results of Frieze (1983) indicated that even within a nonbattered group, over a third of women acknowledged that they had experienced being pressured to have sex by their partners. The estimates obtained indicate that marital rape may be the most frequently occurring type of rape. In addition, with regard to the relatively lower frequencies of marital rape in the general population, Frieze (1980) suggested that a problem that may be experienced by from 3 to 6% of married women is a significant societal problem.

Victim Characteristics

Before beginning this section it should be noted that generalizability of findings in this area is necessarily limited to the extent that the samples studied are truly representative of marital rape victims. As noted in the previous section, there are several factors that may affect victims' perceptions and acknowledgment of marital rape, and several of the studies conducted thus far have employed fairly select sample populations. It should also be noted that problems inherent in rape research also apply to attempts in some of these studies to examine incidence rates of childhood sexual assault and nonspousal rape.

In a review of the marital rape literature, Hanneke and Shields (1985) observed that results related to demographic characteristics have been mixed. For example, an early study by Doron that was cited indicated no significant differences in demographic characteristics in marital rape victims, aside from a higher likelihood of being employed outside the home. Frieze (1980), however, in her sample of 137 women who had experienced nonsexual violence, and matched control groups, found that marital rape victims had married at a younger age, were *less* likely to be employed, were more likely to be dependent on welfare or child support, had more children, and showed lower levels of education than nonvictimized women. Frieze suggested that these factors might relate to a lower likelihood of having the option to leave the marital relationship.

In addition to demographic characteristics, the occurrence of previous childhood sexual victimization and other adult victimization in association with marital rape has been examined. In the Doron (1980) study, cited by Hanneke and Shields (1985), marital rape victims reported higher rates of childhood sexual assault and nonpartner sexual assaults than did nonvictims. Similarly, Frieze (1983) found that marital rape victims reported significantly higher rates of nonpartner adult rapes. However, the sequence of occurrence of these rapes in relation to marital rape was not reported. Thirty-two percent of the victims of repeated marital rape had also been raped as adults by someone other than the husband. The rapist was a stranger in 43% of the cases, and a close relative or father in 43% of the cases. In 16% of the cases the assailant was a neighbor. These women also reported a higher incidence of childhood sexual abuse, although the rate was not significantly different from that reported by control group women.

Shields and Hanneke (1984) attempted to examine various hypotheses about increased rates of childhood sexual abuse among marital rape victims. Subjects were women who had experienced rape and nonsexual violence ($N = 44$), women who had experienced only nonsexual violence ($N = 48$), and a nonvictimized group of 45 women. Although the highest rates of childhood sexual abuse were reported in the rape and battery group (50%), this was not significantly higher than the rate of 33% reported in the battery-only group. The rate observed in the third group was 22%.

Hypotheses examined included the possibility of greater tolerance of the use of sexual violence, sexual dysfunction prior to marriage, or the assumption of a "victim" identity as a consequence of labeling of childhood victimization. The results did not support the first two hypotheses. Victims of marital rape were not different from others on severity ratings of sexually violent behaviors, nor was there evidence of differences in sexual functioning prior to sexual victimization occurring in the marital relationship. Victims of marital rape were more likely to have disclosed the childhood sexual abuse to a parent. The authors suggested that possibly disclosure of childhood abuse may indirectly relate to later victimization, such that the response to the victimization by the parent and the environment may have an influence on development of normal sexual identity and/or self-identity. No attempt was made to actually test this latter hypothesis in this study.

The results of the studies examining previous and other adult sexual victimization in association with marital rape victimization are provocative. Results indicate an increased rate of adult sexual victimization by nonpartners associated with presence of marital rape. Results related to childhood victimization have not indicated consistently significant associations thus far. Future studies should incorporate assessment of previous or other nonsexual victimization, as well as careful assessment of psychological and behavioral reactions to early victimization, along with factors such as positive or negative family or societal reactions or legal consequences to disclosure of childhood sexual abuse, to gain further understanding of possible relationships between early trauma and risk for later victimization.

Psychological and Behavioral Indices Associated with Marital Rape

Hanneke and Shields (1985) suggested that since the study of reactions to marital rape is a relatively new and small area, it would be beneficial to examine findings related to the effects of spouse abuse and rape in general. Their summary of psychological and behavioral variables associated with battery indicated that decreased self-esteem, increased rates of suicide attempts, alcohol use, psychosomatic symptoms, social isolation, physically abusive behavior toward children, help seeking, divorce or separation, and initiation of other legal actions, as well as negative attitudes toward men, sex, marriage in general, and toward their spouses, specifically, had been associated with nonsexual violence in general.

Results obtained in the rape literature indicate that rape victims report increased levels of general psychological distress, including depression and anxiety, as well as problems associated with later sexual functioning. The results of Kilpatrick, Veronen, and Resick (1979), in a longitudinal study of psychological functioning of rape victims and nonvictimized women, indicated that at assessment periods immediately following assault, rape victims displayed significantly higher levels of distress on virtually all standardized measures included to evaluate psychological distress, compared with scores displayed by nonvictims. However, by 3 months postassault, indices of general distress had decreased in the rape victim group, but indices of specific and general fear and anxiety remained at significantly higher levels than those observed in the control group. These differences were maintained through the 6-month assessment period as well.

More recently, interest in this area has focused on the presence of posttraumatic stress disorder (PTSD) following rape trauma. Although their early work was conducted prior to the introduction of the DSM-III (American Psychiatric Association, 1980) criteria for PTSD, Kilpatrick, Veronen, and Best (1985) noted that the most frequently observed symptoms in rape victims, including fear and anxiety, intrusive cognitions, avoidance behavior, and sleep disturbance, are consistent with the diagnostic criteria. In addition, Kilpatrick, Saunders, Amick-McMullan, Best, Veronen, and Resnick (1989) found that PTSD was associated with the crime of rape at a higher rate than that observed for other crimes. In that study, 57.1% of victims of completed rape met criteria for PTSD.

Only one study to date (Kilpatrick et al., 1988) assessed current frequency of major psychiatric disorders in a group of rape victims that included a marital rape subgroup. Rates of disorders were not reported separately for the marital rape subgroup. However, as previously noted, the marital rape subgroup did not significantly differ from the subgroups of date and stranger rape victims on any of the disorders assessed, while the rape victim group displayed significantly higher rates of all disorders, except obsessive-compulsive disorder, than women who were not crime victims. Specifically, the current rates of sexual dysfunction, obsessive-compulsive disorder, social phobia, and major depressive episode were 30.2%, 7.2%, 14.0%, and 11.6%, respectively, within the rape victim group. Rape victims were 11 times more likely to be clinically depressed, 6 times more likely to display criteria for social phobia, and 2.5 times more likely to currently meet criteria for sexual dysfunction than were nonvictims.

Frieze (1983) examined specific emotional and behavioral factors associated with marital rape in her group of 137 women who had experienced marital violence, and in control groups of battered and nonbattered women. To examine associated emotional and behavioral indices (acknowledging the problem of order of occurrence, which is not controlled for in the methodology of the study), she conducted a regression analysis using marital rape as the predicted variable, and the other indices as predictors.

Results indicated that trying to leave the husband, filing legal charges, having lesbian affairs, having a husband who would not seek emotional or psychological treatment, and wanting to leave the husband were significantly associated with marital rape, in that order. A second regression analysis, including marital rape as a predictor variable, and leaving the husband as the predicted variable, was conducted. Results indicated that marital rape was not significantly associated with leaving the husband, but presence of the wife's finding sex unpleasant because of force or pressure was significantly related, and followed presence of violence, which was the most significant variable, in order of significance. Frieze concluded that behavioral reactions were more common than emotional reactions in association with marital rape. She raised the issue that studies of effects associated with marital rape need also to examine and attempt to control for the effects of violence in general.

Shields and Hanneke (1983) attempted to examine factors that might be uniquely associated with marital rape after controlling for levels of violence in their sample of women, which included a group that had experienced rape and battery and a group that had experienced battery only. Initial analyses indicated that women who had experienced rape had been exposed to higher levels of violence, and that violence was significantly associated with several psychological and behavioral indices. Results of correlational analyses, controlling for level of nonsexual violence, indicated that presence of marital rape was significantly associated with lower self-esteem, negative attitudes toward men, use of alcohol, having husband arrested, withholding sex, and wanting sex less frequently.

Within the subgroup that had experienced marital rape, correlational analyses were conducted between frequency of marital rape and other variables, controlling for level of violence. These analyses indicated significant relationships between frequency of marital rape and lower self-esteem, negative attitude toward own marriage, psychosomatic reactions, suicide attempts, and not wanting sex. The authors suggested that both marital rape and violence appeared to be possibly jointly related to depression and filing for divorce.

Results of analyses of variance that included a third nonbattered group indicated that the group that had experienced rape and battery had significantly lower ratings of self-esteem than the battered and nonbattered controls, which were not significantly different on this measure; use of retaliatory violence and alcohol was significantly more frequent in both battery groups. The authors noted that without a separate rape-only (without battery) group, the effects of marital rape alone remain unclear, since there may be interactive effects of rape and battery.

A final study by Shields and Hanneke (1987) was an attempt to test the hypothesis that marital rape victims experience less serious psychological reactions than stranger rape victims. The groups consisted of 44 women who had experienced rape and battery, 48 who had experienced battery only, and 45 nonvictimized women. In this study, standardized measures of general psychological distress, anxiety, and questions about sexual functioning that had previously been used with general rape samples were administered. Scores on these measures were compared across these three groups and were also compared with scores obtained with general rape victims from previously published reports in the rape literature.

The authors noted that results of any differences between their sample and the previously conducted studies need to be interpreted cautiously, because there were significant demographic differences between the samples that could relate to other findings. Similarly, they acknowledged that in the cases of rape and battery, there may be an ongoing problematic marital relationship that may include chronic victimization rather than acute victimization, which might account for differences on symptom measures across groups.

In general, the results indicated that marital rape victims reported significantly higher levels of distress than stranger rape victims on several indices, including some measures of anxiety, paranoid ideation, psychoticism, and impairment in sexual functioning. In addition, the battery-only group also reported high levels of distress on several measures, in some cases as high as or greater than those observed in the stranger rape samples. The authors concluded that contrary to some hypotheses, occurrence of marital rape and battery is associated with serious mental health effects, and that battery alone is also associated with severe effects. They suggested that these results highlight the need to also be aware of possible separate and interactive effects of battery in association with marital rape.

Finally, the results of Kilpatrick *et al.* (1989), although not specific to the question of marital rape, are relevant to the question of whether rape is associated with psychological distress, apart from other components of violence. Their study of factors associated with presence of PTSD in a group of 294 victims of different types of crime indicated that victims whose crimes included completed rape, perceived life threat, and physical injury were 8.5 times more likely to meet criteria for PTSD than other crime victims. In addition, only the crime of rape was significantly associated with PTSD, even after controlling for the effects of life threat and injury. The authors concluded that rape may involve separate elements that are important in the development of PTSD.

In summary, the area of assessment of psychological distress and behavioral reactions associated with marital rape is very limited. Few studies have been conducted to date that have used standardized assessment instruments. The results of the studies reviewed here indicate that marital rape is associated with low self-esteem, elevated levels of psychological distress on standardized psychological assessment measures, and increased rates of major psychiatric disorder. The results also indicate that marital rape is associated with presence of nonsexual violence, and that both marital rape and nonsexual violence may have separate as well as interactive effects. Perhaps one useful paradigm for examining these effects would be to compare groups of subjects who have experienced rape only, battery only, and rape plus battery, controlling for relationship with assailant and chronicity of exposure (i.e., serial versus single-incident assaults).

Case Descriptions

Two case descriptions are presented here to illustrate the range of characteristics that may be associated with marital rape. In the first case, the woman presented for treatment but did not maintain contact following an initial decrease in symptoms of acute distress. The first case also illustrates issues related to the current legal status of marital rape. The second case history illustrates the use of a behavioral treatment approach designed to facilitate adaptive coping with stress and problems associated with marital rape trauma.

Case 1

L.C., a 29-year-old white female who worked part time, initially presented for evaluation and treatment following an assault that had occurred approximately a month earlier. During the assault, the perpetrator physically pinned her down and forcibly inserted a bottle into her vagina. The assault took place at 3:30 a.m., while her children were asleep in the next room. During the incident, she feared that she might be killed or seriously injured. In response to the attack, L.C. kicked her assailant, screamed, verbally argued, and finally was able to run from him and terminate the assault.

At initial evaluation, L.C. met criteria for posttraumatic stress disorder (PTSD). Symptoms included recurrent thoughts of the assault, psychological distress to reminders, efforts to avoid related thoughts or feelings, feelings of detachment from others, numbing of affect, sleep disturbance, and startle response. Nightmares had occurred initially following the assault but had decreased in frequency by the time of the evaluation. The results of assessment with standardized psychological measures indicated a high level of distress on all indices of anxiety, depression, and intrusion and avoidance symptoms of PTSD.

L.C. reported a victimization history that included six years of repeated physical and sexual assaults by the same assailant. In the past she had been beaten, threatened with a gun, and at times tied to the bed for 24-hour periods and forced to have sexual intercourse. Although L.C. had called the police in the past, she had never formally brought charges against her assailant until the most recent incident. The only charge that was allowed in this case was assault and battery. When asked for her appraisal of the incident, L.C. indicated that the incident was not rape or attempted rape but was a sexual crime.

From a legal standpoint in the southern state where this incident occurred, the victim's appraisal was partially incorrect. Despite the fact that the incident consisted of forced vaginal penetration, in this and several other states it is not considered to be rape or attempted rape *nor* is it classified as a sexual crime, because the assailant was the victim's husband, and they were living together at the time of the assault.

Case 2: Illustration of a Behavioral Treatment Approach

The case study utilized stress inoculation training (SIT; Veronen & Kilpatrick, 1983), a behavioral treatment designed to facilitate adaptive coping with fear and other symptoms of distress following rape trauma. This is accomplished primarily through instruction in active coping techniques for modification of responses to rape- and non-rape-related stressors that may occur in physiological, cognitive, and behavioral response channels. In addition to SIT, cognitive restructuring, tailored after the model proposed by Janoff-Bulman (1985), was included in the treatment of PTSD symptoms in a rape victim, approximately 4 months postassault. Treatment consisted of weekly individual and group sessions that followed the SIT framework described in further detail in the treatment options section of the chapter. Standardized assessment measures were used pre- and posttreatment to assess levels of psychological distress.

J.L. was a 26-year-old single white female who was referred for assessment and treatment by the local rape crisis center. She had been raped by her former live-in boyfriend. During the same week that the rape occurred, she was physically assaulted by her boyfriend on a second occasion. The assaults had occurred 4 months prior to assessment. The assaults occurred shortly after J.L. had asked her boyfriend to move out. During the assaults, in which J.L.'s boyfriend broke into her apartment, J.L. reported that she feared that she might be killed or seriously injured. She reported that she sustained moderate injury. During the rape, her assailant forced her into the bedroom, tore her clothes off, bloodied her nose by hitting her in the face several times, and raped her repeatedly. On the second occasion, her boyfriend repeatedly threw J.L. down onto a wood floor and forcibly robbed her of $40. The second assault was terminated when J.L. was able to phone the police, and her boyfriend fled. Both assaults were reported to the police. The assailant was arrested, but he left the state after posting bond, and remained at large throughout the course of treatment.

J.L. reported no prior history of psychological treatment. She did have a history of previous physical victimization by another boyfriend, which she had never disclosed. J.L. had an associate arts degree from college and had worked as a waitress since high school. At assessment she had a waitressing job, as well as a supervisory job in food services. J.L. had recently moved here from another state and had no family in this area. She had begun to develop a network of friends. J.L. had a history of ulcers, which she reported were exacerbated following the assaults.

Assessment and Treatment

Assessment included symptom data gathered at initial interview, and weekly throughout treatment, as well as administration of standardized psychological assessment measures, including the Impact of Events Scale (IES; Horowitz, Wilner, & Alvarez, 1973), a 15-item scale designed to assess current intrusion and avoidance components of PTSD following trauma, and the Veronen-Kilpatrick Modified Fear Survey (MFS, Veronen & Kilpatrick, 1980), a 120-item inventory of potentially fear-related items and situations. Rated on a 5-point scale, the MFS yields scores on the following subscales: (1) animal fears, (2) classical fears, (3) social interpersonal fears, (4) tissue damage fears, (5) miscellaneous fears, (6) failure/loss of self-esteem, and (7) rape fears. Also used was the Derogatis Symptom Checklist 90-R (Derogatis, 1977), a 90-item self-report inventory designed to assess current psychological distress, in which items are rated on a 5-point scale ranging from no discomfort to extreme discomfort related to each problem during the past week. In addition, at the beginning of weekly group sessions, J.L. assigned subjective units of discomfort ratings (SUDS) for the past week to each of three target fears.

At initial interview, J.L. met criteria for PTSD, including reexperiencing, avoidance, and increased arousal symptoms. Reexperiencing symptoms included frequent nightmares and recurrent intrusive thoughts of the assaults several times per day. Symptoms of avoidance included reports of reduced range of emotions since the assault, feeling distant or cut off from others, and decreased interest in activities that were previously considered enjoyable. Symptoms of increased arousal included sleep disturbance with initial, middle, and terminal insomnia, and physical symptoms of anxiety, including increased heart rate in association with assault-related cues (e.g., being in the apartment alone, and men who resembled her ex-boyfriend). J.L.'s self-selected target fears were darkness, being at home alone at night, and sleep/nightmares.

Treatment following the SIT model (and the additional cognitive restructuring component) was conducted both individually and in a group format over the course of 16 weeks. The total number of treatment sessions was 26, with 12 conducted in group format. The basic group format consisted of 1½ sessions covering education and treatment overview, 1½ sessions devoted to specific physiological relaxation techniques, 4 sessions focused mainly on cognitive techniques, and 4 sessions focused on learning and practice of behavioral techniques. Of the three other group members, two had been victims of stranger rape and one had been the victim of acquaintance rape. Possible benefits of the group modality include the opportunity to hear other victims' experiences, thereby normalizing reactions to the rape, and provision of support and modeling throughout the skills acquisition phase. Individual therapy was used to address unique aspects of the clients' experience in greater depth, using the same therapeutic model.

A comparison of IES intrusion, avoidance, and total mean scores before and after treatment is displayed in Figure 1. The most striking change from pretreatment to posttreatment was obtained in mean intrusion scale scores, while mean avoidance score did not appear to change greatly.

Mean MFS subscale scores pretreatment and posttreatment are displayed in Figure 2. It can be observed that mean scores on the rape subscale showed the greatest decrease from pretreatment to posttreatment levels. J.L. also displayed the highest elevations on this subscale both before and after treatment.

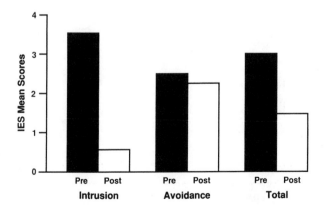

Figure 1. IES mean scores pre- and posttreatment.

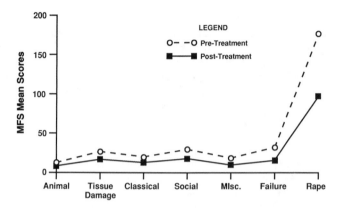

Figure 2. MFS mean scores pre- and posttreatment.

SCL-90-R subscale *T* scores from pretreatment and posttreatment assessments are displayed in Figure 3. In general, scores on all subscales were decreased at posttreatment assessment. At pretreatment assessment all but the hostility subscale score were above a *T* score of 70, the cutoff for clinical significance. At posttreatment, all subscale scores were below this level. Finally, SUDS ratings (scale of 0 to 100) for the three target fears across weeks of group treatment are displayed in Figure 4.

These results indicate that subjective distress decreased following the initial treatment sessions that focused primarily on education and information about reactions to rape, in addition to relaxation training in the group setting. After that point, subjective distress related to darkness and being home alone at night remained stable, while fear of sleep/dreams fluctuated but did not return to initial levels.

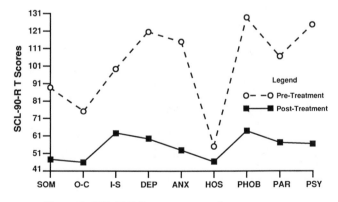

Figure 3. SCL-90-R *T* scores pre- and posttreatment.

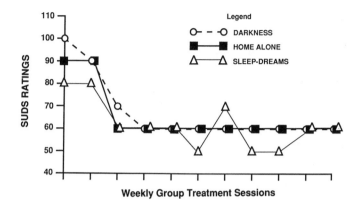

Figure 4. SUDS ratings of target fears over the course of treatment.

Discussion

Decreases in psychological distress were observed as indicated by measures of intrusive and avoidance components of PTSD, specific fears, and general psychological distress following treatment with SIT and cognitive restructuring. No controlled comparison was conducted, and it is not possible in this case to assess possible differences in effectiveness of group or individual treatment modalities.

Medical Issues

As noted in the literature review, marital rape has been observed to occur at a high rate in subgroups of women who experience nonsexual battery. Further, rape in marriage has been found to be positively associated with level of nonsexual violence (Frieze, 1983; Shields & Hanneke, 1983). Finally, in addition to psychological sequelae, increased rates of psychosomatic symptoms have been observed in victims of marital rape (Shields & Hanneke, 1983). Therefore, it may be the case that marital rape victims may seek medical treatment for physical injury or for other physical symptoms.

Results of a study by Hilberman and Munson (1978) indicated that fully half of all female referrals for psychiatric evaluation from a medical clinic over a 1-year period had histories of victimization, including battery and marital rape. In all but four cases, the referring clinic staff were unaware of the victimization history. Hilberman and Munson noted that physical symptoms in this group of women included somatic complaints, headaches, back and pelvic pain, and gastrointestinal problems. Reasons for psychiatric referral included long-term use of pain killers or tranquilizers and persistence of problems despite treatment. It was also observed that in some cases stress exacerbated preexisting medical conditions. In addition, some women reported histories of abortions and premature births following physical abuse. The authors noted that many of the women who were referred had past psychiatric as well as past medical histories, but that their victimization histories had not been previously assessed during those prior contacts.

These findings highlight the importance of thorough assessment of victimization history for female clients by medical personnel as well as by mental health professionals.

Legal Issues

Currently, marital exclusion laws, which exempt the husband from prosecution in cases in which the partners are living together at the time of the assault, exist in 22 states. In the sate of Alabama, the exclusion also extends to situations in which the marital partners are living apart (Gelles & Straus, 1988). For a thorough review of legal issues related to the marital rape exemption, including the history of the legal definition of rape, as well as legal arguments in favor of or against retention of the exclusion law, the reader is referred to Barshis (1983). She noted that one of the most prominent current arguments in favor of retention of the exemption is the notion that when a woman marries she engages in a contractual agreement that includes perpetual sexual availability and consent. In general, Barshis suggests that these laws reflect societal attitudes. As she points out at the beginning of her review, actions are classified as crimes under the law "on the basis of their harm to society and to the individual" (p. 383). As Kilpatrick *et al.* (1988) suggest, one of the important implications of their results is the need to promote public education on this issue and to provide information as a basis for legal policy making.

Social and Family Issues

This section focuses on the literature related to partner and relationship characteristics that provide descriptive information about the context in which marital rape may occur.

Partner and Relationship Characteristics

The major focus of research within the marital rape area has been the reaction of the victim. No study, to date, has utilized a methodology of partner/perpetrator as respondent in the research. What is known about the partner as the perpetrator of marital rape has been acquired from studies of the marital rape victim and from studies of rapists.

Bowker (1983) conducted in-depth interviews with 146 women who were long-term victims of marital violence. Twenty-three percent of her sample had experienced marital rape. The violence in the other 113 relationships did not include marital rape. One-half of those married at the time of the violence were no longer married. Focusing on the partner's characteristics and the relationship's characteristics, data analyses revealed the following: (1) No significant differences existed between demographic characteristics of the raped wives and nonraped wives; (2) participation in joint recreational activities was significantly less frequent in marriages where rape occurred than in other violent marriages, and raped wives found what participation occurred to be less satisfying; (3) significantly lower marital satisfaction was reported by raped wives for time spent together, sexual relations, affection, quality of spousal communication, and overall marital satisfaction; (4) significantly greater disagreements and marital violence was reported among raped wives; (5) perpetrators of marital rape placed lower value on children and on spousal understanding than other batterers; (6) raping husbands were more likely to have witnessed assaults between their parents; (7) raped wives were less likely than the other battered women to be living with partners at the time of the interview.

This study appears to have no explicit or implicit theoretical base. All subjects were volunteers, responding to media notices. No standardized assessment measures were utilized and no comparison group was used. The author acknowledged the limitations of the victim-only perspective in studying the abusing partner and the relationship. However, the strength of this study is its attention to relationship factors (e.g., social embeddedness, marital satisfaction, and value dissimilarity, which have not previously received attention in the marital rape literature).

Frieze (1980) investigated the causes and consequences of marital rape. A sample of 137 women who reported physical violence were interviewed about the violence and about marital rape. A matched control group was also interviewed utilizing the same schedule. As previously noted, 48 of these women had experienced marital violence and formed a separate "battered control" group. Frieze examined the characteristics of men who rape their wives versus those that do not, given the wives' reports of husband characteristics. She found that "raping" men earned less, spent more time away from home, had fewer close friends, drank more, and disagreed with their wives about drinking. Family of origin differences included having had more sisters, parents who were less affectionate and children who were less affectionate to one another, and parents who were violent to one another. Couple characteristics included less time spent together, less enjoyment of the time spent together, and less expression of affection. In regard to relationship dominance, men who raped were more likely to decide where the couple would go when they went out together, the couple was more likely to visit his friends than hers, and the husbands went out alone more frequently.

In terms of ways of influencing their wives, "raping" men were more likely to try to get their way by use of emotional withdrawal, restricting wives' freedom, threatening to leave them, and using physical force against their wives and children. In regard to arguments, "raping" men were more likely to get angry and fight verbally or physically, and were more likely to get their way. Regarding the history of violence in the relationship, "raping" husbands started violence earlier in the relationship, and the violence was more severe and more frequent than the violence of men who did not rape their wives. Husbands who raped were more likely to be drinking when violent and to beat their wives when they were pregnant. While conducting subsequent analyses of men who rape, particularly focusing on their use of violence toward their wives, a correlation of .34 was found between the husband's worst violence and the frequency of marital rape. Furthermore, men who raped were significantly more likely to want to have sex after being violent, although the frequencies were low. Sexual abuse most often occurred as a result of physical violence.

Analyses were conducted to determine if there were differences in "battering" men versus those who were "battering" and "raping" men. "Raping" men were reported as having more children, more dominant in the marital relationship, and more likely to have greater drinking problems. "Raping" husbands were more violent generally, and experienced fights outside the home as well. Violence included sexual abuse (often associated with injuries resulting from forced anal intercourse) as well as rape and violence toward their wives when they were pregnant. They were also more often drunk when violent.

This investigation has several strengths, including use of comparison groups that strengthen the interpretations and the use of appropriate data analyses.

The research into the marital rape perpetrator from the standpoint of rape research has serious sampling problems. Rape research has mainly been done with incarcerated rapists or court-referred rapists. Since marital rape has not been a punishable offense, only rapists who are convicted of nonmarital rapes are incarcerated. A few of these rapists have also reported having raped their wives. Groth (1979) reported four case histories of marital rape. He discussed five different situations of marital rape wherein sex was equated with power, sex was equated with love and affection, sex was equated with virility, sex was equated with debasement, and sex was seen as a panacea. These marital rape descriptions are highly simplistic and are based upon interpretations of an observer/researcher guided by psychodynamic theory. There were no specific descriptions of samples, standard observations, or treatment of data.

In summary, the partner as perpetrator is a frightening entity who may be violent both physically and sexually. Generally, little research has been done on either perpetrator or relationship characteristics. This area could benefit from research that includes standardized psychological and behavioral assessment measures, aimed at assessment at the different levels of the victim, partner, and relationship as units of analysis.

With regard to treatment issues, it has been noted that because of the nature of the relationship between victim and perpetrator, marital rape contains a number of components not present in stranger rape (including betrayal of intimacy and trust, and the victim's continued contact with her assailant) that warrant special attention. With regard to the relationship with the assaultive partner, Kilpatrick et al. (1988) stressed the importance of assessing the victim's attitudes rather than ignoring or making assumptions about the relationship in a judgmental way. In addition, Kilpatrick (1983) urged that therapists take into consideration the considerable impact that rape may have on the significant others in the victim's life, including children and parents. Assessment of family functioning and family therapy may be warranted in addition to individual treatment of the marital rape victim. Lystad (1982) recommended the assessment of the physical, psychological, social, and legal needs of family members subsequent to disclosure of sexual abuse within the family.

Assessment of Psychopathology

Major issues in assessment include the importance of conducting a thorough victimization history as well as use of standardized assessment instruments to assess psychological distress and functioning. Many rape victims may not seek psychological treatment immediately after their assault (Koss, 1983), and when they do, the focus may be on presenting symptoms, such as anxiety or depression, rather than the rape incident per se. In addition to possible failure to associate an assault with later symptoms, many victims may not label or acknowledge the incident as rape. Hanneke and Shields (1985) suggested that women who experience both marital rape and battering may define the rape as another instance of violence, and they may not specifically report the occurrence of rape. Also, these women may be more likely to focus on nonsexual violence or general marital problems in treatment, rather than marital rape specifically.

To address these issues, Kilpatrick (1983) recommended that thorough assault histories of female clients be done routinely by mental health providers. In addition, use of specific, operational language in questions about the occurrence of concrete behaviors, versus labels such as "rape," "sexual abuse," or "battery," is recommended to avoid biases about what actually constitutes rape (Kilpatrick, 1983, Weingourt, 1985). Kilpatrick also recommended obtaining a careful assessment of chronological sequencing of victimization incidents and psychological distress to formulate hypotheses about the association between specific traumatic events and symptoms in the individual's history. This may be particularly important with marital rape victims in cases in which the abuse has been chronic and has included both sexual and nonsexual violence, and/or cases in which previous or extramarital sexual assaults or other types of victimization have also occurred.

Thorough interviewing to assess the impact of the rape is also necessary. Douglas (1982) in light of her work with victims of domestic violence, recommended that a mental status examination be done if the victim was recently assaulted by her husband, with attention paid to risk of suicide, homicidal intent toward the assailant, and assessment of capacity to care for herself and her children. In addition, we recommend use of standardized instruments to assess psychological functioning, such as those in the Shields and Hanneke (1987) study. Included are several standardized measures of general psychological distress as well as specific fears that have previously been used with rape victim samples. Finally, structured diagnostic interviews are available that allow for comprehensive clinical assessment across diagnostic categories.

Treatment Options

The literature on marital rape has focused mainly on assessment issues rather than on specific techniques to be used in treatment, and there are no controlled outcome studies of effectiveness of different treatment approaches with this particular population. On the basis of the marital rape literature reviewed in this chapter, it is evident that a first step necessary for conceptualization of treatment is a thorough description of problems or reactions to marital rape. Because research in this area is still at the stage of problem description, the relevant literature on treatment is limited.

This section contains a summary of suggestions for treatment based primarily on the literature related to spouse abuse and stranger rape. This will be followed by a brief summary of behavioral treatment approaches used with rape victims and posttraumatic stress disorder in general, and an overview of stress inoculation training (SIT). SIT is a behavioral approach developed by Veronen and Kilpatrick (1983) that employs instruction in anxiety management techniques for the treatment of rape-related fear and anxiety. Finally, the use of SIT in a combined group and individual therapy format with a marital rape victim will be described.

As previously noted, Hanneke and Shields (1985) suggested that reactions to marital rape may be similar to reactions to battering and stranger rape. Thus, cognitive therapy approaches and the use of support groups derived from work with battered women, as well as systematic desensitization, behavioral treatments based on instruction in skills for coping with anxiety, and treatment of sexual dysfunction that have been used for reactions following stranger rape, may be useful tools in dealing with victims of marital rape. However, a major difference between marital rape and stranger rape victims is the chronicity of exposure to stress, which indicates that crisis intervention may be helpful with marital rape victims, but would probably not be sufficient.

Kilpatrick (1983) noted treatment issues relevant to therapist interactions with rape victims in general that may also apply to marital rape victims. These include the need for the therapist to guard against displaying a judgmental attitude toward the victim, owing to possible personal biases, or allowing inconsistent or disorganized behavior on the part of the victim to cause frustration and anger. Similarly, in terms of possible attitudinal biases that may effect the therapeutic interaction, Hanneke and Shields (1985) suggested that the ambiguous legal and social atmosphere in which marital rape victims are considered may cause some therapists to doubt the validity of the victims' claims and problems. Also contributing to this is a tendency in our society to blame the victim (Weingourt, 1985). It is clearly important that therapists be knowledgeable about the prevalence of marital rape and the serious impact it can have on victims.

Finally, treatment suggestions made by Douglas (1982), based on her work with domestic violence victims, argue for the importance of empowering the victim and modeling a more balanced relationship with the client (including facilitation of autonomous decision making and acquisition of more adaptive responses to stress).

Behavioral Approaches to Treatment of Rape and Other Posttrauma Reactions

As previously underscored, marital rape differs from stranger rape in several ways, especially the chronicity of exposure to the stressor, the ongoing nature of the relationship with the perpetrator, and the woman's individual interpretation of the event. However, some similarities in psychological symptomology have been reported for victims of marital and nonmarital rape. These include the observations of similar levels and patterns of distress on standardized assessment instruments and similar rates of specific psychiatric diagnoses across the two victim groups. This section includes a brief discussion of treatment approaches that have been used in rape victim reactions, along with the suggestions outlined above to address factors unique to marital rape trauma. As Fairbank and Brown (1987), and Foy, Resnick, Carroll, and Osato (1990) noted, major behavioral treatment approaches that have been used with posttrauma reactions have included mainly exposure-based techniques. Included are flooding or skills training approaches that focus more heavily on instruction in adaptive coping techniques. These are to be used in coping both with current trauma-related stress reactions, and with future stressful situations.

The exposure-based technique of flooding involves either imaginal or in vivo exposure to trauma-related stimuli or cues, with the goal of extinction of the physiological anxiety response and associated maladaptive cognitive and behavioral responses.

Skills approaches which may include components such as cognitive restructuring, assertion training, and relaxation training, are also aimed at facilitating new and adaptive responses to trauma-related stimuli, by teaching the client active skills to be used in the fact of anxiety-related cues, rather than maladaptive coping responses such as avoidance. The process of application of these new skills to trauma-related stimuli also includes the element of exposure.

In a review of the literature on treatment effectiveness, Foy *et al.* (1990) noted that, in general, no single treatment appeared to be clearly most effective; however, most approaches did include some component of exposure to trauma-related cues.

A third major treatment approach suggested by Foy *et al.* (in press) primarily focuses on global changes in attitudes or cognitions that may relate to the experience of a traumatic event. For example, Janoff-Bulman (1985) argues that basic life assumptions may be altered following trauma, including views about invulnerability to harm, life fairness, and a positive view of self. Janoff-Bulman theorized that trauma victims may reject these assumptions in the face of experiences that are radically inconsistent with these views, and that new extreme assumptions that may be adopted as a result (e.g., self-blame, or sense of global unfairness) may be maladaptive. Treatment may then involve identification of the relationship between the effects trauma and the client's attitudinal views, with the goal of reformulating assumptions that are both more valid and more functional. This is a theoretical model that remains to be tested as an effective treatment approach. Foy *et al.* (1990) reported the use of a cognitive restructuring treatment based on this model with a Vietnam veteran, following initial treatment with flooding.

Stress Inoculation Training

Stress inoculation training (SIT) is a comprehensive coping skills training approach, developed at the Medical University of South Carolina, to treat anxiety-related symptoms following rape (Veronen & Kilpatrick, 1983). The treatment, which was patterned after Meichenbaum's stress inoculation procedures, includes instruction in coping skills for management of anxiety in physiological, cognitive, and behavioral response channels. It is to be applied to rape-related fears as well as to anxiety related to other stressful situations. SIT includes an initial educational phase in which clients are provided with information about typical reactions to rape, as well as a learning theory formulation of the development of rape-related fears that may be expressed in the three response channels. Clients actively participate in the process of identifying fear-eliciting cues related to the rape (target fears), as well as identification of their own unique responses experienced in each of the three channels. The rationals for application of various component skills is outlined, and treatment is presented as an active strategy for the management of anxiety in a variety of situations. This phase of treatment may serve to normalize reactions and to promote a sense of control by assisting clients to discriminate particular situations that are more or less anxiety producing.

In the next phase of treatment, a variety of strategies are taught to the client for each of the three channels in which anxiety is expressed. Clients are encouraged to select those techniques that they find most useful.

Physiological Channels. For application in the physiological channel, tension relaxation, muscle relaxation, and controlled breathing techniques are taught. Clients are instructed to practice relaxation techniques at home and to apply them with both rape-related (target) and nontarget fear stimuli. For example, a target fear might be staying home alone at night, while a nontarget fear might be a job interview.

Cognitive Channel. The techniques of thought stopping and guided self-dialogue are taught to address the cognitive expressions of anxiety. Self-dialogue is a cognitive restructuring technique that includes identification of irrational or dysfunctional cognitions and adoption and use of more adaptive cognitions to cope with a stressor.

Behavioral Channel. Finally, role-playing, covert modeling, imaginal progression through anxiety-producing situations, and assertion techniques are applied to decrease behavioral avoidance.

Veronen and Kilpatrick (1983) reported improvement on measures of anxiety and mood in a small group of rape victims following SIT treatment. Kilpatrick and Amick (1985) also reported positive results in a single case study, in which cognitive, physiological, and behavioral assessment measures were used pre- and posttreatment. Resick, Jordan, Girelli, Huter, and Marhoefer-Dvorak (1987) found that SIT was associated with significantly greater reduction in anxiety-related symptoms, compared with a waiting list control group, but results indicated that there were no significant differences between SIT and assertion training or supportive/educational psychotherapy group treatments. Finally, Foa, Olasov-Rothbaum, and Steketee (in press) reported preliminary results of a controlled comparison study of SIT and exposure treatments with rape victims, indicating that SIT was associated with symptom improvement on measures of PTSD, anxiety, and depression.

Summary and Conclusions

The two cases included in this chapter are examples of the variety of characteristics that may be observed in marital rape. In one case, the woman was married and had children, and the rape occurred in the context of an ongoing marital relationship. In the second case, the rape occurred following the breakup of a live-in relationship. Although both cases consisted of forced vaginal penetration, only in the second case was the crime subjectively defined as rape by the victim. In both cases, nonsexual violence was present in the relationship, and the women were not interested in maintaining the relationship with their partners following the rapes. Finally, both of these women feared that they might be killed or injured during the assault, and both women met criteria for posttraumatic stress disorder following the assault.

In other cases, threatening or pressuring may be less overtly violent, victims may not acknowledge or identify the incident as rape, and the victims may not be at a decision point with regard to their relationships. These factors highlight the need for clinicians and researchers to carefully assess both objective and subjective factors involved in individual cases, to assess treatment needs of individual clients, as well as to obtain accurate prevalence rates of marital rape. As Kilpatrick *et al.* (1988) noted, on the basis of the results of their study of marital rape in a community sample, the data directly contradict common assumptions about marital rape. The literature on marital rape indicates that this may be the most frequently occurring type of rape, that it is often associated with nonsexual violence, and that it is subjectively perceived by victims as dangerous or threatening.

Results related to effects of marital rape indicate that marital rape is associated with increased levels of psychological distress, rates of major psychiatric disorder, and violence comparable to those observed in stranger rape victims.

At this time, the findings appear to be limited primarily to cases in which marital rape is associated with nonsexual battery. Thus, an important component of research in this area is the assessment of characteristics associated with nonsexual violence as well as marital rape to clarify possible unique and interactive effects.

It appears that SIT, a learning theory-based treatment approach that includes education about the client's modes of responding and instruction in coping techniques, may be useful in the amelioration of psychological reactions associated with marital rape.

References

American Psychiatric Association. (1980). *Diagnostic and statistical manual of mental disorders* (3rd ed.). Washington, DC: Author.

Barshis, V. R. G. (1983). The question of marital rape. *Women's Studies International Forum, 6,* 383–393.

Bowker, L. H. (1983). Marital rape: A distinct syndrome? *Social Casework,* 347–352.

Derogatis, L. R. (1977). *SCL-90: Administration, scoring and procedure manual I for the R (revised) version.* Baltimore: Johns Hopkins University School of Medicine.

Doron, J. (1980, August). *Conflict and violence in relationships: Focus on marital rape.* Paper presented at the American Sociological Association Annual Meeting, New York City.

Douglas, M. A. (1982). *Behavioral assessment with battered women.* Paper presented at the 90th annual convention of the American Psychological Association, Washington, DC.

Fairbank, J. A., & Brown, T. A. (1987). Current behavioral approaches to the treatment of posttraumatic stress disorders. *The Behavior Therapist, 3,* 57–64.

Finkelhor, D., & Yllo, K. (1983). Rape in marriage. A sociological view. In D. Finkelhor, R. J. Gelles, G. T. Hotaling, & M. A. Straus (Eds.), *The dark side of families* (pp. 119–130). Beverly Hills, CA: Sage.

Foa, E. B., Olasov-Rothbaum, B., & Steketee, G. S. (in press). Treatment of rape victims. *NIMH Monograph Series. State of the Art in Sexual Assault Research.*

Foy, D. W., Resnick, H. S., Carroll, E. M., & Osato, S. S. (1990). *Behavior therapy with PTSD.* In M. Hersen & A. Bellack (Eds.), *Handbook of comparative treatments for adult disorders* (pp. 302–315). New York: Wiley.

Frieze, I. H. (1980, September). *Causes and consequences of marital rape.* Paper presented at the Annual Meeting of the American Psychological Association, Montreal, Canada.

Frieze, I. H. (1983). Investigating the causes and consequences of marital rape. *Signs, 8,* 532–533.

Gelles, R. J., & Straus, M. A. (1988). *Intimate violence.* New York: Simon & Schuster.

Groth, N. A. (1979). *Men who rape: The psychology of the offender.* New York: Plenum Press.

Henneke, C. R., & Shields, N. M. (1985). Marital rape: Implications for the helping professions. *Social Casework,* October, 451–458.

Hanneke, C. A., Shields, N. M., & McCall, G. J. (1986). Assessing the prevalence of marital rape. *Journal of Interpersonal Violence, 1,* 350–362.

Hilberman, E., & Munson, K. (1978). Sixty battered women. *Victimology, 2,* 460–470.

Horowitz, M., Wilner, N., & Alvarez, W. (1979). Impact of event scale: A measure of subjective stress. *Psychosomatic Medicine, 41,* 209–218.

Janoff-Bulman, R. (1985). The aftermath of victimization: Rebuilding shattered assumptions. In C. R. Figley (Ed.), *Trauma and its wake* (pp. 15–35). New York: Brunner/Mazel.

Kilpatrick, D. G. (1983). Rape victims: Detection, assessment, and treatment. *Clinical Psychologist, 36,* 92–95.

Kilpatrick, D. G., & Amick, A. E. (1985). *Rape trauma.* In M. Hersen & C. G. Last (Eds.), *Behavior therapy casebook* (pp. 87–103). New York: Springer.

Kilpatrick, D. G., Veronen, L. J., & Resick, P. A. (1979). The aftermath of rape: Recent empirical findings. *American Journal of Orthopsychiatry, 49,* 658–699.

Kilpatrick, D. G., Best, C. L., Saunders, B. E., & Veronen, L. J. (1988). Rape in marriage and in dating relationships: How bad is it for mental health? *Annals of the New York Academy of Sciences, 528,* 335–344.

Kilpatrick, D. G., Veronen, L. J., & Best, C. L. (1985). Factors predicting psychological distress among rape victims. In C. R. Figley (Ed.), *Trauma and its wake* (pp. 113–141). New York: Brunner/Mazel.

Kilpatrick, D. G., Saunders, B. E., Amick-McMullan, A., Best, C. L., Veronen, L. J., & Resnick, H. S. (1989). Victim and crime factors with the development of crime-related disorder. *Behavior Therapy, 20,* 199–214.

Koss, M. P. (1983). The scope of rape: Implications for the clinical treatment of reactions. *Clinical Psychologist, 36,* 88–91.

Lystad, M. H. (1982). Sexual abuse in the home: A review of the literature. *International Journal of Family Psychiatry, 3,* 3–31.

Resick, P. A., Jordan, D. G., Girelli, S. A. Hutter, C. K., & Marhoefer-Dvorak, S. (1987). A comparative outcome study of group therapy for sexual assault victims. Unpublished manuscript, University of Missouri, St. Louis.

Russell, D. E. H. (1982). *Rape in marriage.* New York: Macmillan.

Shields, N. M., & Hanneke, C. R. (1983). Battered wives' reactions to marital rape. In D. Finkelhor, R. J. Gelles, G. T. Hotaling, & M. A. Strauss (Eds.), *The dark side of families* (pp. 131–148). Beverly Hills, CA: Sage.

Shields, N. M., & Hanneke, C. R. (1984, November). *Multiple sexual victimization: The case of incest and marital rape.* Paper presented at the Second National Conference on Family Violence Research, Durham, NH.

Shields, N. M., & Hanneke, C. R. (1987, July). *Comparing the psychological impact of marital and stranger rape.* Paper presented at the National Conference on Family Violence Research, Durham, NH.

Veronen, L. J., & Kilpatrick, D. G. (1980). Self-reported fears of rape victims: A preliminary investigation. *Behavior Modification, 4,* 383–396.

Veronen, L. J., & Kilpatrick, D. G. (1983). Stress management for rape victims. In D. Meichenbaum & M. E. Jarenko (Eds.), *Stress reduction and prevention* (pp. 341–373). New York: Plenum Press.

Weingourt, R. (1985). Wife rape: Barriers to identification and treatment. *American Journal of Psychotherapy, 39,* 187–192.

19

Elder Abuse

Rosalie S. Wolf and Edward R. McCarthy

Description of the Problem

Despite the advances that have been made over the past decade in public awareness of elder abuse, service delivery, training, and social policy, family violence toward older adults remains a relatively obscure phenomenon. Definitions of elder abuse are not uniform, the causes are not fully understood, and the intervention programs are untested. Yet hundreds of elder abuse workers are called upon daily to respond to situations that are among the most challenging facing the human service system. The medical, psychological, social, legal, and ethical problems embodied in these cases require the most skillful and experienced case managers in addition to a cadre of other professions and paraprofessionals for consultation and intervention. The case that is the subject of this chapter is a typical example. To place it in context, we will begin with a brief review of the nature and scope of elder abuse, followed by the case study and a concluding discussion.

Definitions

From the very beginning of scientific investigation into the nature of elder abuse, definitions have been a controversial matter. Even though there appeared to be agreement regarding the broad categories—physical abuse, psychological abuse, material abuse (or financial exploita-

Rosalie S. Wolf • Institute on Aging, The Medical Center of Central Massachusetts, Worcester, Massachusetts 01605.   **Edward R. McCarthy** • Elder Home Care Services of Worcester Area, Worcester, Massachusetts 01603.

tion), and neglect—there was less consistency in what those terms represented. While researchers struggled with capturing the essence of the problem in a single phrase (Fulmer & O'Malley, 1987; Hudson, 1988; Johnson, 1986), the 50 states passed elder abuse legislation using their own definitions (APWA/NASUA, 1986). Some laws include abuse against oneself (self-abuse) as well as abuse perpetrated by others. Some consider physical and psychological harm as abuse; others designate only physical harm. Some states do not use the term *abuse* at all. The definitions of neglect have been even more diverse, with some describing the condition and others the intent. The lack of uniformity has hindered efforts to determine the scope of the problem and to build the knowledge base necessary for the development of intervention and prevention programs.

Risk Factors

In trying to understand why elder mistreatment occurs, researchers turned to the child abuse, family violence, psychological, sociological, and gerontological literatures for guidance. Five theoretical explanations seemed the most persuasive, although certainly not the only possible ones: (1) psychopathology of the perpetrator, (2) dependency and exchange relations between the abused and the abuser, (3) external stress, (4) social isolation, and (5) intergenerational transmission of violence. Subsequent research found strong support for psychopathology of the perpetrator and dependency as risk factors, some proof for social isolation, but less conclusive evidence for external stress factors or the intergenerational transmission of violence (Anetzberger, 1987; Bristowe & Collins, 1989; Phillips, 1986; Pillemer, 1986; Wolf, Godkin, & Pillemer, 1984).

Characteristics of Victims and Perpetrators

While the early investigators showed that the victims were likely to be disproportionately female and "old-old," there was no agreement about other aspects of the problem, including the degree of physical and mental impairment of the victims, the characteristics of the perpetrators, and the dynamics of the relationships (Block & Sinnott, 1979; Lau & Kosberg, 1979; O'Malley, Segars, Perez, Mitchell, & Kneupfal, 1979; Sengstock & Liang, 1982). Criticism of these pioneer studies for using small, unrepresentative samples, relying only on retrospective case records, omitting control groups, and lumping together the various types of maltreatment (Callahan, 1982; Pedrick-Cornell & Gelles, 1982) led to the utilization of more rigorous methodologies by the next group of researchers. Emerging from these latter works was a more complicated representation of the problem than had been described before (Anetzberger, 1987; Bristowe & Collins, 1989; Crouse, Cobb, Harris, Kopecky, & Poertner, 1981; Giordano & Giordano, 1983; Pillemer, 1986). From the earlier depiction of elder abuse as a very dependent and impaired elderly woman mistreated by a well-meaning but overburdened adult child caregiver, the concept evolved into a much more complex set of players and relationships. A comparative analysis of the various types of abuse (physical, psychological, financial) and neglect (active/intentional, passive/unintentional) revealed at least three different profiles (Wolf & Pillemer, 1989). Victims of physical and psychological abuse were relatively independent in their activities of daily living, but they suffered from emotional problems. The perpetrators in these cases had a history of alcoholism and/or mental illness and were dependent on the victim for financial resources. Victim and perpetrator were more likely to live together than in other types of elder maltreatment. Neglect cases often involved a very old victim with cognitive and functional impairments and little social support. The perpetrators neither had psychological problems nor were financially dependent on the victim. They found the victim to be a source of stress. Another distinct pattern was associated with material abuse (financial exploitation). The victims were generally unmarried with a very limited social network. The perpetrators had financial problems, sometimes traceable to a history of substance abuse. For them, the single, lonely elder was an easy target for exploitation. These sparse findings represent a decade of investigations into the causes of abuse and neglect. Even fewer attempts were made to determine the extent of the problem.

Scope

Although 4% and even 10% have been widely quoted in the literature (Block & Sinnott, 1979; U.S. House Select Committee on Aging, 1981) and the popular press as estimates of the extent of elder abuse, just two prevalence studies have been carried out in the 10-year history of research into the problem. One was based on interviews of 342 elders (a random probability sample) in New Jersey using a structured questionnaire that included vignettes about four different types of abuse: physical, psychological, financial, and neglect (Gioglio & Blakemore, 1983). The five cases that were identified were too small a number with respect to the confidence limits of the analysis to generalize to the state's elder population. The second was done in the metropolitan Boston area, using a methodology that has been validated in national surveys of child and spouse abuse (Straus & Gelles, 1986). Contacts were made with 2020 community-dwelling persons either by telephone or in person to inquire about their experience with three types of maltreatment (physical, psychological, neglect). Slightly more than 3% of the 65-and-over population had been so mistreated: 20 per 1000, physical abuse; 11 per 1000, verbal aggression; and 4 per 1000, neglect. If a national survey yielded similar numbers, there would be between 701,000 and 1,093,560 abused elders. These results differed markedly from previous findings. First, spouse abuse was more prevalent (58%) than abuse by adult children (24%); second, there were roughly equal numbers of men and women among the victims; and third, the study showed that economic status and age were not related to the risk of abuse (Pillemer & Finkelhor, 1988). If financial exploitation had been included in the study questions (Wolf et al., 1984), the percentage would have been higher, perhaps closer to the 4% figure.

The state reporting systems are another potential source of data for estimating incidence. All 50 states have established a system for collecting statistics on cases of elder abuse, but, because of the lack of uniformity in definitions and criteria and inclusion in some instances of unsubstantiated cases, the state data cannot easily be aggregated to provide a national picture. Using a methodology based on grouping states with similar, but not identical, reporting criteria, Tatara (1988) has estimated that between 51,000 and 186,000 persons aged 60 years were reported to public agencies as victims of abuse and neglect during the FY 85, an increase over FY 83 and FY 84. Clearly, the number of reports represented only a fraction of the cases in the community. With increasing public awareness and service development, we can anticipate more cases of abused and neglected elderly persons in the coming years even if strong preventive and treatment measures are undertaken.

Treatment Models

At this point in the history of elder abuse, there are probably as many treatment "models" as there are organizations working in this area. The early researchers (Block & Sinnott, 1979; O'Malley et al., 1979) found that social and medical services, civil sanctions, and criminal proceedings were utilized in treating these cases, but often removal of the victim from the home situation was thought to be the only remedy.

Although a number of theories, such as "social exchange theory" (Pillemer, 1986), "symbolic interactionism" (Phillips, 1986), and "environmental press model" (Ansello, King, & Taler, 1986), have been proposed as the basis for formulating intervention strategies, no empirical studies have been conducted to validate them. Practitioners have been left to rely on field experience and professional training.

One of the first treatment strategies to be described is the "Elder Abuse Diagnosis and Intervention Model" of Quinn and Tomita (1986), which makes use of traditional psychosocial casework and incorporates crisis, short-term, and long-term intervention methodology. Counseling is at the heart of the model, but it also encompasses the utilization of legal instruments, including those that do and do not require court involvement, and the criminal justice system. Fulmer and O'Malley (1987) approach intervention from a different perspective. Using "inadequate care" as the paradigm, they have designed decision trees for various categories of cases based on (1) the needs of the client, and (2) the significance of the caretaking role of the individual believed to be responsible for the inadequate care. Still another method, the Staircase Model (Breckman & Adelman, 1988), is based primarily on the receptivity of the victims to helping themselves. The staircase has three stages representing the process of change: reluctance, recognition, and rebuilding. Counseling is a major aspect of treatment, along with the use of victim self-help groups.

Programs dealing with elder abuse have been organized in three ways (Crouse *et al.,* 1981). The first is the "child abuse or mandatory reporting" model that is an adaptation of the service system used for abused and neglected children, and probably the most common version. The second is the "legal intervention model," which considers the legal system a primary source of assistance for case resolution through such means as restraining orders, civil and criminal complaints to the police and courts, and collection of case data for use in possible prosecution. The "advocacy model," the third type, assumes that the service provider will not intrude unnecessarily in the lives of the elder victims but will use a broad range of formal and informal services to assist them in meeting their goals. Many programs use a combination of techniques, such as the protective service unit of Elder Home Care Services of Worcester Area, the home agency of the case presented in this chapter.

Elder Home Care Services

One of 27 "home care corporations" in the commonwealth with which the Massachusetts Executive Office of Elder Affairs has contracts, Elder Home Care Services (EHC) serves persons who are 60 years and older living in the city of Worcester and 15 surrounding towns. It provides case management and information and referral services directly, and social services through subcontracts with local vendors. When individuals request services, they are prescreened by an intake worker. If they meet basic eligibility guidelines regarding functional status, income, and informal supports, they are referred to a case manager, who performs a detailed assessment of the client, develops a plan of care, monitors the situation, and conducts periodic reassessments.

With the passage by the Massachusetts General Court of the 1982 "Act providing further protection of elderly persons," protective service units were established within each of the home care corporations to receive reports of suspected cases of abuse and neglect, assess the situation, and provide services. Under Massachusetts law, elder abuse is defined as "acts or omissions resulting in serious physical or serious emotional injury to an elderly person." They include physical and emotional abuse and neglect (but not self-neglect). While medical and social personnel are mandated to report suspected cases of elder abuse under the law, anyone who has reasonable cause to believe an elder has been abused may report. In the case study to be presented, it was the victim's pastor.

Case Description

Harriet Fields is an 88-year-old widow who lives in her own single-family home in a pleasant middle-class neighborhood. She shares the home with her only child, Bernard, 55, who apparently has lived with his mother all of his life. He worked in a steel mill for many years, but the plant closed about 5 years prior to the opening of the case, and he has been unemployed ever since. Mrs. Fields is a very religious woman, but she is no longer able to attend services, so her pastor comes to visit her at least monthly. During the course of one of these visits the pastor noticed that one of her legs was badly cut and bruised and had obviously not been treated. When questioned, Mrs. Fields reluctantly admitted that her son had thrown a cooking utensil at her. Further questioning revealed that there had been other such incidents, but Mrs. Fields made it clear that she did not want her visitor to report the matter. Nevertheless, on his return to the rectory, the pastor called a protective services worker at EHC, who agreed to accompany him on a visit to Mrs. Fields the following morning.

Mrs. Fields was clearly upset at the course that events were taking and hesitated, at first, about admitting her visitors. However, she finally relented. The scene inside was very depressing: dark, shabby, and grimy. The house had obviously not been cleaned or cared for in many years. Mrs. Fields blended into this bleak picture. She was unkempt, her dress dirty and ragged, and it was evident that she had not bathed in some time. Her vision was poor, one eye was red and watery, and she had difficulty hearing. Her legs were swollen and badly bruised, and there were lacerations around one ankle and foot that were obviously infected. Despite the early hour, Bernard had already left for the day—part of his usual routine, according to Mrs. Fields.

After some small talk, she became somewhat more relaxed and finally agreed to answer some questions. Her injury, it seems, had occurred a few days before when her son became irritated that the food she had cooked for him was not hot enough, and he threw a heavy iron pot at her. She conceded that there had been other such instances. He was often "mean" and used foul language when she suggested that he find a job or criticized him for leaving her alone all day. She admitted that she was sometimes fearful when he came home late at night and often barricaded her bedroom door. In describing all this, however, Mrs. Fields seemed both embarrassed at what had occurred and somewhat protective of her son. While his pattern of behavior seemed clearly to indicate a drinking problem, Mrs. Fields steered clear of any mention of alcohol. She protested that she did not want to "cause trouble" or be a "bother" and became quite agitated when the worker explained that he had a responsibility to call for medical treatment for her and to make a report to the police.

While waiting for a response to the calls, Mrs. Fields described for her visitors a lonely existence. Her husband had died "years ago." She had outlived all the members of her own family, but three of her husband's siblings were still in the area. One elderly brother-in-law stopped by weekly to do her grocery shopping and pay her bills, and a sister-in-law called her on the phone periodically to check on her. Except for her pastor, there were no other visitors. She rarely left the house. She had no personal physician and could not remember when she had first received any medical attention. She liked to read and watch television, but increasing problems with vision and hearing had lessened her enjoyment. However, she had never considered having an eye examination or a hearing test.

In spite of her lack of interest in seeking medical care, she made no serious objection when a visiting nurse arrived to treat her wounds and give her a preliminary physical examination. The nurse noted the edema in her legs and her elevated blood pressure and recommended a complete examination by a physician. She also recommended follow-up visits to check on her infected legs, to help with bathing, and to see about her nutritional needs. Mrs. Fields' reaction indicated that there might be a problem carrying out these recommendations, but her objections were phrased with a wry good humor.

This changed abruptly when the police arrived. The officers had been briefed beforehand and handled the interview sensitively, but Mrs. Fields was clearly upset at the whole procedure. After questioning her about the episode, they patiently explained that she could file charges of assault and battery against her son for this infraction, or any subsequent ones. She could also seek an order of protection, which would enjoin him from further harming her, and this could include a requirement that he vacate the premises. Mrs. Fields was clearly not interested in taking any action against her son. She tried to discount the seriousness of the abuse and seemed much more worried about "the disgrace to the family" that even this visit would cause. After they had left, however, she agreed that it might serve as a deterrent to her son and did not object when the worker proposed an early visit the following morning to talk with him.

The worker tried not to prejudge Bernard, but the reception he received made it difficult for him to remain objective. Bernard was initially unwilling even to open the door, but after some shouting in the background from his mother, he finally did so, reluctantly. He was a burly, slovenly-looking man, unshaven and apparently "hung over" from the evening before. The worker tried to explain his role and the reason for his intervention the previous day, but Bernard made it clear that he resented the "interference" and felt that everyone was badly overreacting to a minor family problem. He and his mother had arguments; she "does nothing around the house," constantly nagged him, and, out of frustration, he may have pushed her to "get off his back," but there had been nothing to justify all this attention. During this conversation, Mrs. Fields kept up a string of criticism from the background, and the effect was bizarre. The worker had to remind himself that he was not listening to an obstreperous teen-ager and the shrill complaints of a middle-aged mother.

Attempts to empathize with Bernard and his difficulties in trying to find work in his mid-50s were unsuccessful, and so were the efforts to involve him in obtaining more assistance for his mother. He made it clear that he was terminating the interview, wanted his visitor to leave immediately, and wished no further visits from anyone. Only then did the worker spell out for him that, from the point of view of the community and the law, his mother, whatever the provocation, had been physically abused and, probably more important, badly neglected, and that intervention was required for her safety and health. He could either cooperate or an order of protection would be obtained, one effect of which might be that he would be forced to move from his home. Bernard continued his harangues, but the last point clearly had an intimidating effect.

Later, Mrs. Fields' sister-in-law Marion agreed to talk with the worker, but she was very guarded in her responses to questions about the Fields. She was in her early 80s, cared for her frail older brother, George, and rarely left the house, but she said she talked to Mrs. Fields regularly on the phone. In fact, Mrs. Fields, sometimes confused, had called her at times in the middle of the night for reassurance. Marion minimized the reports of physical abuse. She described Bernard as a "roughneck" who was sometimes "off his rocker," but hastened to say that this did not mean that he had serious mental problems or was necessarily an alcoholic. Admittedly, he was not supportive of his mother, but, then, Mrs. Fields had never been much of a mother to him. It was because Bernard did not drive that Marion's brother Paul stopped by weekly to shop for her. He cashed her retirement checks and paid her bills, and Harriet kept the balance in her purse. From this, she doled out an allowance to her son.

Medical Issues

Although the physical abuse of Mrs. Fields had the most dramatic impact and generated the most emotion, more disturbing was the physical neglect that was evident to those encountering her for the first time. The contrast between her relatively attractive home in a genteel neighborhood and the interior of that home was marked. Passing through the front door was to enter a time warp; nothing had been maintained inside for more than a decade, neither the furnishings nor Mrs. Fields herself. There was only deterioration. This was so despite the fact that Mrs. Fields, though experiencing some confusion, seemed intelligent and competent enough to recognize her problems and cope with them. She also had adequate financial resources, though she herself might not have made the same evaluation. Her supports, particularly her brother-in-law, seemingly could have functioned more effectively, had she cooperated.

The temptation on the part of those who intervened was to try to remedy all the shortcomings at once: to protect her from further harm, to deal with her physical ailments, to improve her environment and the quality of her life, and to make her remaining years happier than those that had preceded. Mrs. Fields, though, seemed bent on denying them this satisfaction. She was wary of each proposal, agreed, then hesitated, or changed her mind. She was not going to be stampeded into anything, however logical it seemed, and yielded control reluctantly. The visiting nurse was accepted, but Mrs. Fields had to be persuaded that regular bathing with the help of a nurse's aide was necessary. (Later, the aide was instrumental in detecting more bruises and other evidence of further abuse.) Additional persuasion was required before she finally agreed to leave the house to receive a complete physical examination and establish a relationship with a geriatric specialist. Remarkably, considering her age and lack of care, she had relatively few serious problems. Hypertension was verified; she had arthritis in her legs, and there was some evidence of malnutrition. It was also suggested that she see an ophthalmologist.

One way of dealing with the nutrition issue was to introduce a homemaker, who would ensure that she received at least one balanced hot meal daily. This also was a way to reduce her isolation, make her more secure, monitor her medications, and observe her functional state. Needless to say, Mrs. Fields did not readily accept the idea, and the first experiment failed. The homemaker was frightened by Bernard, seemed overwhelmed by the housekeeping challenge, and found Mrs. Fields too difficult. After an interval, however, Mrs. Fields agreed to try another worker, and this time the match was successful. Later, Mrs. Fields agreed to have home-delivered meals on those days when the homemaker was not scheduled, but only after complaining about "all these people" coming into her house.

It was obvious to the homemaker and others that vision and hearing problems were affecting Mrs. Fields' safety and well-being. She also complained about a loose-fitting dental plate that interfered with her eating. It took several visits, however, before she agreed to make appointments to see if she could be helped. To reduce the work load and attempt to keep the family involved, the worker tried to enlist Bernard and Paul in the task of getting Mrs. Fields to these appointments. Not surprisingly, Bernard proved completely unreliable, and Paul seemed wary about being drawn any further into the situation and unwilling to deal with Mrs. Fields' inevitable last-minute vacillations. As a result, there were many cancellations and much rescheduling. She finally was seen by an ophthalmologist, who immediately made arrangements for surgery to remove a cataract. An audiologist verified a severe hearing loss but felt that she was a good candidate for amplification. The dental appointments were never kept.

Mrs. Fields had some last-minute reservations about her surgery but finally entered the hospital. She claimed that this was her first such experience, and she was very frightened. Possible because of this, her vital signs were dangerously low for a short period in the operating room, so that her return home was delayed. Nevertheless, her recovery was complete; her vision improved measurably, and she was very pleased. She could not be persuaded to try a hearing aid. She joked that she might "hear too much."

Thus, many of Mrs. Fields' physical and medical problems were addressed. Her situation improved, but it was accomplished at *her* pace and not without setbacks and failures. Her care managers became frustrated at times; Mrs. Fields, like most abuse clients, would not fit neatly into a daily or weekly schedule, and the care plan was constantly being revised. However, the workers reminded themselves that they were dealing with a frail and very old person who had adapted to a routine and an environment with which she was familiar. It was not a pleasant situation in which she found herself, but she was not convinced that the changes that were being suggested would necessarily improve matters. Her apprehension about medical personnel was evident. Clinics and technology frightened her; she required reassurance before she would agree to any procedure. The extent of the fear and the lack of any medical history, in fact, contributed to the suspicion that Mrs. Fields had neglected her health care even when she was younger and completely functional.

Legal Issues

Because physical abuse was the precipitating cause of the referral and intervention in Mrs. Fields' case, the first legal remedies considered were those described to her by the police: initiating a complaint for assault and battery against her son or seeking an order of protection to enjoin him from further harming her. The latter might include ordering him to vacate the home they shared. Her negative reaction to these proposals was both typical and understandable. Taking such a step would have meant that she had failed as a mother. Even having the police show up at her door was a "disgrace." She could only imagine the reaction of the neighbors. Apparently, Mrs. Fields never gave it any further thought, but it would be difficult to envision her following through on such a complaint, enduring the turmoil of the courthouse, and facing her son in open court. Then, the consequences for her if he were cleared, or released after minimal punishment as a first offender, would have to be considered.

The order of protection, which can be handled in a civil action, might have been somewhat less traumatic for Mrs. Fields from the standpoint of process, but the effect would have been the same. The order would have required Mrs. Fields, if threatened or actually abused, to telephone the police and report that her son had violated the injunction and was in contempt of court. Knowing Mrs. Fields and her son, it is difficult to believe that she would actually have carried through such a procedure. As for vacating the premises, it should be remembered that Bernard had apparently lived with his mother all his life and was, presumably, completely dependent on her for financial support. No matter what the provocation, this would have been a most serious step for her to take. The result, too, would have left her completely alone. Bernard was not much of a son or a companion, but Mrs. Fields, given the opportunity to be free of him, clearly chose not to take advantage of it.

There were always concerns about Mrs. Fields' competence to manage her affairs. She sometimes displayed confusion, did not remember names, forgot that she had made an appointment—though sometimes it seemed that this might have been a ploy. Still, in the care manager's experience, there was never a question about her judgment being affected to the degree that she required a legal guardian, even had there been someone willing to accept the responsibility. A possible conservatorship was another matter. When she discussed her finances, as she did rarely, she was quite vague and revealed her naivete in these matters. As noted earlier, she kept a relatively large amount of cash in her purse and had a number of long-standing passbook savings accounts that added up to a substantial amount (certainly enough for her remaining years). When the worker examined these books, he noted a pattern of small withdrawals, none of which Mrs. Fields could explain. It appeared that, ideally, the appointment of a conservator was appropriate. The problem was the lack of candidates. Certainly, Bernard would not qualify, and Paul's integrity could at least be questioned. However, if someone else were to be appointed—a lawyer, for example—it seemed probable that Paul would be upset and withdraw from the scene, resulting in the loss of vital, even though tenuous, support. The relationship between Mrs. Fields and the worker would also be jeopardized. Even if she fully understood the concept, she would not have agreed to a voluntary conservatorship; an involuntary one, which would require the cooperation of the worker, her new physician, and the court system, would have confirmed her worst fears about what "all these people" were up to. The situation was uncomfortable for those involved, but the remedy appeared to create more problems that it would solve.

Social and Family Issues

One of the problems of obtaining social supports for the frail elderly is that they have outlived most of their friends and relatives and, because of their needs or demands, have discouraged or estranged many of those who remain. Even their children, approaching retirement status themselves, because of their geographical separation or their preoccupation with their own or their children's problems are not always the resources that they are assumed to be. In Mrs. Fields' case, the potential supports were further limited by the fact that she had only one child, and he remained a bachelor. In many such instances, conscientious digging will produce blood relatives, one or more of whom may feel at least a moral obligation to step forward and help with decision making, even to the point of accepting a conservatorship or guardianship. Mrs. Fields mentioned none, and neither did her in-laws.

Bernard not only was a problem because of the threat he presented and his failure to contribute to the household or to accept a caregiver role, but he seemed, by his attitude and personality, to discourage anyone who might want to help. Their neighborhood seemed the kind that would have rallied round a woman like Mrs. Fields, but apparently it did not do so. One has to surmise that the presence of Bernard was a factor. He also seemed to be at least one of the reasons for the limited involvement by the in-laws. Paul appeared to feel a moral obligation to do the grocery shopping and pay the bills, but he probably resented the fact that he had to assume Bernard's role. That he did little beyond this—take care of household repairs, or meet more of Mrs. Fields' personal needs, for example—was undoubtedly because he had been rebuffed before and did not want to become more immersed in the Fields' problems than necessary.

Protective service workers, if they are to be effective over the long run, must avoid the tendency to "take over" from whatever supports exist. Instead, they must work with them, encourage and reinforce those efforts so that professional help can eventually be phased out. But too much pressure cannot be applied either, or a fragile support system might collapse—and assuredly Mrs. Fields' supports fitted that description. Since neither Paul nor Marion was very forthcoming, it was never clear how close their relationship was to the Fields, even when Mr. Fields was alive. Their disinclination to help out was probably indicative of a lack of affection for their sister-in-law. Even if they had been close, their increasing age, declining health, and reduced mobility would probably have resulted in a concentration of their remaining energy on their own survival and that of their siblings. Recognizing this, the workers were careful not to press them and limited the requests that they made of them. When Mrs. Fields balked at buying new clothes to replace her rags, Marion's help was enlisted, and a shopping trip was arranged with positive results. Marion basked in the praise she received, and Mrs. Fields, despite her protestations, seemed to enjoy her new image. As noted previously, Paul, by his inaction, demonstrated that his help could not be taken for granted. Requests were made of him selectively and reinforced by letter. The workers were careful to recognize his contributions.

It was ironic that Mrs. Fields, also, could not be pressed too hard to accept the help that seemed so reasonable to those who were concerned about her safety and welfare. She yielded grudgingly to each proposal and occasionally took what seemed a symbolic stand against "those strangers." She had articulated her fears, complained about her ailments, and lamented her isolation, yet when steps were proposed to address each of these concerns, she saw them as an invasion of her privacy and an attempt to disrupt the familiar pattern of her existence.

For those accustomed to dealing with elders at risk, this reaction is not very surprising. Workers may see themselves operating on the side of the angels, "saving" or "rescuing" a beleaguered victim and improving the quality of her life, but the person at risk often has a different perspective. The worker may instead be seen as a threat, an agent of change, someone who wants to impose his/her own values on an individual who is too helpless to object. The care managers in this case were sensitive to this problem, but it was complicated by the difficulty in communicating with Mrs. Fields. Her hearing loss and her episodes of confusion led to shouted exchanges and inevitable misunderstandings. It was difficult, for example, to determine what her own values were and what the quality of her life had been previously. Earlier it was noted that she may not have set high standards for herself in the area of health care and nutrition. She had to be coerced, for sanitary reasons, into purchasing new clothes. Suggestions that the dungeon-like atmosphere of her living spaces be brightened and enlivened with new curtains, lamp-shades, and rugs were dismissed out of hand; her objections had to be overridden to take care of necessary plumbing and electrical repairs. Part of the problem, admittedly, was her belief that she was poor, and she resisted those who "just want to spend my money."

The ultimate threat presented by any "stranger," of course, is nursing home placement. While this may never have been considered as an option by the worker, the fear of being removed from one's home and institutionalized is usually uppermost in the mind of the vulnerable elder, and, therefore, every proposal or suggestion, innocuous though it may be, is looked upon suspiciously. To overcome this barrier, those working with Mrs. Fields, from the beginning, treated the subject with candor. The option of nursing home placement was discussed, but she was assured that no one considered this to be appropriate for her. However, there was a well-managed and attractive rest home close by, and she was asked to give some thought to this if her safety became more of a concern. Later, when there was, in fact, evidence of further abuse, the option was discussed again; at one point, she seemed to consider making a test visit. Another opportunity presented itself following her eye surgery, when a temporary placement would have simplified her recovery and possibly removed her apprehension about such a home. Mrs. Fields would have none of it; she insisted on returning to her own house. As an individual who was still legally competent, she could make that choice.

Assessment of Psychopathology

The conventional wisdom is that in most cases of elder abuse there are two victims: the person abused and the perpetrator, and both need help. Mrs. Fields, of course, was unarguably a classic victim of abuse and neglect. Bernard, on the other hand, because of his actions, attitude, and personality, was seen by most observers as the "villain of the piece." It would have been difficult for the care managers to consider him to be a victim as well. They were certainly in agreement, however, that he was in desperate need of help.

That a physically able man would strike and cause visible damage to a vulnerable old, old woman would appear to be a pathological act. Bernard disputed this characterization; he was merely flailing out at someone who was "bugging" him; there was no beating involved. The distinction would seem to have been an academic one; the effect of abuse on the victim was the same. Evidence of at least four different episodes was found, and in one instance Mrs. Fields' ribs were bruised and vaginal bleeding was discovered. Anyone capable of such anger and so lacking in control obviously needed treatment.

The problem in this case was that it was necessary to take sides to protect the endangered victim, and any opportunity there may have been to help the perpetrator had to be sacrificed. The worker making the intervention attempted, as much as he could under the circumstances, to take an evenhanded approach, to withhold judgment, and keep the lines open to Bernard. Often in abuse cases the original assessment is changed drastically after more facts are assembled, so that this is always a wise approach to take. But Bernard's response soon indicated that he was not interested in these overtures and that there would be no time for further fact gathering. The primary objective, then, became Mrs. Fields' safety and welfare. In focusing on this, any realistic chance of helping Bernard deal with his problems was essentially forfeited.

Because there were relatively few contacts with Bernard after this point, and those were usually abrupt and contentious, it was not possible to learn much more about him. The workers on the case could only speculate about his personal problems and about the relationship with his mother that eventuated in such violence. He gave every evidence that he was an angry, unstable, violent person, but he had no prior police record and apparently no record of treatment for mental disorder. His reputation was that of a heavy drinker, but his drinking seemed to be confined to downtown bars; there was no indication that he drank at home. He had no job and presumably was dependent on his mother for shelter and spending money. Yet, until a few years before, he had held a steady, physically demanding job that paid well, and he undoubtedly must have contributed to the support of the household. When the company and industry closed down, and he lost his job and trade, he claimed to have kept up his efforts to find work, but was unsuccessful. This could have been because of his age and, possibly, his unwillingness to work for a lesser wage.

Those listening to the heated exchanges between mother and son wondered whether such antagonism was recent or long-standing. Bernard was an only child, not born until his mother was 33, and there was a question about how much he was wanted. Yet he seemingly stayed with his mother all his life. He expressed at times his unhappiness at others' taking over the family responsibilities. Nevertheless, he never cooperated when challenged to share part of that burden. Had Bernard been amenable to help, all agreed that he would have presented a daunting challenge to any therapist.

Treatment Options

Mrs. Fields posed the classic dilemma faced repeatedly by protective service workers (i.e., balancing the rights of the client against the need to protect that client from harm). The pressure from the community, friends, or neighbors is to "do something" about the elder at risk, even though that person may not want anything "done." That pressure aside, service workers themselves feel a great deal of personal anxiety about their clients and are tempted to override the latter's wishes and remove them to safety, or take some other action, so that they can sleep at night. The question, then, is: How well do the clients sleep?

The problem is complicated when the competence of the client comes into question, and Mrs. Fields' competence periodically became an issue: when she appeared confused or when she was resistant or ambivalent about a course of action that seemed not to be controversial (e.g., the introduction of a nurse's aide or home-delivered meals). At this point, the border between persuasion and coercion became a very blurred line. When, for example, the news was received that Mrs. Fields had almost died on the operating table, the worker felt guilty, reviewing in his mind his role in helping to convince Mrs. Fields that she should undergo the operation. Or again, when yet another instance of abuse surfaced, he wondered whether he should have been more persuasive in presenting the option of moving to a rest home. When the question hung in the balance, the worker tried to resolve the doubt in favor of the client's rights, but this resolution was never a comfortable one. Seeking a legal determination of competence would have been, if anything, more discomforting. Bringing the client to a physician or a psychiatrist, usually on some pretext, for an evaluation of competence always raises self-doubt in anyone who is sincerely concerned about infringing on the client's rights.

While the protective service worker often agonized over these decisions, he was not alone in his concerns for Mrs. Fields; protecting and caring for her was basically a team effort. The worker formulated the basic plan and served as coordinator, but there were a number of caregivers, and each had a role to carry out: visiting nurses, nurse's aides, physicians, homemakers, home-delivered meals volunteers, friendly visitors, police detectives, and relatives. The plan, basically, was to introduce as many caregivers as Mrs. Fields would tolerate, not only to perform their expected functions but also to monitor her status and report to the coordinator anything out of the ordinary. Thus, the homemaker not only cooked meals and performed household tasks, but she served as companion, monitored Mrs. Fields's functional state, watched Bernard, and checked on medications. The nurse's aide reported any signs of abuse; the home-delivered meals volunteer reported when she could not gain entry. There were no formal meetings of the entire group, but there were several informal sessions with parts of the team when crises occurred or plans needed to be changed. In general, given the parameters Mrs. Fields had herself established, the plan can be said to have been successful. Her health and quality of life improved, though not to the degree her caregivers had hoped. And the physical abuse, though not eliminated, was appreciably reduced. Best of all, from Mrs. Fields' viewpoint, she was able to remain in the familiar surrounding of her own home.

Postscript

Slightly over a year after the case was opened, Bernard was killed, apparently during a robbery, while returning home from his usual haunts late one evening. The case was never solved. Mrs. Fields was quite depressed following this shocking incident. She remained alone in her home, but services were reduced to some degree when she refused to pay even a nominal fee. She became more confused and was persuaded to move in temporarily with her sister-in-law (Marion). She stayed for about 3 months and appeared to be thriving under Marion's care, but then she became restive and kept trying to return home. When Marion could no longer handle the situation, Mrs. Fields was moved back home and services were resumed. She remained there for about 1 year in a marginal status, experiencing a number of crises before finally collapsing and being hospitalized with an inoperable tumor on her lung. She was transferred to a nursing home, where she died about 3 months later at 90 years of age.

Mrs. Fields died without a will. Her estate consisted of her house and a substantially reduced bank account. Five first cousins appeared from another state and received the bulk of the estate. Her brother-in-law sued, claiming he had been promised that he would receive all proceeds in return for services rendered to the family. He was awarded a nominal amount.

Summary

From many perspectives, the case study of Mrs. Fields and her son is a characteristic elder-abuse situation, involving multiple types of mistreatment over an extended period of time. Physical abuse was the primary form of mistreatment in this case, accompanied by psychological abuse, although the latter was more difficult to substantiate. Neglect was also evident but, perhaps, more correctly defined as self-neglect, since in no way could the son be considered a "caregiver." In fact, he was dependent on the victim for the basic necessities of life, giving little in return, neither affection nor companionship.

The attributes associated with physical-abuse cases are to a great extent in evidence here: the victim's and perpetrator's poor emotional health, the shared living arrangement, and the mutual dependency. While there was no history of mental illness or alcohol abuse on the part of the perpetrator, his uncontrolled behavior, immaturity, dependency, and alcohol consumption suggest an unhealthy mental state. Since the perpetrator denied the severity of his actions and was unwilling to discuss the matter with the caseworker, we can only speculate as to the reasons for his actions. Finkelhor (1983), in an attempt to identify common features of family abuse, notes that abuse can occur as a response to perceived powerlessness. Acts of abuse, he writes, "seem to be acts carried out by abusers to compensate for their perceived lack or loss of power" (p. 19). In her study of the physical abuse of elderly parents by adult children, Anetzberger (1987) found the typical abusing adult offspring to be burdened by close contact with the elder parent, the parent's disturbing behaviors, lack of time for personal pursuits, and absence of support from other family members. With regard to those offspring who were financially dependent, she writes that "they never achieved the social, economic or emotional status expected of American adults. Rather, they seemed to remain attached to the elder parent in a child-like dependency, impassive in their desire to alter the present situation" (p. 90).

The details of the case fit Pillemer's (1986) hypothetical causal model that has the abuser's mental and emotional difficulties, including alcohol abuse, directly leading to violence and indirectly to dependency. Dependency, according to exchange theory (powerlessness), can also lead to physical abuse. The situation is exacerbated by the social isolation of the family, which forms a sort of "negative feedback loop" with dependency. Not only is social isolation a causal factor of the abuse, since outsiders are not present to see and stop the abuse, but it is also the abuser's behavior that keeps outsiders away.

The case also illustrates the dilemma that workers face in preserving the client's right to self-determination. The social worker arranged for and monitored an array of services that involved health care, social service, aging, and law enforcement agencies, but only after considerable persuasion and negotiation with the victim. Other possible solutions through legal, judicial, or mental health means had to be abandoned because of the refusal of the victim and the abuser to consider them.

Although a single case study, the subject matter lends itself to some thoughts about the future of elder-abuse treatment programs and practice. As this case has shown, spouse abuse may be a more appropriate frame of reference than the child-abuse model. Finkelhor and Pillemer (1984) argue that it may be useful to start examining elder abuse, particularly physical mistreatment, for parallels with spouse-abuse situations rather than child abuse. This is suggested because the individuals involved are legally independent adults and because the model allows for consideration of the dependency of the abuser on the abused. If this is so, then treatment for elder abuse can include not only protection of the victim but some of the responses used in cases of spouse abuse, such as legal sanctions and control of offenders. One district attorney recently stated that prosecution aids in therapy since it provides the leverage needed to bring the perpetrators into treatment and to acknowledge wrongdoing. Similarly, victim support groups that enable battered persons to gain self-esteem and courage to confront their abusers can be successfully used with older persons (Breckman & Adelman, 1988).

Elder-abuse cases are particularly troublesome, and sometimes dangerous, for practitioners. They require special skills in investigating the problem and assessing the client, orchestrating the many service providers, counseling the victim and perpetrator, preparing testimony for court proceedings, working with law enforcement and other professionals, and strengthening the informal support system. But learning how to deal with the client's refusal or reluctance to accept lifesaving or life-enhancing services is, perhaps, the most difficult aspect of the work. So far, there have been very few studies that have examined the effectiveness of treatment. As this case study has demonstrated, in the final analysis, "successful treatment" and "case resolution" are relative terms.

References

American Public Welfare Association and National Association of State Units on Aging. (1986). *A comprehensive analysis of state policy and practice related to elder abuse*. Washington, DC: Authors.

Anetzberger, G. (1987). *The etiology of elder abuse by adult offspring*. Springfield, IL: Charles C Thomas.

Ansello, E. F., King, N. R., & Taler, G. (1986). The environmental press model: A theoretical framework for intervention in elder abuse. In K. A. Pillemer & R. S. Wolf (Eds.), *Elder abuse: Conflict in the family* (pp. 314–330). Dover, MA: Auburn House.

Block, M. R., & Sinnott, J. D. (1979). *The battered elder syndrome: An exploratory study.* College Park, MD: University of Maryland, Center on Aging.

Breckman, R. S., & Adelman, R. D. (1988). *Strategies for helping victims of elder mistreatment.* Newport Park, CA: Sage.

Bristowe, E., & Collins, J. B. (1989). Family mediated abuse of noninstitutionalized frail elderly men and women living in British Columbia. *Journal of Elder Abuse & Neglect, 1*(1), 45–64.

Callahan, J. J. (1982). Elder abuse programming: Will it help the elderly? *Urban and Social Change Review, 15,* 15–19.

Crouse, J. S., Kobb, D. C., Harris, B. B., Kopecky, F. J. & Poertner, J. (1981). *Abuse and neglect of the elderly in Illinois.* Springfield: Illinois Department on Aging.

Finkelhor, D. (1983). Common features of family abuse. In D. Finkelhor, R. J. Gelles, G. Hotaling, & M. Straus (Eds.), *The dark side of families: Current family violence research.* Beverly Hills, CA: Sage.

Finkelhor, D., & Pillemer, K. A. (1984). *Elder abuse: Its relationship to other forms of domestic violence.* Paper presented at the Second National Conference on Family Violence Research, Durham.

Fulmer, T. T., & O'Malley, T. A. (1987). *Inadequate care of the elderly: A health care perspective on abuse and neglect.* New York: Springer.

Gioglio, G. R., & Blakemore, P. (1983). *Elder abuse in New Jersey: The knowledge and experience of abuse among older New Jerseyans.* Trenton: New Jersey Department of Human Services.

Giordano, N. H., & Giordano, J. A. (1983). *Individual and family correlates of elder abuse.* Paper presented at the Annual Scientific Meeting of Gerontological Society of America, San Francisco.

Hudson, M. (1988). *Schematic version of elder mistreatment taxonomy.* Durham, NC: University of North Carolina, School of Nursing.

Johnson, T. (1986). Critical issues in the definition of elder mistreatment. In K. A. Pillemer & R. S. Wolf (Eds.), *Elder abuse: Conflict in the family* (pp. 167–196). Dover, MA: Auburn House.

Lau, E., & Kosberg, J. (1979). Abuse of the elderly by informal care providers. *Aging,* 10–15.

O'Malley, H., Segars, H., Perez, R., Mitchell, V., & Kneupfel, G. M. (1979). *Elder abuse in Massachusetts: A survey of professionals and paraprofessionals.* Boston: Legal Research and Services for the Elderly.

Pedrick-Cornell, C., & Gelles, R. J. (1982). Elder abuse: The status of current knowledge. *Family Relations, 31,* 457–465.

Phillips, L. R. (1986). Theoretical explanations of elder abuse: Competing hypotheses and unresolved issues. In K. A. Pillemer & R. S. Wolf (Eds.), *Elder abuse: Conflict in the family* (pp. 197–217) Dover, MA: Auburn House.

Pillemer, K. A. (1986). Risk factors in elder abuse: Results from a case-control study. In K. A. Pillemer & R. S. Wolf (Eds.), *Elder abuse: Conflict in the family* (pp. 239–263). Dover, MA: Auburn House.

Pillemer, K. A., & Finkelhor, D. (1988). The prevalence of elder abuse: A random sample survey. *Gerontologist, 28*(1), 51–57.

Quinn, M. J., & Tomita, S. (1986). *Elder abuse and neglect: Causes, diagnosis and intervention strategies.* New York: Springer.

Sengstock, M. C., & Liang, J. (1982). *Identifying and characterizing elder abuse.* Detroit: Wayne State University, Institute of Gerontology.

Straus, M. A., & Gelles, R. A. (1986). Societal change and change in family violence from

1975 to 1985 as revealed by two national surveys. *Journal of Marriage and the Family, 48,* 465–479.

Tatara, T. (1988). Toward the development of estimates of the national incidence of reports of elder abuse based on currently available state data: An exploratory study. In R. Filinson & S. R. Ingman (Eds.), *Elder abuse: Practice and policy* (pp. 153–164). New York: Human Sciences Press.

U. S. House of Representatives, Select Committee on Aging. (1981). *Elder abuse: An examination of a hidden problem.* Washington, DC: U.S. Government Printing Office.

Wolf, R. S., & Pillemer, K. A. (1989). *Helping elder victims: The realities of elder abuse.* New York: Columbia University Press.

Wolf, R. S., Godkin, M. A., & Pillemer, K. A. (1984). *Elder abuse and neglect: Report from three model projects.* Worcester, MA: University of Massachusetts Medical Center, University Center on Aging.

20

Domestic Homicide

Daniel G. Saunders and Angela Browne

Introduction

> WHEATON (AP) A 22-year-old woman who feared a former boyfriend might
> kill her was shot to death early Friday at her father's home in the town of
> Wheaton. . . . The shooting came just three days after a temporary restrain-
> ing order was issued against the suspect. . . . "Last Friday he told me that he
> was going to kill me if I didn't find a house and let him move in with me," the
> victim wrote in the court document. (*Capital Times*, 1988)

Could anything have been done to prevent this tragedy? Professionals
and the public alike ask themselves such questions when they hear
about a case of homicide in an intimate or spousal relationship. Attempts to generalize about spousal homicide raise a number of questions. Are there clear risk factors? What are the motives? Is the pattern of
spousal homicide different from that of other homicides?

Although our present state of knowledge makes it difficult to answer these questions with precision, in this chapter we will describe the
scope of domestic homicide and present the available evidence on its
patterns and dynamics. We draw from the small number of studies that
exist on this topic, as well as from our courtroom and empirical work
with spousal homicide cases. Our major emphasis will be on the differences in the dynamics of male and female perpetrators.

We refer to "domestic" or "spousal" homicide as the murder of a
spouse or other intimate partner. Knowing the risk factors for domestic

Daniel G. Saunders • Department of Psychiatry, University of Wisconsin–Madison Medical School, and Family Service Program to Prevent Woman Abuse, Madison, Wisconsin
53792. **Angela Browne** • Department of Psychiatry, University of Massachusetts
Medical School, Worcester, Massachusetts 01655.

homicide may prove useful for preventing it in future generations. Prevention may also occur in current relationships by identifying those at greatest risk of being victims or offenders and by recognizing high-risk situations. Although the prediction of rare events like homicide is always difficult, many in the mental health and criminal justice fields are required to make such predictions, and the seriousness of the problem alone means that we should take advantage of our growing, if imprecise, knowledge (Gottfredson & Gofftredson, 1988).

Until recently, domestic homicides have been relatively ignored as an area of study. Most studies of criminal homicide focused on stranger and acquaintance killings, with only brief statistical descriptions of other categories. Clinical case studies existed on homicide between partners or other family members. However, reporting on a case-by-case basis contributed to the impression that homicides between intimates were exceedingly idiosyncratic and isolated events. The epidemiological and case studies both failed to identify trends and dynamics that might link these cases together and provide a basis for understanding, intervention, and the construction of effective legal and social responses.

Despite its relative unpopularity as an area of study, partner homicide forms a major component of our national homicide picture. During the years 1980 through 1984, the deaths of over 17,000 people resulted from one partner assaulting the other. Within the category of domestic homicide, spousal homicide is by far the most prevalent type. For the years 1976 through 1984, the rates of spousal homicide were four times higher than those for child homicide (Plass & Straus, 1987).[1] Women are at particular risk. In an analysis of national homicide rates for 1979 through 1984, Plass and Straus (1987) note that women have a one-third higher risk of being murdered by their spouses. Indeed, it is in the home, at the hands of their partners, that women are most likely to be assaulted and injured, raped, or killed (Finkelhor & Yllo, 1985; Langan & Innes, 1986; Lentzner & DeBerry, 1980; Russell, 1982).

Homicides between partners rarely happen "out of the blue." What studies exist indicate that such homicides are more typically the end point in a series of assaultive incidents and/or threats (Browne, 1987; Chimbos, 1978; Daniel & Harris, 1982; Totman, 1978), and many domestic homicides are preceded by a series of attempts to gain intervention. A review of records for spousal homicide in Detroit and Kansas City in the mid-1970s revealed that, in approximately 90% of the cases, police had

---

[1]Compared with nonlethal forms of domestic violence, however, domestic homicide is still a relatively rare event. Over 12 million husbands and wives admit to using aggression every year, making it over 5400 times as likely as domestic homicide. This does not mean that 1 out of 5400 domestic violence cases ends in homicide, because homicide may not always be preceded by other marital violence (cf. Campbell, 1981; Scott, 1974).

been called to the same residence at least once during the 2 years before the lethal incident (Breedlove, Kennish, Sandler, & Sawtell, 1976). Similar reports come from other police studies and from battered women incarcerated for the deaths of their partners (e.g., Campbell, 1981; Lindsey, 1978).[2] Therefore, studies of nonlethal violence may be useful in understanding homicide, because the difference between lethal and nonlethal violence can arise merely from the availability of a weapon or the lack of medical care (e.g., Mulvihill & Tumin, 1969). Building accurate models of prediction based on these factors, however, is difficult because severe assaults rarely end in death. About 108,000 men and an equal number of women had a gun or a knife used against them by a partner in 1985 (Straus & Gelles, 1986), yet homicide rates constitute only a fraction of these cases (less than 2%).

One of the risk factors consistently found for being a victim or a perpetrator of domestic homicide in the United States is belonging to a racial minority group, especially black. Between 1976 and 1985 the rates for domestic homicide among blacks averaged five to eight times higher than for whites (Mercy & Saltzman, 1989; Plass & Straus, 1987). This finding is consistent with the high rates of nonfamily homicide (e.g., O'Carroll & Mercy, 1986) and nonlethal family violence among blacks (Cazenave & Straus, 1979). Fortunately, over the decade from 1976 to 1986 there was a steady and substantial decrease of domestic homicides among blacks, totaling 52% (Mercy & Saltzman, 1989).

Explanations for the high rate of black homicides are beginning to be uncovered. The theory that blacks constitute a subculture that accepts violence has largely been rejected. Hampton (1987), for example, points out that black homicide rates are highly associated with social structural factors, especially poverty. Similar findings exist for nonlethal violence, where income explains the higher rates for blacks (Cazenave & Straus, 1979). Hampton also describes broader ecological models that include poverty, the stress of urban living, and certain high-risk environments where expressive violence is the norm. Hawkins (1987) provides an equally broad analysis when he links the devaluation of black life in American society to the reluctance of social agents to intervene to aid victims and punish offenders. The relative lack of medical help, for

[2]Even when we know some of the risk factors, it remains difficult to predict homicide, simply because it is a rare event. In the above studies of prior police contact, one needs to consider the large number of police calls that did *not* result in homicide. Rosen (1954) first pointed out the problem of predicting rare events. A highly accurate prediction formula may identify most of the "true positives" but may not be useful because of the exceedingly high rate of "false positives" it also selects. Thus, the science of predicting the most dangerous forms of behavior is still rudimentary and may never be very good (Monahan, 1981).

example, can make the difference between serious injury and death. Hawkins also presents evidence that assaults and homicides among blacks are not taken as seriously by the criminal justice system, and thus, he speculates, there may be less of a deterrent for homicide.

One of the more puzzling findings is that for many years the rate of domestic homicide by black women has been even higher than for black men, although recently their rates have been about the same (Mercy & Saltzman, 1989). A major factor causing black women to use lethal violence seems to be the need to protect themselves from severe assaults by their partners. It appears likely that they are the scapegoats of the anger and frustration felt by black males in our society (Harvey, 1986; White, 1985). They usually have to resort to the use of a firearm if they are to equalize the severe force they face from their partners. For example, in one study of women who killed their partners (96% were black), 71% did so in response to violence from their partners (Goetting, 1987); self-defense was much less likely a motive for nonspousal homicides. Hawkins's (1987) observations of society's response to black violence are especially pertinent here. Black women cannot rely as much as white women on the criminal justice system for protection. Harvey (1986) notes that black women are especially vulnerable to violence because of racism and meager incomes.

The self-defense motive for homicide found in black wives has also been found in white wives and is one of the gender differences revealed in a number of studies. Failure to study or to report findings on homicide by gender, therefore, runs the risk of fostering misconceptions that have serious implications for intervention and services. For example, the recently reported finding of an overall downward trend in lethal violence in couples from 1976 through 1984 (e.g., Plass & Straus, 1987) fails to reveal that much of the decrease appears to be from a reduction in homicide by wives, ex-wives, and girlfriends (Browne & Williams, 1989). Among white husbands, ex-husbands, and boyfriends, there appears to be an increase in homicide (Browne & Williams, 1988, 1989).[3]

The motivational differences between men and women have been found in regional and small-sample studies (e.g., Browne & Flewelling,

[3]Mercy and Saltzman (1989) found a less dramatic increase in homicides by white husbands and a somewhat greater decrease in homicides by white wives. The major difference in their findings was a very large decrease in homicides by black husbands found in the Mercy and Saltzman study. Their study differs from that of Browne and Williams (1989) primarily in its exclusion of ex-spouses and boyfriends/girlfriends, and in not using weighting and adjustment procedures for nonreporting by police departments and missing data for relationship status. Since many black couples do not marry, the Browne and Williams study may be more representative of trends among blacks. The two studies also used different populations in the denominator to calculate rates. Browne and Williams' study is more likely to include many not-at-risk persons because it includes the total population, not just couples.

1986; Browne & Williams, 1989; Daly & Wilson, 1988; Daniel & Harris, 1982; Silverman & Kennedy, 1987a, 1987b; Silverman & Mukherjee, 1987). As far back as Wolfgang's classic (1958) study of criminal homicide in Philadelphia, the importance of self-defense in female-perpetrated homicides was noted. In analyzing police and court records, Wolfgang found that at least 60% of husbands killed by their wives had "precipitated" their own deaths—i.e., were the first to use physical force, strike blows, or threaten with a weapon, compared with only 9% of wife victims (Wolfgang, 1967). These figures were based on "provocation recognized by the courts," and do not necessarily reflect the number of wives who had actually experienced physical abuse or threat from their partners. Wilbanks (1983) found similar results in his study of all men and women arrested for homicide in Dade County, Florida, in 1980. Men were much more likely to have been the first to use physical force or threat, and thus to have precipitated the lethal assault.

Research on more specialized samples also indicates that a substantial proportion of female mate slayings are in response to the partner's aggression and threat. Chimbos (1978), in a review of available police records on spousal homicide in Canada, noted that nearly all of the women charged with the death of their mates had been physically assaulted by them. Totman (1978), studying women serving time in a California prison for killing of their mates, noted that 93% of the women who had killed partners reported being physically abused by them, and 67% said that the homicide was in defense of themselves or a child (see also Daniel & Harris, 1982; Jones, 1980). Studies of abused women who kill indicate that they often feel hopelessly trapped in a desperate situation from which they see no avenue of safe escape. The homicide occurs as part of an attempt to stop their partner from harming them or a child any further, or to prevent an attack they believe to be imminent and life-threatening (Browne, 1986, 1987; Jones, 1980).

Self-defense is not nearly as common a motive for husbands who kill, being 7 to 10 times less frequent than for wives (Campbell, 1981; Wolfgang, 1958). In analyzing responses from men who were interviewed as a part of a psychiatric evaluation following a fatal incident, Barnard and his associates (Barnard, Vera, Vera, & Newman, 1982) noted that the precipitating event in male-perpetrated partner homicide was usually related to some type of perceived rejection on the part of the woman. Separation or threat of separation was especially threatening, being interpreted by the men to represent "intolerable desertion, rejection, and abandonment." In killing their wives, offenders believed they were responding to a previous "offense" against them (e.g., leaving on the part of their mates).

Dutton (1988a) found that a consistent theme underlying nonlethal aggression against wives is a perception of loss of control by the male, especially the fear of being abandoned (see also Coleman & Straus, 1986; Dutton & Browning, 1987; Dutton & Strachan, 1987; Hamberger & Hastings, 1986). In a review of the empirical literature, Wilson and Daly (1987) reached similar conclusions about male-perpetrated homicides, contending that possessiveness explains their motivations. They note that "in fatal conflicts, men are remarkably possessive of their wives" and are prone to kill out of jealousy or because of their "inability to control their wives' . . . decision to quit the marital relationship" (p. 1).

While Daly and Wilson (1987) make a sociobiological interpretation of their literature review, Campbell (1981) places these men's possessiveness and jealousy within the context of patriarchal culture. She reviews studies linking "machismo" culture with greater violence toward women. She notes, "Because women are considered the possession of men in patriarchy, real or imagined sexual infidelity is the gravest threat to male dominance" (p. 78). In her study of homicide in one city, she found that most of the men killed out of jealousy, whereas most of the women killed in response to violence from their partners.

The possessiveness of the men may explain why they seem more likely to kill a partner who leaves than are women (Campbell, 1981; Daly & Wilson, 1988). In a more detailed analysis of the impact of loss and jealousy on male-perpetrated partner homicide, Rasche (1988) found that men who kill because their relationship has ended are more likely to commit suicide after the homicide, whereas men who kill out of jealousy are more likely to kill only their partners. The losses suffered by the homicide-suicide perpetrator have also been investigated by Humphrey and Palmer (1982). They found that the losses could include childhood losses, such as abandonment by or death of a parent.

Because of the differences commonly noted in the motives of husbands and wives, we will present a case in which each is the perpetrator.[4] Risk factors for lethal—and for severe, nonlethal—partner violence will be highlighted and discussed in a following section. Each case illustrates only some of the possible risk factors, and the reader is cautioned that there is no single type of domestic homicide offender.

Case Description: A Man Who Killed His Wife

His friends and relatives described him as quiet, gentle, and kind. What mattered most to him were his children, his small business, and his home in the country. He believed that he stood to lose all three if his divorce became final.

---

[4]The two cases examples had many facts changed in order to hide the identities of the families.

Steve and Sally had been married for 6 years and had two children, ages 4 and 6. They had met in a class on nonviolent civil disobedience in the protest movement during the Vietnam war. She was attracted to him by his gentleness and good looks. She could not see his insecurities and his tendency to become dependent on and possessive of women.

He worked as a nurse for a grade school and she was a special education teacher. The early years of their marriage were stressful but exciting for both of them. Having a child immediately and paying off school debts put pressure on them, but they shared many dreams and worked toward fulfilling them. They built a home in the country and started a business raising goats and selling goat cheese.

The seeds of conflict between them and for his sense of threat were planted early in the relationship. She had more education and made more money than he did. Despite his liberal views about new roles for women, the disparity between them would sometimes aggravate him. He wanted to quit his job to expand their business into a full-time operation. She was frightened that their income would be too little and gave him ultimatums about leaving him if he followed through with his plans. He took this as a put-down of his abilities. He also felt she was abandoning him and their dreams.

Another common argument concerned what each thought was best for the children. The rigidity of his upbringing surfaced at these times. His temper flashed if the children did not eat the "right" food or pick up their toys by bedtime. The strictness of his own father could be seen in him. He hated the way his father had treated him. He was frequently made to feel "small" when he did not live up to expectations, and his father had threatened him with a belt. Yet Steve found that he sometimes acted exactly like his father. Steve's anger doubled whenever he felt that Sally's parents were interfering in their lives, especially with raising their children. He never felt accepted by his in-laws because he did not share their fundamentalist religious background.

Occasionally when they argued, Steve would yell at Sally. At first he only raised his voice, but later he would call her "stupid" or "bitch"—and accuse her of only marrying him for his paycheck or to have children. Although Steve's yelling was infrequent, when combined with his much greater size it enabled him to intimidate Sally. She became more passive in hopes that his outbursts would stop. He learned that a hard stare or storming out of the house was enough to get his way. Secretly, she began to wonder if she should leave him. She finally developed enough courage to ask for a temporary separation, explaining to him that it could get their marriage back on track. He reacted by begging her not to "throw him out." He held her by the shoulders and shook her. He stopped suddenly and they were both surprised by what he had done. He cried and apologized, saying that he would never use force again.

About a week later, when they were talking alone in the bedroom, she again told him that she thought it would be best if they separated temporarily. She said she felt extremely tense near him, that he was sullen all the time, and that he needed help. He again grabbed her by the shoulders and said that he could not leave—his "whole life was here." His fear switched into rage and he began to choke her. He pushed her onto the bed and shouted, "No! No! No! " The shouting brought the children to the door and he stopped. He left the house quickly and called later to say he was moving out. She obtained a restraining order to try to keep him away. A preliminary divorce hearing established that Steve was allowed to visit the children twice a week, which provided an exception to the restraining order's no-contact provision.

In his desperation to maintain the relationship, Steve violated the restraining order several times. The judge found him in contempt of court. At the time, however, there were no criminal penalties for such a violation. One time, after dropping the children off, he yelled to Sally through the window that he had a gun in the car and would kill her and burn down the house if she did not take him back. On another occasion, she let him in the house, thinking that it would lower the risk of violence. She told him she was going ahead with the divorce. He carried her into the bedroom, slapped her, and raped her. She went to the battered women's shelter with the children and stayed for a week. The police took no action because marital rape was not a criminal offense. They also felt that by letting him into the house, Sally was partly responsible for what had occurred.

About a month before the divorce, while returning the children, Steve pushed his way into the house, beat Sally up, and attempted to rape her. To her, the sexual violence was his statement that she belonged to him and that she would not get away. She felt totally degraded by it. She went to the police and told them she wanted the violence stopped. Because she said she did not want him to go to jail, they took no action. They were also tired of her "complaining." Her fears made her abrasive and shrill at times.

As the divorce date approached, the violence escalated. Steve shoved her against a wall so hard that she struck her head. Another time he held her arms so tightly that they were bruised for a week. He called her repeatedly at home and work to either plead with or threaten her. Her attorney and co-workers saw her bruises and difficulty walking due to the beatings and rapes. They called the police and the prosecutor to ask them to take action, but they were told there was insufficient evidence for an arrest. Sally's spirit collapsed, and she told a counselor that she felt resigned to more violence, including her death. She considered relocating to another state but feared she could not get as good a job and did not want to move the children away from their relatives.

Two days before the divorce, Steve returned the children from a visit. He made a last attempt to reconcile. Sally became frightened that he would become violent and screamed for him to leave. She went toward the phone. He got their first and tore it off the wall. She ran into the garage and was headed for the car when he caught her. He struck her repeatedly on the head with a board that he had picked up from the floor. When he saw that she was no longer breathing, he went to the neighbors and told them to call the police because someone had killed his wife.

This case illustrates some of the structural components of violent marriages, the psychology of the offender and the victim, and the response of social agencies. The nature of Steve's upbringing was another notable risk marker. All of these areas will be expanded upon in later sections.

The next case is an example of a woman who killed her husband. We illustrate the motive of self-defense, which we noted previously to be the most common motive among women who kill their partners.

Case Description: A Woman Who Killed Her Husband

Nicole met Gary when she was 26, a few months after an acrimonious divorce from her first husband. She had two small children and was feeling overwhelmed and vulnerable. Gary was warm and charming, and quickly became involved with the details of her life. They dated for 6 months before living together, and were married by the time they had known one another a year. Gary had a family by a previous marriage. They resided in another state and Nicole knew very little about them.

The first incident of physical aggression occurred when Nicole and Gary had been dating 5 months. They were at a party at which another man had repeatedly asked Nicole to dance, although she refused him each time. Gary drank quite a bit that night. (Nicole discovered later that he also used amphetamines daily.) As they left the party, he turned and hit her in the stomach with his fist, asking if she wouldn't rather leave with her "new friend." He apologized by the time they reached home, and the next day he admitted that he was mainly frightened by how much he had come to care about her and how deeply he wanted her to be his. Gary didn't drink heavily during the rest of their courtship, and there were no further assaultive incidents. He was the most charming and affectionate man Nicole had ever known, and his involvement with her and the children seemed an invaluable support.

The next assault occurred about 4 months after the wedding. Nicole had been in a car accident in which she was thrown into the windshield, and she was hospitalized for head and facial injuries. Gary became suspicious of the medical procedures and the length of her hospital stay. The tension was exacerbated by the fact that Nicole did not have adequate insurance and the bills mounted quickly. When Nicole returned home, Gary remained upset and on edge. The second assault was triggered when Nicole had her mother drive her to a doctor's appointment while Gary was at work. Gary returned home before they got back and went out in the car looking for her. When Nicole and her mother returned, he was waiting. He demanded to know where Nicole had been and refused to believe her story of going to the doctor. He ripped the bandages from her forehead and chin, accusing her of spending their money on plastic surgery so that she could look beautiful for another man. When her mother attempted to intervene, Gary dragged Nicole into the bathroom and began hitting her repeatedly with the back of his hand. The assault ended when Gary realized that Nicole was bleeding. He became concerned and gentle, washing her face with his hands, applying ice packs, reassuring her that everything would be alright.

Nicole went to her mother's with the children the next day. However, she was unable to come up with enough money for a deposit and first month's rent on an apartment and was frightened about the medical bills. Gary confessed that he had been using "pills" and made an appointment at the Mental Health Center for counseling. He told Nicole that his first wife had left him for another man, and attributed his irrational fears to his past bad experiences. Nicole and the children returned home, although against Nicole's better judgment. She was withdrawn and depressed for several months, and Gary attributed the next assault to her refusal to "forgive" him and to meet his sexual needs.

Arguments in the relationship usually started over the children or over sex. Early on, Gary assumed a father role with the children, establishing his own rules and disciplining them harshly for infractions. He overruled Nicole on her decisions and accused her of attempting to turn the children against him. Although initially they adored him, the children began to fear Gary, and would jump up on the couch and sit very still whenever they heard his truck turning into the driveway at night. When Gary got upset, he became increasingly verbal, escalating from lectures to accusations. Verbal abuse quickly turned into physical violence. Gary would throw Nicole to the floor or down on the bed, hit her in the face, or begin to choke her. Nicole couldn't reason with Gary once an attack began. Gary would suddenly stop himself, becoming concerned over Nicole's injuries, and telling her how "precious" she was to him. The next day he would be loving and contrite, and the household would be peaceful for a few weeks until his anger escalated again.

After the first year of marriage, Gary also became sexually abusive. Sexual attacks typically began late at night when Nicole had fallen asleep and sometimes continued for several hours. These assaults were quite severe and involved the use of other physical violence as well. Nicole nearly always sustained injuries. She began to suffer from sleep disorders and severe stomach cramps, and eventually developed ulcers. While having sex with Nicole, Gary would sometimes verbally fantasize about sexual experiences with his ex-wife's daughter. After his death, Nicole found out that charges had been filed against him for sexual molestation and for assault of his first wife, but they had been dropped when he left the relationship. Gary also had fantasies about killing his first wife, and Nicole became increasingly afraid.

As Gary's violence became more severe, Nicole became increasingly desperate. She called the police for help if she could reach a phone during an assault. She also left Gary several times. However, her leaving or attempts to gain help seemed to escalate the danger. Gary shifted his homicidal fantasies about his ex-wife to homicidal threats toward Nicole. He warned her that he could find her wherever she went, and that he would kill her if she tried to leave him or called the police again. He came after her the few times she left, and her family became so frightened by his behavior that Nicole no longer turned to them for help. The police did not arrest Gary when they were called to the house, since wife assault was categorized as a misdemeanor, although they did transport her to the hospital several times when she needed treatment. Nicole felt her love for Gary had ended, and she wanted only to find safety for herself and her children. She talked to the prosecutor about pressing charges or filing for divorce, but gave up when she found that Gary would remain free in the community during the long months it would take for legal action to be completed. His threats were so severe that Nicole was sure she would be killed.

The most severe assault occurred when Nicole attempted to talk with Gary about a separation. Gary became enraged and attacked Nicole, beating her over the head with a heavy vase. A neighbor intervened and the police were called. Gary was jailed, and Nicole was hospitalized for surgery. This time Nicole agreed to file charges and, after she left the hospital, found an apartment for herself and the children. She filed for divorce and obtained a restraining order. However, upon his release from jail, Gary followed the children home from school and quickly learned their location. Several times he intimidated her daughter into letting him into the apartment and refused to leave when Nicole got home. Nicole attempted to have the restraining order enforced, but the police informed her it was no longer valid since Gary had been allowed on the premises. Although Gary was not assaultive during this period, Nicole lived in constant fear.

When Gary was awarded weekly visitation rights in the divorce settlement, Nicole took the children and left the state. It took Gary several months, but he quit his job and found them. Again Nicole moved, but again Gary found them. This time the police assisted him since he had reported them all missing and claimed that he feared foul play. Nicole and the children had been on the run for nearly a year at this point. Nicole was ill and unable to find steady employment, and the children were falling behind in school. Gary moved in, and Nicole felt she no longer had the strength to fight back. He found work quickly and began to pay the bills, insisting that Nicole stay home and regain her strength. Assaultive incidents were less frequent now. Nicole tried to resist recurring fantasies about suicide and told herself that the situation was best for her kids.

Gary lost his job after 3 months, and the only work Nicole could find was on the swing shift. Since he stayed at home all day, Gary's drinking increased, as did his abusive behavior. Increasingly, much of his verbal abuse was directed toward the children. Nicole was especially worried about her daughter Sarah, who had become withdrawn and silent, rarely leaving her room unless Gary made her come out and join the family. There was something menacing in his behavior toward Sarah. Again, Nicole began thinking about leaving. Ten months after Gary moved in, Nicole came home at midnight to find her daughter hiding in the garage. Sarah was crying and disheveled, and admitted that Gary had been sexually abusing her but had threatened to kill her if she told. It was a Friday night, and Nicole promised her that they would be gone by Monday, before she had to be alone with Gary again. They spent the weekend making what plans they could with Gary in the house.

Gary always spent Sundays playing pool at a favorite bar. As soon as he left the house Sunday afternoon, Nicole called a friend to come over and pick up the children, and they packed as much as they could while they waited. When the friend arrived, they loaded the children and their belongings in her car, with Nicole insisting that they leave immediately. Nicole stayed behind to pack papers related to her divorce and gather some things for herself. She was barely back in the house when she heard Gary's pickup truck pull into the driveway. He slammed on the brakes and ran toward the door, yelling that she had better let him in. He had never come back that early. Nicole realized he must have been watching the house all along.

Nicole fastened the chain lock and ran toward the kitchen to call the police, but Gary was already trying to force the door. Gary's .22 was in the hall closet. Nicole dialed 911 and then grabbed the gun and ran back toward the front window. She hoped if Gary saw her with the gun it would hold him off until help arrived. As Gary pushed through the door, Nicole backed up into the dining room, facing Gary but holding the gun toward the floor. She told him that she had called for help and that they would be there any minute, but he still came toward her, raging at her about leaving, grabbing a suitcase that was standing in the living room, and throwing it aside, flushed red in his anger. He kept saying, "You've had it now"—a phrase Nicole remembered as preceding the beating with the vase. Gary picked up a dining room chair, held it over his head, and came toward her, and Nicole lifted the gun and fired once. Gary died at ten o'clock that evening, and Nicole was arrested and charged with murder.

This case illustrates some dynamics of homicide in which a woman kills a mate in self-defense, on the basis of her assessment of danger from previous assaults and threats from her partner. Although relatively little is known about female-perpetrated homicide in general, homicides by abused women have been studied, and some precipitating factors identified. Crucial factors include the severity of the assaults and threats and the effectiveness of the woman's attempts to gain help or stop the violence. The severe and chronic violence produces desperation in the woman and a sense of "being on one's own with the danger" when all attempts to alleviate the violence fail. In her study of women incarcerated for the deaths of their partners, Totman (1978) reported that a major contributing factor was a perceived lack of effective alternatives to an "overwhelming and entrapping life situation."

In the above example, Nicole's attempts to use legal alternatives, and repeated attempts at separation, convinced her that there was no escaping Gary and that police responses would be inadequate to protect her from serious injury or death. The severity of the violence and threats also forms an important component, both psychologically and legally, in the perceptions leading to homicide by an abused woman. These perceptions will be explained further in the section on assessment.

Medical Issues

Among professionals who are in a position to detect and prevent domestic homicide, medical practitioners are especially pivotal. Straus (1986) points out that medicine can become more active in identifying high-risk cases and promoting public health campaigns to reduce risk factors. Case identification can occur in all medical settings. Emergency room staff are most likely to spot the precursors of domestic homicide, however, because the best predictor of homicide is likely to be prior severe violence (Kelso & Personette, 1985; Monahan, 1981). For example, one emergency room study found that 21% of the injured women seen were battered women (Stark, Flitcraft, & Zuckerman, 1981).

Straus (1986) sees the public's trust in the medical field as another important reason for its involvement. He warns, however, that the medical community can exceed public expectations if it makes pronouncements about marital roles or if it begins to "medicalize" the problem as a disease, resulting in less responsibility assigned to the offender. In an effort to intervene in the problem of family violence, the surgeon general's office has begun a public health campaign to combat family violence by making public pronouncements and supporting physician training. For example, his office helped the Academy of Obstetrical and Gynecological Physicians send informational packets to all of its members.

Legal Issues

Legal and Extralegal Alternatives for Abused Spouses

In both of the cases we presented in this chapter, separation—or the discussion of separation—played a major role in the escalation of aggression by the male partner. This dynamic becomes "catch-22" for abused women. Particularly in relationships in which the violence escalates in severity over time, women perceive that remaining in the relationship may lead to serious injury or death; yet they fear that leaving the violent partner may bring about equally serious reprisals. Faced with this dilemma, women may vacillate between staying and leaving, frustrating and confusing outsiders who fail to understand these competing forms of risk.

Further, until recently, there were virtually no alternatives available to women experiencing assault from their male partners. In most jurisdictions, assault by a man toward his wife could be charged only as a misdemeanor unless it was attempted murder, even if the assault would have been considered a felony if perpetrated against an acquaintance or a stranger (Lerman, 1981; Lerman & Livingston, 1983). Police could not arrest on a misdemeanor unless they witnessed a part of the offense. And if women pressed charges and the case was carried forward to trial, it rarely resulted in a conviction or sentence. Marital rape was a specific exemption, and the self-defense plea was not used to help women who took protection into their own hands (see Field & Field, 1973; Lerman, 1981; Lerman & Livingston, 1983; U.S. Commission on Civil Rights, 1978, 1982).

Only since the late 1970s have legal protections become available to abused women, although such protections still vary widely by jurisdiction, in both content and implementation. By 1980 nearly all states had passed some type of domestic violence legislation. Battered women's shelters and other extralegal resources for the protection of women and their children were established in most major urban areas (Schechter, 1982), and there was an increase in public awareness of the legitimacy of the problem. Women were encouraged to use available resources and were faulted if they chose to remain with or were afraid to leave a man who abused them.

Given the finding that a history of violence and threat usually precedes domestic homicides, and the frequent evidence for a self-defense motive, such resources should act to reduce the rate of homicides that occur between partners. In fact, for women this has been the case. From 1976 through 1984, there was over a 25% decrease in the number of women killing their male partners. This decline began in 1979, about the time that domestic violence legislation and extralegal resources for abused women were coming into place (based on supplementary homicide data for all one-on-one partner homicides involving individuals over the age of 15). In further analyses, Browne and Williams (1989) confirmed that those states having more domestic violence laws and other resources for abused women (e.g., shelters, crisis lines, support groups) had lower rates of female-perpetrated homicide, and that the presence of such resources was associated with the decrease in homicides. Although national homicide figures do not give us information about the histories of the individuals involved, it seems reasonable to assume that some women—given the alternatives to violence—are turning to these alternatives. Stout (1989) obtained similar results in her state-by-state analysis. The number of programs for men who batter, on the other hand, was not correlated with the rate of women killed.

Practitioners' Duty to Warn

Once a practitioner detects some of the risk factors for lethality, a question is raised about the obligation to report the case. An increasing concern for practitioners, based on recent court decisions, is the duty to warn or protect potential victims of homicide. Many of these court cases have involved battered women. Sonkin and Ellison (1986) reviewed the court cases as they have evolved and noted that courts gradually broadened the scope of the duty. Some recent rulings take the definition of potential victim beyond an identifiable victim to include potential physical and mental harm to family members and to the general public (Koocher, 1988).

These court actions have been curtailed, however, by laws in over 10 states (American Psychological Association, 1988). For example, a California law granted therapists immunity from lawsuit unless "the patient has communicated a serious threat of violence against a reasonably indentifiable victim" (Sonkin & Ellison, 1986). In California, the therapist must try to inform the victim and the police of the threat. Clinicians were at first concerned that the rulings would create a reluctance to treat dangerous patients and that patients, upon hearing of the duty to warn, would drop out of treatment. Apparently, such consequences have not occurred (McNeill, 1987).

McNeill (1987) points out some of the benefits of the ruling that clinicians often overlook. For example, when the principle case (*Tarasoff v. Regents of the University of California*, 1974) went before the court for a rehearing, the court broadened the options for psychotherapists. The duty to warn was broadened to the "duty to protect," which means that detaining the client for observation becomes an option. McNeill encourages therapists to inquire about patients' violent propensities and to use the history of violence as an indicator of future violence. She suggests that the following indicators be considered:

1. The extent to which the client appears to have a plan as distinguished from a fantasy.
2. The specificity with which the client describes the plan.
3. Whether the client has targeted a victim or a victim is reasonably foreseeable with knowledge in the therapist's possession.
4. Whether triggering events are attached to the plan that will cause the client to activate it upon the occurrence of some conditions.
5. Whether a dramatic or sudden change in the client's circum-

stance has occurred, such as divorce, loss of job, infidelity of spouse, romantic rejection, failure in an educational setting, humiliation caused by a known person, or death of a loved one.

6. Whether any steps have been taken to execute the plan, such as purchasing a weapon or other dangerous material, buying an airplane ticket to visit the intended victim, saving money toward the objective, sending threats to the victim directly or through third parties, or performing minor acts as a prelude to the intended "grand finale."

Legal Sanctions as Deterrence

The police training in family crisis intervention that occurred in the early 1970s claimed to reduce the incidence of family homicide (Bard, 1970). However, further analyses of these studies shows inconclusive results (Elliot, 1989; Liebman & Schwartz, 1973). The Minneapolis Police Experiment (Sherman & Berk, 1984), which found that arrest lowered the recidivism rate of offenders more than separation of the parties or advice and mediation, has had a tremendous influence on shaping police policies. Fagan (1989), among others, has pointed out the limitations of the study, including the short-term nature of the follow-up and the fact that only misdemeanor cases were studied. He presents evidence to show that perpetrators of more severe violence are not as affected by arrest or prosecution. Thus, the deterrent effects may exist only for certain types of offenders.

Social and Family Issues

Many social and family issues associated with domestic homicide were present in the two case descriptions. We will highlight a few of those issues here.

Social Issues

All too often, the social agencies that could balance the power between the couple consider the violence a "private matter," part of a domestic squabble to which the two partners contribute equally. Fortunately, the community in which the case of Steve and Sally took place has seen some changes in the criminal justice response. The state now has a law that makes marital rape and restraining order violations criminal offenses. There is a mandatory arrest law for spousal battery, and the local prosecutor does not usually drop complaints at the request of the victim. There is also a special detectives unit trained to deal with sexual and domestic crimes. Although these responses have not been conclusively shown to prevent homicide, there is evidence that battered women usually need a firm response from the criminal justice system if the violence is to stop (Bowker, 1983, 1986).

The social response to domestic homicide is further illustrated by the events following Sally's death. The case was plea-bargained from first- to second-degree murder and a guilty plea was entered. At Steve's sentencing hearing, a psychiatrist testified that violence was very uncharacteristic of the defendant. However, the psychiatrist used limited and biased accounts of events in the marriage because he relied primarily on Steve's story. He also stated that Steve had been pushed to the "breaking point" by Sally's "taunting." The propensity to blame female victims of crime, especially those intimately involved with their attackers, is still sometimes found in our disciplines of law and mental health.

Steve was sentenced to 10 years in prison but was released after only 3 years. While he was in prison, the children lived with his parents. Upon his release, he was awarded custody of the children. Apparently the decision-makers viewed the murder as caused by Steve's emotional distress and the victim's behavior and did not think that more prison time would act as a specific or general deterrent. They also did not seem to take into account the emotional trauma that Steve caused the children by repeatedly physically abusing their mother and then killing her. The emotional abuse suffered by children in violent marriages is now well documented (e.g., Rosenberg, 1987). Unfortunately, there is little in the way of research or policy regarding the children who survive domestic homicide.

Family Issues

Steve and Sally's case also illustrates some of the factors arising from the family of origin and the nuclear family. Steve's harsh upbringing was one clear risk marker of husband-to-wife violence (Hotaling & Sugarman, 1986), especially of severe violence (Saunders, 1988). Sally's greater educational attainment, although not much greater than Steve's, was another risk marker (Hornung, McCullough, & Sugimoto, 1981). Her status was likely to threaten the traditional sex-role beliefs from Steve's upbringing. Their different religious backgrounds was another such indicator (Hotaling & Sugarman, 1986).

The above case also illustrates some of the relationship dynamics of wife abuse, not all of which end in murder. Despite the man's wish for a nonviolent, egalitarian marriage on a cognitive level, the structure and stresses of the marriage brought out his socially reinforced "need" for control. The controlling behavior is a repetition of what he himself felt as a child. This further alienated Sally, and she eventually sought a temporary separation because she was not in a powerful enough position to negotiate change in the relationship. Over time, the negative spiral accelerates, with the man seeking more control and the woman seeking more freedom from the abuse and coercion.

Assessing Psychopathology and the Risk of Homicide

A common reaction to the news of a spousal killing is to think of the perpetrator as mentally "deranged." What else would explain a gruesome murder by someone who professed to love the victim? However, measures of psychopathology in themselves are not very good predictors of dangerousness and usually need to be combined with environmental indicators (Monahan, 1981). Large, well-controlled studies of psychopathology in domestic homicide perpetrators have yet to be conducted. In one small-sample study, the profile of men who killed their wives was very similar to that of men who killed strangers, although the latter group had a greater tendency toward psychopathic traits and impulsivity (Kalichman, 1988). The psychopathic deviate scale was the most elevated in both groups. Most of the women who killed their partners did not have significant scale elevations (69%). In-depth case studies often "uncover" some form of dissociative reaction among perpetrators (Berkman, 1980; Blinder, 1984). However, standardized measures are rarely used in these studies.

If men who kill their partners are similar to men who assault without killing, then they are seldom likely to suffer from severe mental disorders. In an MMPI study of men who batter, they were characterized as irritable, erratic, and unpredictable. They had signs of being distrustful of others, isolated and severely alienated, with a personality disorder and excessive concerns about their own masculinity (Bernard & Bernard, 1984). Even when measures of personality disorders are administered to men who batter, the majority do not meet the criteria for such a disorder, although many are "negativistic," "narcissistic," and "borderline," with alcohol-prone tendencies (Hamberger & Hastings, 1986). On rare occasions, alcoholism in these men can cover up other, physiologically based disorders, such as bipolar affective disorder or hypoglycemia. In a study of men who killed their partners, most of whom had alcohol-abuse problems, many showed an impaired ability to metabolize glucose and at the same time had normal MMPI profiles (Virkkunen & Kallio, 1987).

If measures of psychopathology do not prove useful in predicting homicide in the family, then behavioral and background characteristics probably will. Risk factors identified in studies of battered women who killed their partners may also apply to cases of men killing female partners because these women perceived that they were about to be killed. In a multivariate analysis comparing battered women who killed their partners with those who had not, Browne (1987) found seven variables that distinguished the homicide from the nonhomicide groups: (a) frequency of assault by the man, (b) severity of the woman's injuries, (c) frequency and severity of sexual assault, (d) frequency of the man's intoxication, (e) his drug use, (f) the man's threat to kill, and (g) suicide attempts or threats by the woman. By the end of their relationships, women who killed their mates were often experiencing frequent and severe attacks from men who were also sexually assaulting them, drinking heavily and/or abusing substances, and threatening to kill them or others. The case of Nicole and Gary illustrates, to some extent, all of these variables.

There are no similar studies on factors associated with men who kill their wives. However, since most of the women in the studies were about to be killed, the same risk factors are likely to apply to men who kill. Campbell (1986) relied on this logic when developing the initial version of her danger assessment instrument for use with battered women. It is a 15-item checklist, still in the development stages, that correlates significantly and moderately with the severity of violence and injuries reported by a sample of battered women. In addition to the factors listed by Browne, Campbell asked women about the presence of guns in the home, whether their partners are violent outside the home, whether they control all aspects of the woman's life, and whether their income is below the poverty level.

Less direct evidence of risk factors can be derived if studies of severe, nonlethal violence are assumed to have characteristics similar to lethal violence. Some recent studies of types of men who batter provide this evidence (for a review, see Dutton, 1988b). For example, Saunders (1988) empirically derived three types of men who batter. The most severe violence was used by men who were severely abused or witnessed abuse in childhood, who abuse alcohol and other drugs, and who are violent outside as well as inside the home.

Gondolf (1988) used a more behaviorally based typology of men who batter. The two types with the most severe forms of violence are men who threatened to kill, used drugs, blamed the partner for the abuse, threatened to abuse again, abused the children, and sexually abused their wives. They also destroyed property and were violent outside of the home. Note that many characteristics of the most severe abusers are the same as those in cases in which battered women killed their partners.

Treatment Options

Perpetrators of domestic homicide often do not receive treatment while in prison. Men who batter and are incarcerated for killing their partners are usually not ordered by courts to receive treatment for their violence. As in the case of Steve, the homicide is seen as an isolated "act of passion" that will never occur again. These men often make "model prisoners," and treatment referrals are more likely to be made for those who are aggressive while in prison. Some perpetrators refuse treatment because they fear that any information they reveal in treatment will be used against them and will lengthen their time in prison. Aside from states, like Alaska, that have prison batterers' programs, it appears that the men are more likely to be referred for treatment by a parole officer after they are released.

Battered women incarcerated for killing their partners need a great deal of support. A number of communities have established advocacy programs for these women (e.g., Bauschard, 1986). Support groups within prisons can be sponsored by prison human service workers, formerly battered women, or community shelters. A major need of these women is to have their emotional, physical, and sexual abuse experiences validated. Even though their abuser is dead, they may continue to fear him and to show evidence of posttraumatic stress. Grief work may be necessary because, despite the end of an abusive life, they have lost someone with whom they have been intensely involved, and they have lost their dreams and hopes for a happy relationship. Resolution of feelings of fear and grief may sometimes be cut short if the woman becomes too quickly immersed in political advocacy and is a rallying point for changing society's response to battered women.

Finally, more attention needs to be directed toward helping the children who survive these tragedies. Little is known about the suffering they endure and their potential for being violent later in life. If the studies of nonlethal violence can be a guide, then we have reason for great concern. Two potent risk factors for later violence are combined: being exposed to violence (Hotaling & Sugarman, 1986) and the sudden, traumatic loss of a parent (Humphrey & Palmer, 1982). The immediate and long-term emotional turmoil these children experience is likely to be great. They may experience guilt that they did not do more to stop the killing and may have split loyalties between the parents if they hear differing accounts of who was to "blame."

Summary

In this chapter we presented two cases that illustrate some of the common risk factors and dynamics involved when a spouse or lover takes the life of his or her partner. Our choice of examples stresses the differing backgrounds and motives of men and women. Although clinicians are obligated to warn and protect potential victims in some circumstances, the science of risk prediction is in its infancy. The ability to prevent any particular person from committing homicide may remain a difficult task because homicide is a relatively rare event. The discovery of risk markers, however, can lead to prevention programs on a social and family level that will decrease all forms of marital violence, including its most extreme form—spousal homicide. It will be through the lessons taught to the children in our present generation, however—through example and words—that the most effective prevention will take place.

Acknowledgments

The authors would like to thank Patricia Cumbie and Nancy Newton for their helpful comments on an earlier version of this chapter.

References

American Psychological Association. (1988, June). New laws limiting duty to protect (John Bales) (p. 18). *APA Monitor.* Arlington, VA: Author.

Bard, M. (1970). *Training police as specialists in family crisis intervention.* National Institute of Law Enforcement and Criminal Justice. Washington, DC: U.S. Government Printing Office.

Barnard, G. W., Vera, H., Vera, M. I., & Newman, G. (1982). 'Til death do us part: A study of spouse murder. *Bulletin of the American Academy of Psychiatry and the Law, 10,* 271–280.

Bauschard, L. (1986). *Voices set free. Battered women speak from prison.* St. Louis, MO: Women's Self Help Center.

Berkman, A. S. (1980). The state of Michigan versus a battered wife. *Bulletin of the Menninger Clinic, 44,* 603–616.

Bernard, J. L., & Bernard, M. L. (1984). The abusive male seeking treatment: Jekyll and Hyde. *Family Relations, 33,* 543–547.

Blinder, M. (1984). The domestic homicide. *Family Therapy, 11,* 185–198.

Bowker, L. (1983). *Beating wife-beating.* Lexington, MA: D. C. Heath.

Bowker, L. (1986). *Ending domestic violence.* Holmes Beach, FL: Learning Publications.

Breedlove, R. K., Kennish, J. W., Sandler, D. M., & Sawtell, R. K. (1976). Domestic violence and the police: Kansas City. In Police Foundation (Ed.), *Domestic violence and the police* (pp. 23–33). Washington, DC: Police Foundation.

Browne, A. (1986). Assault and homicide at home: When battered women kill. In M. J. Saks & L. Saxe (Eds.), *Advances in applied social psychology* (pp. 57–79). Hillsdale, NJ: Erlbaum.

Browne, A. (1987). *When battered women kill.* New York: Free Press.

Browne, A., & Flewelling, R. (1986, November). *Women as victims or perpetrators of homicide.* Paper presented at the Annual Meeting of the American Society of Criminology, Atlanta.

Browne, A., & Williams, K. R. (1988, November). *Race, resources, and the reduction of partner homicide.* Paper presented at the Annual Meeting of the American Society of Criminology, Chicago.

Browne, A., & Williams, K. R. (1989). Exploring the effect of resource availability and the likelihood of female-perpetrated homicides. *Law and Society Review, 23,* 75–94.

Campbell, J. C. (1981). Misogyny and homicide of women. *Advances in Nursing Science/Women's Health, 3,* 67–85. '

Campbell, J. C. (1986). Nursing assessment of risk of homicide with battered women. *Advances in Nursing Science, 8,* 36–51.

Capital Times. (1988). "Woman lived in fear, and now she is dead" (December 2, p. 1b). Madison, WI: Capital Times, Inc.

Cazenave, N., & Straus, M. A. (1979). Race, class, network embeddedness and family violence. *Journal of Comparative Family Studies, 10,* 281–300.

Chimbos, P. D. (1978). *Marital violence: A study of interspousal homicide.* San Francisco: R & E Associates.

Coleman, D. H., & Straus, M. A. (1986). Marital power, conflict, and violence in a nationally representative sample of American couples. *Violence and Victims, 1,* 141–157.

Daly, M., & Wilson, W. (1988). Evolutionary social psychology and family homicide. *Science, 242,* 519–524.

Daniel, A. E., & Harris, P. W. (1982). Female homicide offenders referred for pretrial psychiatric examination: A descriptive study. *Bulletin of the Academy of Psychiatry and Law, 10,* 261–269.

Dutton, D. G. (1988a). *The domestic assault of women: Psychological and criminal justice perspectives.* Boston: Allyn & Bacon.

Dutton, D. G. (1988b). Profiling of wife assaulters: Preliminary evidence for a trimodal analysis. *Violence and Victims, 3*(1), 5–30.

Dutton, D. G., & Browning, J. (1987). Power struggles and intimacy anxieties as causative factors of violence in intimate relationships. In G. Russell (Ed.), *Violence in intimate relationships.* New York: Spectrum.

Dutton, D. G., & Strachan, C. E. (1987). Motivational needs for power and spouse-specific assertiveness in assaultive and nonassaultive men. *Violence and Victims, 2,* 145–156.

Elliot, D. S. (1989). Criminal justice procedures in family violence crimes. In L. Ohlin & M. Tonry (Eds.), *Family violence: Crime and justice, a review of research* (Vol. 11, pp. 427–480). Chicago: University of Chicago Press.

Fagan, J. (1989). Cessation of family violence: Deterrence and discussion. In L. Ohlin & M. Tonry (Eds.), *Family violence: Crime and justice, a review of research* (Vol. 11, pp. 377–426). Chicago: University of Chicago Press.

Field, M. H., & Field, H. F. (1973). Marital violence and the criminal process: Neither justice nor peace. *Social Service Review, 47,* 221–240.

Finkelhor, D., & Yllo, K. (1985). *License to rape: Sexual abuse of wives.* New York: Holt, Rinehart & Winston.

Goetting, A. (1987). Homicidal wives. *Journal of Family Issues, 8,* 332–341.

Gondolf E. W. (1988). Who are those guys? Toward a behavioral typology of batterers. *Violence and Victims, 3,* 187–204.

Gottfredson, D. M., & Gottfredson, S. D. (1988). Stakes and risks in the prediction of violent criminal behavior. *Violence and Victims, 3,* 247–262.

Hamberger, L. K., & Hastings, J. E. (1986). Personality correlates of men who abuse their partners: A cross-validational study. *Journal of Family Violence, 1,* 323–341.

Hamberger, L. K., Hastings, J. E., & Lohr, J. E. (1988, November). *Cognitive and personality correlates of men who batter: Some continuities and discontinuities.* Symposium presented at the meeting of the Association for the Advancement of Behavior Therapy, New York.

Hampton, R. L. (1987). Family violence and homicide in the black community: Are they linked? In R. L. Hampton (Ed.), *Violence in the black family* (pp. 135–156). Lexington, KY: Lexington Books.

Harvey, (1986). Homicide among young black adults: Life in the subculture of exasperation. In D. F. Hawkins (Ed.), *Homicide among black Americans* (pp. 153–157). Lanham, MD: University Press of America.

Hawkins, D. F. (1987). Devalued lives and racial stereotypes: Ideological barriers to the prevention of family violence among blacks. In R. L. Hampton (Ed.), *Violence in the black family* (pp. 189–206). Lexington, KY: Lexington Books.

Hornung, C. A., McCullough, B. C., & Sugimoto, T. (1981). Status relationships in marriage: Risk factors in spouse abuse. *Journal of Marriage and the Family, 43,* 675–692.

Hotaling, G. T., & Sugarman, D. B. (1986). An analysis of risk markers in husband to wife violence: The current state of knowledge. *Violence and Victims, 1,* 101–124.

Humphrey, J. A., & Palmer, S. (1982). *Stressful life events and intra and extra-familial homicide.* Unpublished manuscript, University of North Carolina.

Jones, A. (1980). *Women who kill.* New York: Fawcett Columbine Books.

Kalichman, S. C. (1988). MMPI profiles of women and men convicted of domestic homicide. *Journal of Clinical Psychology, 4*(6), 847–853.

Kelso, D., & Personette, L. (1985). *Domestic violence and treatment services for victims and abusers.* (Available from Abused Women's Aid in Crisis, 100 W. 13th Avenue, Anchorage, Alaska, 99501.)

Koocher, G. P. (1988). A thumbnail guide to "duty to warn" cases. *Clinical Psychologist, 41,* 22–25.

Langan, P. A., & Innes, C. A. (1986). Preventing domestic violence against women. Washington, DC: U.S. Department of Justice, Bureau of Justice Statistics.

Lentzner, H. R., & DeBerry, M. M. (1980). *Intimate victims: A study of violence among friends and relatives.* Washington, DC: U.S. Department of Justice, Bureau of Justice Statistics.

Lerman, L. G. (1981). Criminal prosecution of wife beaters. *Response, 4*(3), 1–19.

Lerman, L. G., & Livingston, F. (1983). State legislation on domestic violence. *Response, 6,* 1–27.

Liebman, D., & Schwartz, J. (1973). Police progress in domestic crisis intervention: A review. In J. Snibbe & H. Snibbe (Eds.), *The urban policeman in transition* (pp. 421–472). Springfield, IL: Charles C Thomas.

Lindsey, K. (1978). When battered women strike back: Murder or self-defense? *Viva, 58–59,* 66–74.

McNeill, M. (1987). Domestic violence: The skeleton in Tarasoff's closet. In D. J. Sonkin (Ed.), *Domestic violence on trial: Psychological and legal dimensions of family violence* (pp. 197–217). New York: Springer.

Mercy, J. A., & Saltzman, L. E. (1989). Fatal violence among spouses in the United States, 1976–85. *American Journal of Public Health, 79,* 595–599.

Monahan, J. (1981). *Predicting violent behavior. An assessment of clinical techniques.* Beverly Hills, CA: Sage.

Mulvihill, D. J., & Tumin, M. M. (1969). *Crimes of violence* (Vol. 2). Staff report to the National Commission on the Causes and Prevention of Violence, Washington, DC.

O'Carroll, P. W., & Mercy, J. A. (1986). Patterns and recent trends in black homicide. In D. F. Hawkins (Ed.), *Homicide among black Americans* (pp. 29–42). Lanham, MD: University Press of America.

Plass, P. S., & Straus, M. A. (1987, July). *Intra-family homicide in the United States: Incidence, trends, and differences by region, race and gender.* Paper presented at the Third National Family Violence Conference, University of New Hampshire, Durham.

Rasche, C. (1988, November). *Domestic murder-suicide: Characteristics and comparisons to nonsuicidal mate killing.* Paper presented at the 40th Annual Meeting of the American Society of Criminology, Chicago.

Rosen, A. (1954). Detection of suicidal patients. *Journal of Consulting Psychology, 18,* 397–403.

Rosenberg, M. (1987). Children of battered women: The effects of witnessing violence on their social problem-solving abilities. *Behavior Therapist, 10,* 85–89.

Russell, D. E. H. (1982). *Rape in marriage.* New York: Macmillan.

Saunders, D. G. (1988). *A typology of men who batter their wives: Three types derived from cluster analysis.* Unpublished manuscript, Department of Psychiatry, University of Wisconsin-Madison.

Schechter, S. (1982). *Women and male violence.* Boston: South End Press.

Scott, P. D. (1974). Battered wives. *British Journal of Psychiatry, 125,* 433–441.

Sherman, L. W., & Berk, R. A. (1984). The specific deterrent effect of arrest for domestic assault. *American Sociological Review, 49,* 261–272.

Silverman, R. A., & Kennedy, L. W. (1987a). Relational distance and the law: The role of the stranger. *Journal of Criminal Law and Criminology, 72,* 272–308.

Silverman, R. A., & Kennedy, L. W. (1987b, November). *The female perpetrator of homicide in Canada.* Paper presented at the American Society of Criminology, Montreal.

Silverman, R. A., & Mukherjee, S. K. (1987). Intimate homicide: An analysis of violent social relationships. *Behavioral Sciences and the Law, 5,* 37–47.

Sonkin, D. J., & Ellison, J. (1986). The therapist's duty to protect victims of domestic violence: Where have we been and where we are going. *Violence and Victims, 1,* 205–214.

Stark, E., Flitcraft, A., & Zuckerman, D. (1981). *Wife abuse in the medical setting: An introduction for health personnel.* National Clearinghouse on Domestic Violence Monograph Series, No. 7. Washington, DC: U.S. Department of Health and Human Services.

Stout, K. D. (1989). "Intimate femicide": Effect of legislation and social services. *Affilia, 4,* 21–30.

Straus, M. A. (1986). Domestic violence and homicide antecedents. *Bulletin of the New York Academy of Medicine, 62,* 446–465.

Straus, M. A., & Gelles, R. J. (1986). Societal change and change in family violence from 1975 to 1985. *Journal of Marriage and the Family, 48,* 465–479.

Tarasoff v. Regents of the University of California. (1974). 118 Cal. Rptr. 129, 529 P 2d 553.

Totman, J. (1978). *The murderess: A psychological analysis of violent behavior.* San Francisco: R & E Research Associates.

U.S. Commission on Civil Rights. (1978). *Battered women: Issues of public policy.* Washington, DC: U.S. Government Printing Office.

U.S. Commission on Civil Rights. (1982). *Under the rule of thumb: Battered women and the administration of justice.* Washington, DC: U.S. Government Printing Office.

Virkkunen, M., & Kallio, E. (1987). Low blood sugar in the glucose tolerance test and homicidal spouse abuse. *Aggressive Behavior, 13,* 59–66.

White, E. C. (1985). *Chain chain change: For black women dealing with physical and emotional abuse.* Seattle, WA: Seal Press.

Wilbanks, W. (1983). The female homicide offender in Dade County, Florida. *Criminal Justice Review, 8*(2), 9–14.

Wilson, M., & Daly, M. (1987, July). *Spousal homicide in Canada.* Paper presented at the Third National Conference for Family Violence Researchers, University of New Hampshire, Durham.

Wolfgang, M. E. (1958). *Patterns in criminal homicide.* New York: Wiley.

Wolfgang, M. E. (1967). A sociological analysis of criminal homicide. In M. E. Wolfgang (Ed.), *Studies in homicide.* New York: Harper & Row.

Index